# Beyond the Gymnasium

# Beyond the Gymnasium

## *Educating the Middle-Class Bodies in Classical Germany*

Heikki Lempa

LEXINGTON BOOKS

A division of
ROWMAN & LITTLEFIELD PUBLISHERS, INC.
*Lanham • Boulder • New York • Toronto • Plymouth, UK*

LEXINGTON BOOKS

A division of Rowman & Littlefield Publishers, Inc.
A wholly owned subsidiary of The Rowman & Littlefield Publishing Group, Inc.
4501 Forbes Boulevard, Suite 200
Lanham, MD 20706

Estover Road
Plymouth PL6 7PY
United Kingdom



Chapter 3 includes passages from Heikki Lempa's article "The Spa: Emotional Economy and Social Classes in Nineteenth-Century Pyrmont."

British Library Cataloguing in Publication Information Available

**Library of Congress Cataloging-in-Publication Data**

Lempa, Heikki.
Beyond the gymnasium : educating the middle-class bodies in classical Germany / Heikki Lempa.
p. cm.
Includes bibliographical references and index.
ISBN-13: 978-0-7391-2089-7 (cloth : alk. paper)
ISBN-13: 978-0-7391-2090-3 (pbk. : alk. paper)
ISBN-10: 0-7391-2089-1 (cloth : alk. paper)
ISBN-10: 0-7391-2090-5 (pbk. : alk. paper)
1. Physical education and training—Germany—History—19th century.
2. Middle class—Germany—Social life and customs—19th century. 3.
Blood—Social aspects—Germany—History—19th century.
I. Title.
GV251.L46 2007
613.70943—dc22 2006102796

Printed in the United States of America

™ The paper used in this publication meets the minimum requirements of American National Standard for Information Sciences—Permanence of Paper for Printed Library Materials, ANSI/NISO Z39.48–1992.

# Contents

# List of Tables and Figures

# Preface

This book is about the body. But it is also about the ways the body forms what we call our selves. The beginning of this work is in my earlier life, as an undergraduate student in Finland. In the 1980s, I, as many in my disillusioned generation, turned away from those great political projects that had shaped the lives and aspirations of my elders and mentors in the 1970s. We were not fascinated by social upheavals but tended to look for our personal and political identity in groups of friends and in our selves. It was the techniques of the self, we thought, that would ultimately help build a better world. What was the self? What was subjectivity? Can we learn to be good selves? These were the questions that occupied my mind and inspired my individual and communal activities. I was particularly drawn by an idea that suggested a radical autonomy of the self. The self, its advocates claimed, is not a thing, not a skill that can be taught by somebody. The formation of one's self is possible only through the actions of the self. Education and university education in particular were only possible through the struggles of the self to embrace the world as knowledge. In the end of the 1980s, I made a personal discovery. The techniques of the self was the unfinished project of Michel Foucault. But much closer to a Finn were the German sources. In the first decade of the nineteenth century, German intellectuals formulated an agenda that was based on the discovery of the autonomous self. Was it a political agenda? Did it promote social revolution? We do not know. But we do know that these intellectuals invested intellectual energy in an institution that seemed rather unimportant—university. They gave birth to the modern concept of university. And, as I soon discovered, it was the very foundation of all Finnish universities. I started to dig where I stood. German education would give an answer to the question of the self. Followed years on eighteenth-century German education and, to my dismay, the original question was fading away.

It took a radical change in my life, an emigration to the United States, to remind that the question of self still had some relevance. In 1993, I landed in Chicago in a graduate seminar of Alf Lüdtke. My previous work on the eighteenth century and German education was quickly overhauled. I moved from ideas to practices, from philosophies to everyday, from arguments to discreet actions of stubbornness and, as the German word *Eigensinn* so well captures, trajectories of making sense. In this book, there is no reference to Alf Lüdtke's work. In the early 1990s, his interests were already in the twentieth century. But the basic question of this book, the question of forming one's self through the nonverbal techniques of the body, is understandable only in the context of that graduate seminar in 1993. It is hard to overestimate the impact of its members on some of the fundamental decisions in this work. Jim Bjork, Maureen Healy, Paul Steege, and especially the intellectual neighbor of mine, Andre Wakefield have had more influence on this book than they realize. Andre has been a generous and rigorous critic whose sophisticated understanding of the eighteenth century and especially its disciplines has been so valuable for some of its basic arguments.

In two years, I was ready to go to Germany. With a generous help from the Alexander-von-Humboldt Foundation I could start my research at the University of Tübingen. Professor Ulrich Herrmann was a kind and supporting mentor there. While most of the time was spent in numerous archives and libraries, I met two people whose ideas profoundly influenced me. Uwe Zimmermann, who at one point owned one of the largest private collections of nineteenth-century memoirs, made me aware of these underused sources and their importance in tracing continuities that for many historians have gone undiscovered. The eighteenth century, so it seemed, was not so much cut off from the nineteenth as often assumed. I also met Michael Hau whose impeccable command of medical history assured me that medicine is a key to the deeper understanding of German everyday life in the nineteenth century.

In a year, the field work was over. Michael Geyer, who had guided me through the moments of disorientation before my departure for Germany, was now the generous critic that only he can be. It was he who insisted on a comprehensive research rather than a local study. Now, when the manuscript is ready, I can see the wisdom of that advice. Michael has always focused on the context and the main thrust of the argument and this is what one needs in a work like this. I needed context. In 1997 and 1998, I spent fifteen months at the Herzog-August-Bibliothek in Wolfenbüttel, an ideal community of scholars and students of German culture and history. While working on another project, I could finish my dissertation manuscript. The extensive reference collections of the library, friendly and highly professional librarians, and the stimulation of the intellectual community there was so important for my work. Especially to Gilian Bepler and Ulrike Zeuch I will remain in gratitude for their forthcoming and friendly support of my projects.

In the summer of 1999, I was in the envious position to replicate this positive experience in Göttingen at the Max-Planck-Institute, generously funded by a grant from the German Academic Exchange Service (DAAD). It is here that some of the formative ideas for this book started to take shape. I made a personal discovery in spas. They were the sites that best demonstrated the practical ideals and idealistic practices of everyday, so important for middle-class Germans. It is also here that I had the opportunity to meet Anne-Charlott Trepp whose study on the women of Hamburg made me realize the different layers of social formation embedded in private and semi-private activities. These ideas got a clearer shape in the fall of

1999 when I started my postdoc at Columbia University, funded by a grant from the National Academy of Education. Volker Berghahn took me under his wings. In his intellectual *Kränzchen,* there was a unique opportunity to elaborate on ongoing projects and meet kindred souls. One of these was Andrew Zimmerman whose friendly way of making important observations has also left its mark on this work. Over the past five years, I had the great opportunity to join another *Kränzchen*, the Philadelphia Workshop of German Historians. I could present chapters of this work to Paul Steege, Greg Eghigian, Jay Lockenour, David Imhoof, Pieter Judson, Troy Paddock, and Jeffrey Johnson. All they have given their valuable input.

The long journey of tracing the question of self and its formation took a sudden turn when I started in my current position at Moravian College in 2001. I accepted the offer without realizing how much more this place was than a job. It is, in fact, not a job but in a very ancient way a place that recognizes something that is called vocation. And vocation always entails discovery; it does not have a clear job description. What was missing in mine were the multiple connections that this community, the *Herrnhuter* (Moravians), had to my work. Not only Friedrich Schleiermacher, the famous Moravian of higher order, but also Goethe, Schiller, Novalis and so many others were influenced by the ideas and practices of the *Herrnhuter*. And these practices, as Katherine Faull, a good critic of my projects, has shown, revolved around the formation of self. I extend my thanks to many at this college, especially to the colleagues and friends at the Department of History. They have been a great support over the past years. Whenever needed, Anne Dutlinger has helped me with what she knows best: the world of art and design. My special thanks go to those who have taken their time with my chapters. Khristina Haddad, a political theorist, read and gave her detailed comments on the passages on mutual recognition. Kym Morrison read several sections and it was she who suggested the current title of the book. The good soul and a trusted guide for my texts was the late Judith Green. Without her great work this book would not have been possible. It is to my great sadness to realize that Judith has not seen this book finished. Finally, I want to express my gratitude to MacDuff Stewart, Patrick Dillon, and Ryan Quick from Lexington Books. Their professionalism and support has given this book its final shape.

The beginning of this story is a very personal experience. Have I learned something? I and many in my generation moved away from the projects of political transformation. And we turned to personal transformation. Yet the story of the self is not about your self but it is about the ways your self is formed in its social and political environment.

# Chapter One

# Introduction

When Daniel Gottlob Moritz Schreber returned to Leipzig from abroad in 1837, he entertained high hopes for his future. Born the son of a lawyer in Leipzig in 1808 Schreber had gone to the University of Leipzig to study medicine. After defending his dissertation in 1833, he spent three years traveling and working, mostly in Russia. Now, he believed, it was time to settle down and, more important, to put his own stamp on improving his home city, a flourishing commercial and intellectual center of Saxony and East Central Europe. After opening a medical practice, Schreber set his sights on academia. In 1836, he began to lecture at the University of Leipzig on dietetics, a staple of traditional medicine that discussed, in addition to nutrition, a variety of lifestyle practices, including sleep, regulation of the passions, physical exercise, metabolism, the use and impact of air, and the effects of environment on all these.[1] He later added pediatrics and medical gymnastics to the subjects of his lectures.[2] And he produced an array of books on hygienics, balneology, and gymnastics. All this should have impressed the medical faculty of the University of Leipzig—but it did not. Schreber's repeated requests to be nominated a professor were turned down. In 1845, he abandoned his lackluster academic career and turned to practical medicine.

A year earlier, Schreber had taken over Ernst August Carus's orthopedic hospital and redesigned it as a gymnastic-orthopedic institute.[3] The education of the body now became his mission. An avid gymnast (*Turner*) since the late 1820s, Schreber was one of the founders of the local gymnastics club, the Allgemeine Turnverein and in 1846 became its president.[4] The following year he was elected to the city parliament as the representative of the liberal faction.[5] In fewer than ten years, Daniel Gottlob Moritz Schreber had become one of the notables of Leipzig. But without warning, as a result of a severe accident in 1851, he was forced to resign from the city parliament and lay down the directorship of the orthopedic institute.[6] So he embarked on another career. Schreber became a prolific writer whose best-selling tracts on home gymnastics preached "education to beauty through the natural and balanced promotion of normal bodily development."[7] He died in 1861.

Though emblematic of a middle-class man and writer, Schreber's career was neither striking nor exceptional. Yet it has become a symbol and symptom of nineteenth-century Germany in ways he did not intend. His son, Paul Schreber, is a classic case-study of modern psychiatry, discovered and described by Freud in his "Psycho-Analytic Notes upon an Autobiographical Account of a Case of Paranoia."[8] In it, Paul's father is pictured as a paradigmatic authoritarian, even sadistic, father whose orthopedic innovations, such as the infamous *Geradehalter*, a device designed to keep a child erect while sitting, resulted in the nightmares and neuroses of his unhappy son. But Schreber would not have recognized himself in this description, because, as he maintained, "the secret of the most difficult but noble and important art, the art of life, i.e., the art of living correctly, is embedded in the meticulous compliance of . . . two commands, hygienic and ethical."[9] The father of Paul Schreber did not want to impose a regimen on his disciples but to encourage each to find their own "art of life." For Schreber the starting point and ethical model for this art was walking, but its hygienic principles were fully realized in gymnastics, which strengthened and invigorated the muscles.[10]

Who was right: Schreber the idealist, whose goal was to promote beauty and an ethical life? Or the psychoanalytic critics who discovered the terrible side-effects caused by the means of achieving this goal? Interesting as it would be to debate this, the arguments around Schreber raise a larger question of the relationship between the hygienic and the ethical life, between the body and morality. Schreber and his German contemporaries were preoccupied with this question and the answers they found were unique, not in the importance they vested on the relationship between the body and morality but in the social practices that occupied such a central role in their answers. Schreber was interested in dietetics, gymnastics, and walking. Several of his colleagues would have added dancing to this list. In this book, I will probe why and how these theories arose, practices emerged and how they contributed to the relationship between the body and an ethical life.

What did the nineteenth-century Germans mean by "the body"? It is the most obvious presence in our lives and the most nebulous of notions. Germans used two different terms to signify the body: *Körper* and *Leib*. *Körper* was the more generic. Johann Christoph Adelung, a leading lexicographer at the turn of the nineteenth century, associated *Körper* with "any object that consist of materia; in opposition to the spirit."[11] But it could also mean, in a narrower sense, "the body of an animal and especially that of a human being, in opposition to the soul" and was identical with "the natural machine to which the spirit is connected."[12] During the first half of the nineteenth century, the meanings of *Körper* and *Leib* separated. For instance, Krug's *Allgemeines Handwörterbuch der philosophischen Wissen-*

*schaften* (1833) made it clear that there was an underlying difference between physical bodies that are perceptible and bodies that also can perceive. The act of perception made the latter more than mere physical bodies, physical objects; it turned them into animated bodies, *beseelte Körper*.[13] The animated body came to be signified by *Leib*, whereas *Körper* referred to the mere physical body. This distinction had far-reaching consequences for the contemporary understanding of everyday matters—and for politics. Krug himself was convinced that the *Leib* protected individual rights because "who chains, hurts or even kills the animated body of a human being, violates therefore his soul, i.e., the whole human being."[14] In all fields of knowledge, social practice, and politics that shaped or used human bodies, it made a difference to see the body as *Leib*, the animated body with innate rights and its own nature, not just as a physical object or machine that could be subjected to endless manipulation.

Closely associated with the concept of the animated body was the idea of self-formation, *Bildung*. This was anything but an unambiguous notion. Though *Bildung* was predominantly seen as an aesthetic-linguistic action, it was also a term for the body.[15] There were medical doctors such as Christoph Wilhelm Hufeland who sought to prolong human life by enhancing the *Bildungstrieb* (formative instinct) of the human organism[16]; there were advocates of physical exercise such as Johann Christoph Friedrich GutsMuths and Friedrich Jahn, who saw themselves as the preeminent advocates of *Bildung des Körpers* (forming of the body);[17] and finally, there were the dancing masters who polished everyday social life with the skills of elegant conduct.[18] All of them claimed to pursue *Bildung*, the formation of the self.

Two things make it difficult to use and understand the term *Bildung*. It is a key term in the German national self-conception, loaded with ambiguous descriptive meanings and normative intentions.[19] It is also an amorphous historical concept with the potential for continuous re-interpretation. As Aleida Assmann observes in her recent study, *Bildung* always seems to be accompanied by an arcane meaning that increases its tendency to create an imagined social cohesion among those who believed they are initiates.[20] Ever since the 1820s, *Bildung* has framed the fierce contest over the heritage of German nationhood. Through historical writings and especially historical memorials governments and associations sought to shore up their vision of Germanic tradition, be it a romantic-militaristic memorial, such as *Germania* of the Niederwalddenkmal (1877–83) or the neohumanistic statue of Schiller in Stuttgart (1827). *Bildung* was a close political ally of history and historical writing. Given the ambiguous meaning of this term, the question becomes, then, how we should define it to begin our inquiry. The most common option is to adopt the narrow meaning that the Prussian *Gymnasium* coined: the cultivation of skills, personality, and taste through the mastery of ancient languages, ultimately recognized in *Abitur*, the school-leaving exam that qualifies for admission to a university. However, as useful and empirically effective as this definition might be, to use it in all cases would be a mistake, for it would exclude expressions of *Bildung* that were recognized by contemporaries, particularly those aspects that related to the body and its practices. It seems, therefore, advisable to choose an approach that is liberal and broad enough to encompass several of its definitions, namely an historical one.[21]

To understand the idea of *Bildung*, one must start with a certain theological vocabulary that was transferred into social practice and had become part of everyday life by the end of the eighteenth century. In Genesis, it is declared that "God created man in His own image, in the image of God He created him; male and female He created them."[22] This figure, *imago Dei*, an inexhaustible source for the anthropological and theological imagination of the Western world, has been translated in German as *Bild* (image, picture).[23] Yet the theological definition has been balanced all along the way by the primary physiological meaning of *Bildung* whose ever-present connotation goes back to the very root of *bilden* in its meaning of the (beautiful) shape of the body. The combination of physiological and theological meanings increased the appeal of *bilden* to those, such as the natural philosophers, who sought a teleological understanding of nature. A typical and early use of this etymological amalgamation can be found in the works of Paracelsus, the alchemist and physician of the sixteenth century, who maintained that "the human being is created and ordered in another form, image, shape, and substance [than the macrocosm]."[24] Until the end of the eighteenth century, these theological and physiological meanings defined the primary content of *Bildung*.

Around the middle of the eighteenth century, we discover a new usage of *Bildung*. As early as 1752, a text by Johann Gottlob Krüger, a professor of medicine from Halle, promoted a technique for cultivating the soul (*Bildung der Seele*) by transforming "learning into a kind of playing. . . . One should never coerce children to study. Instead one ought to channel their natural inclinations. . . . This is the way to lead children towards Goodness."[25] This conception of education as the prompting of natural inclinations influenced German intellectuals during the following decades. Carl Friedrich Bahrdt's program of 1776 maintained that "we understand by the *Bildung* of customs only the embellishment of decorum. It consists of walking, posture, gestures, facial expressions, and tone—at the dining table, in society, and when distinguished persons are present."[26] Simultaneously with the new physical idea of *Bildung* emerged a linguistic one. In his *Ideen zur Philosophie der Geschichte der Menschheit* Johann Gottfried Herder showed that *Bildung* was connected to language. In their striving for reason, human beings were constantly imitating (*nachbilden*) the model (*Vorbild*) the *imago Dei* realized on the sixth day of Creation. In human tradition, the medium of imitation was language: "We can attain reason," Herder argued, "only through language, we can attain language only through tradition, through our belief in the word of our fathers."[27] Though Herder believed any language fulfilled this role, it was Latin and especially ancient Greek, the primary languages of higher education that he defined as the most effective instruments of *Bildung*.

The fluid definitions of *Bildung* show its evolution to be neither linear nor progressive. A history of this evolution cannot end with the statement that, by 1800, the linguistic notion would have replaced the preceding interpretations.

Instead, many historic connotations of *Bildung* were valid in the beginning of the nineteenth century. As late as 1807, Joachim Heinrich Campe observed that *Bildung* was a biological term of "the Almighty formation of plants and animals. In this formation each part which is added is formed in accordance with the preceding parts (epigenesis). 2) Natural essence and innate order (organization). 3) The shape of a human being, especially its face." But finally it was also "the status of a human being whose heart and spirit has been formed, and who has acquired skills and manners: a human being of sophisticated *Bildung*."[28]

Recent scholarship has started to pay attention how closely the German middle-class identity of *Bildung* was intertwined with the images and practices of the body.[29] Reinhart Koselleck is one of the first to point out that around 1800 *Bildung* was not an exclusively intellectual (linguistic) notion: "on the contrary, the living body (*Leib*), heart, mind, all the senses, and spirit belonged to a conceptual field that was constantly re-thought on the psychological level. It was on this conceptual field that *Bildung* was supposed to be fulfilled."[30] Recent studies on lifestyle, dueling, hygiene, and especially gymnastics have increased our understanding of the German middle-class identity beyond the *Gymnasium*.[31] One of the most focused in following this line of argumentation is Wolfgang Hardtwig's study of *Burschenschaften* (student fraternities). Hardtwig sees the fraternities' code of conduct as a method of controlling instincts, as an expression of what Norbert Elias called civilizing process.[32] Also Henning Eichberg has applied Elias's approach to the history of human conduct by tracing crucial changes in such configurations as dancing and gymnastics between 1770 and 1820.[33] Eichberg, is less interested in social, political, and educational changes than in the civilizing implications of these changes. His work is strong in its conceptual breadth, but it fails to account for developments incited by particular historical situations or the impact of social environments.

How to explain the historical specificity of the body and its history? There is something to learn from Michel Foucault: Human bodies are never mere physical entities but always exist in relation to a conceptual system that has been used to observe and regulate human behavior. Foucault has analyzed, for instance, how the clinic, asylum, and jail as complicated conceptual and political systems have emerged and changed since the sixteenth century. Despite, or perhaps because of, his sensitivity to the pre-modern world, Foucault was interested in how the modern world and its power structures evolved from it. All history, according to Foucault, is ultimately the history of the present.[34] Though it can be argued that both history and the past are only constructions of our mind, it is tempting, consoling, and even necessary to behave as if both were real and had their own right of existence. In this book, I have given in to this temptation and tried to discover the tenacity of the old practices and sciences that shaped the body of middle-class Germans. One should take a step beyond the history of the present and ask about the meaning and scope of old scientific systems. Instead of postulating systemic and conceptual ruptures, as Foucault depicted in his *Discipline and Punish*, this book asks whether and how the sciences of the Old World managed to shape the bodily practices of everyday life beyond the point at which the modern world defined its own path. Around 1800, there seem to be three major areas that fulfilled this function: dietetics, in its older, broader meaning as an organizational plan for lifestyle; dancing, with its social and moral function as a pattern of conduct; gymnastics as a re-enactment of the tribal past. In this study, the body means nothing more or less, except what is defined by these disciplines.[35]

There is no universal history of the body, no codification of sciences and practices that were applied to and applicable to each and everyone equally. The body is that of an individual who is a member of a social class, and that body is the carrier of the signifiers of that class. And for a complete definition, we must look to both sciences and social practices. What was the social meaning of bodily practices in nineteenth-century Germany? A substantial part of an answer to this question is defined by the rise and complex composition of the German bourgeoisie (*Bürgertum*). Much academic energy has been invested recently into detailed scrutiny of the German bourgeoisie in the eighteenth and nineteenth centuries so that the rise of this class has constituted an overarching metanarrative without serious challenges. The specific interpretations vary in describing how the bourgeoisie shared and contributed to the power constellation of the nineteenth century: Either the bourgeoisie failed, showed serious deficiencies (Wehler and Kocka), went through a silent revolution (Blackbourn and Eley), or was the splendid carrier of modernist transformation (Gall).

How should we define the term "bourgeoisie" to make a coherent yet sensitive start in a social history of the body? Mounting evidence testifies to the increasing problems of finding a reasonable nexus for a specifically German bourgeoisie in the late eighteenth and early nineteenth century. Not only did the bourgeoisie lack social cohesion—it had at least three different social functions around 1800—but drastic semantic shifts and social developments also effectively stymie one's efforts to identify a socially unified class.[36] The feudal system of order defined the "burgher" as a person whose position was confined to artisan and merchant groups in cities. During the first decades of the nineteenth century, this group went through a profound change, which resulted in its social disintegration as a feudal formation and gradual incorporation into the broader social constellation of the bourgeoisie, a class of industrialists, merchants, and civil servants. Besides these social notions, a juridical idea of the burgher as citizen (*Staatsbürger*) started to emerge.

If the idea of the bourgeoisie has any empirical relevance for early nineteenth-century Germany, it is in the constantly moving and shifting realm of ideas, norms, and social groups. As Manuel Frey has recently argued, the constitution of the German bourgeoisie was a cultural process in which certain principles, codes of conduct, and cultural patterns created a unified field of values shared by those who called themselves bourgeoisie.[37] But why should we call these values bourgeois? Either we think that these values had become the basis of the common morality of citizens whose home was in civil society, or we attribute those values exclusively to the members of a bourgeois class.[38] Yet neither seems to be true. Though the contours of civil society were visible in Germany in the late eighteenth century—especially in the social clubs and philanthropic societies—it is premature to argue for its universal presence in the early nineteenth century. It is also a mistake to ascribe those virtues and patterns, e.g. hygiene (Frey), just to the bourgeoisie. As recent scholarship shows, the aristocracy had an equal share of the cultural codes and patterns that in the early nineteenth century walked onto the stage of German history. This applies also and especially to the education of the body.[39] To limit this narrative to burghers or the bourgeoisie would lead to a fallacy of social perception. With this in mind, I will use the term "the educated middle class" and not to limit its association to the bourgeoisie but note its multiple social roots.

It is appropriate to be inclusive about and sensitive to all those social segments and groups that carried and shaped the texture of the German body and its education. Wolfgang Kaschuba has suggested an approach that does not take its point of departure from a predetermined description of a social class nor try to adjust it to fit a set of cultural patterns. Instead we should depict the social constitution of the educated middle class "by using the social situations and figurations in which the bourgeois practices of culture also appear as the concrete context for social action."[40] Thus our point of departure must be located in the practices of social classes. Not only schools, universities, and *Gymnasiums* but also the clubs and social circles offered places for bonding among those who aspired to call themselves cultivated (*Gebildete*). Above all, these clubs and social circles were spaces, as Anne-Charlott Trepp and Rebekka Habermas have argued, in which the very content of what it meant to be cultivated, *gebildet*, was defined and shaped.[41] These included not only those who had a diploma from the *Gymnasium* but also women, officers, merchants, aristocrats, and sometimes rich Jewish merchants, bankers, and professionals. By focusing on the process of how various candidates and members were recognized and how they molded and were molded by the principles of these clubs—the process of mutual recognition—we can depict the formation of the educated middle class.

The period of formation is described in many documents, whereas the period of stabilization is relegated to sentences and clauses. This is especially true of the primary sources on bodily practices. The four separate but closely related fields on which I have focused in my study—dietetics, dancing, walking, and gymnastics—reflect this state of affairs in different ways. My original idea was to combine intellectual and social history by, first, carefully reconstructing the specific sciences that shaped certain practices and, second, complementing and contextualizing these findings through an analysis of six cities covering the realm of the Germanic Confederation. This setting determined the kind of sources I could use. Though I purposely reached for a diversity of sources, including autobiographies, private correspondences, diaries, and novels, the main emphasis has been on manuals and handbooks, topographic descriptions and travel guides, journals, and records of social clubs. From a material perspective, the first two categories were the least problematic. Germans wrote a wealth of manuals on dancing, gymnastics, and dietetics between 1700 and 1850. On such material I have based my reconstruction of dietetics, walking, dancing, and gymnastics. Topographic and social descriptions of cities (*Stadtbeschreibungen*) and travel guides were equally important in providing insight into the social and geographic organization of cities, spas, walking spaces, and dancing opportunities.

More problematic than the standardized texts of handbooks and *Stadtbeschreibungen* were those sources that furnished the bulk of the social historical research: the journals and club papers. The journals, especially those with an eye toward broad cultural reflection, gossip, evaluation of tastes, manners and morals, provided rich and vivid descriptions on dancing and walking. Yet only a few journals and newspapers systematically, or even sporadically, discussed or reported on dancing, spa experiences, or promenades. The most important of these were *Journal des Luxus und der Moden* and *Zeitung für die elegante Welt*.[42] While changes in dancing—through the introduction of the waltz—and the shaping of the city environment occasioned intensive discussions from the 1790s until the 1810s, few remarks can be found on the latest masquerades or news from Carlsbad after the Congress of Vienna, and especially after the middle of the 1820s. If anything, this absence of anecdotal material indirectly proves the increasing dominance of intellectual and literary education and the routinization of bodily practices whose presence was as indisputable as it was trivial to mention. Not so with the papers of social clubs from Tübingen, Mannheim, Hamburg, Leipzig, Munich, and Vienna, which I have chosen as my samples. After the 1820s, the number of clubs increased substantially all over Germany, testifying to the reorganization of *Bildung* as everyday practice. However, this material has its limits. Unlike the learned and philanthropic societies, the social clubs hardly ever kept systematic records of their activities.

I argue that a study of the body and its practices tell an important story about the formation of the German educated middle class and that this story is about anachronistic modernization in which social practices and intellectual vocabularies were accommodated to changing socio-economic and political conditions but the willingness to change social conduct and decorum was combined with a reliance on old models and conceptualizations of the body.

In tracing the education of the body among the German educated middle class, I start with the discipline of the six non-naturals, or old dietetics. By focusing on the transformation of dietetics around 1800 from its practice by medical professionals to a domain recommended to lay practitioners and spa regimens by the 1850s, I try to locate the beginnings of a discourse in which the educated middle class became aware of the idea of bodily autonomy. The fourth chapter argues that the main challenge to dietetics was a new form of "tribal" gymnastics developed by Friedrich Ludwig Jahn who introduced an aggressive, dynamic, and socially democratic conception of physical motion. Dancing and walking, which I will discuss in chapters 5 and 6, were paradigmatic examples of dietetic exercise. Unlike gymnastics they retained dietetic elements by teaching moderation and the art of social recognition among unequals. The seventh and eighth chapters indicate that the social and intellectual turbulences of the 1830s caused by cholera epidemics and the controversies over the overloaded curricula of the German *Gymnasium* did not destroy the dietetic tradition, but gave it new momentum; they reinforced the political goal of the educated middle class to defend the autonomy of its body. Dietetics remained an important and peculiar domain of forming one's self, of *Bildung*, until the mid-nineteenth century and beyond.

## Notes

1. "Leipzig. Verzeichniss der Vorlesungen auf der Universität daselbst im Winterhalbjahre 1837." *Intelligenzblatt der Allgemeinen Literatur-Zeitung*. October 1837, 521–26.

2. "Leipzig. Verzeichniss der Vorlesungen auf der Universität daselbst im Winterhalbjahre 1839/40." *Intelligenzblatt der Allgemeinen Literatur-Zeitung* (October 1839): 500; "Leipzig. Verzeichniss der Vorlesungen auf der Universität daselbst im Sommerhalbjahre 1840," *Intelligenzblatt der Allgemeinen Literatur-Zeitung* (Mai 1840): 201–8; "Leipzig. Verzeichniss der Vorlesungen auf der Universität daselbst im Winterhalbjahre 1840/41," *Intelligenzblatt der Allgemeinen Literatur-Zeitung* (October 1840): 397. On his lectures on gymnastics see "Leipzig. Verzeichniss der Vorlesungen auf der Universität daselbst im Sommerhalbjahr 1845," *Intelligenzblatt zur Allgemeinen Literatur-Zeitung* (April 1845): 205.

3. Carus had founded the institute in 1829. Marion Bähr, "Erziehung zur Lebenstüchtigkeit durch harmonische Miteinander von Körper und Geist. Zum 125. Jahrestag der Gründung des ersten deutschen Schrebervereins," in *Leipzig. Aus Vergangenheit und Gegenwart. Beiträge zur Stadtgeschichte* 7 (Leipzig: VEB Fachbuchverlag, 1990), 60. Cf. Han Israëls, *Schreber. Vater und Sohn. Eine Biographie* (Munich: Verlag Internationale Psychoanalyse, 1989), 40–42.

4. Rudolf Gasch, *Festschrift zur fünfzigjährigen Jubelfeier des Allgemeinen Turnvereins zu Leipzig* (Leipzig: Allgemeiner Turnverein, 1895), 5.

5. See Páll Björnsson, "Making the New Man. Liberal Politics and Associational Life in Leipzig, 1845-1871" (PhD diss., University of Rochester, 1999).

6. The accident was a head injury that he suffered while exercising. See Israëls, *Schreber*, 60–61.

7. Schreber's ultimate best seller was the *Zimmer-Gymnastik* (Home Gymnastics) which was reprinted more than forty times and translated into seven languages. Cf. Gerhard Busse, *Schreber, Freud und die Suche nach dem Vater. Über die realitätsschaffende Kraft einer wissenschaftlichen Hypothese* (Berlin: Peter Lang, 1991), 77. See also Daniel Gottlob Moritz Schreber *Kallipädie oder Erziehung zur Schönheit durch naturgetreue und gleichmäßige Förderung normaler Körperbildung, lebenstüchtiger Gesundheit und geistiger Veredelung. Für Aeltern, Erzieher und Lehrer* (Leipzig: Fleischer, 1858).

8. Gasch, *Festschrift*, 5–6; Bähr, "Erziehung," 60–62. There is extensive psychoanalytical literature on Schreber. Against the interpretation of Schreber as a tyrant and vicious educator there has been a recent output of detailed accounts of Schreber's life and his educational activities. See esp. Israëls's *Schreber*, 26–106, which provide the most detailed account of Schreber's life and Busse, *Schreber*, 67–81. On Schreber's educational ideas see Clemens Rethschuhlte's detailed, *Daniel Gottlob Moritz Schreber. Seine*

*Erziehungslehre und sein Beitrag zur Körperbehindertenhilfe im 19. Jahrhundert. Genese und historische Einordnung* (Heidelberg: Edition Schindele, 1995), esp. 59–122.

9. "Denn in der treuen Erfüllung dieser beiden Gebote, des hygienischen und des ethischen, beruht das ganze Geheimniss der schwersten, aber edelsten und wichtigsten aller Künste, der Lebenskunst, d.h. der Kunst, richtig zu leben," Daniel Gottlob Moritz Schreber, *Aertzliche Zimmer-Gymnastik oder Darstellung und Anwendung der unmittelbaren—d.h. ohne Geräth und Beistand, mithin stets und überall ausführbaren—heilgymnastischen Bewegungen für beide Geschlechter, jedes Alter und die verschiedenen speciellen Gebrauchszwecke als ein einfach natürliches System entworfen.* 6th ed. (Leipzig: Friedrich Fleischer, 1859), 21.

10. Schreber, *Zimmer-Gymnastik*, 21.

11. "Ein jedes aus Materie bestehendes Ding; im Gegensatze eines Geistes," Johann Christoph Adelung, *Grammatisch-Kritisches Wörterbuch der hochdeutschen Mundart mit beständiger Vergleichung der übrigen Mundarten, besonders aber der Oberdeutschen*, vol. 2 (Wien: Anton Pichler, 1808), 1727.

12. "Der Leib eines Thieres und besonders eines Menschen, im Gegensatze der Seele ... die natürliche Maschine, mit welcher ein Geist verbunden ist," Adelung, *Grammatisch-kritisches Wörterbuch*, vol. 2, 1728.

13. Wilhelm Traugott Krug, *Allgemeines Handwörterbuch der philosophischen Wissenschaften nebst ihrer Literatur und Geschichte*, vol. 2 (Leipzig: Brockhaus, 1833), 632.

14. "Wer also den Leib eines Menschen fesselt, verletzt oder gar tödtet, vergreift sich dadurch an dessen Seele, mithin am ganzen Menschen," Krug, *Allegemeines Handwörterbuch*, vol. 2, 706.

15. On the classical idea of *Bildung*, see especially Aleida Assmann, *Arbeit am nationalen Gedächtnis. Eine kurze Geschichte der deutschen Bildungsidee* (Frankfurt am Main: Campus Verlag, 1993); Georg Bollenbeck, *Bildung und Kultur. Glanz und Elend eines deutschen Deutungsmusters* (Frankfurt am Main: Insel Verlag, 1994); Walter Bruford, *The German Tradition of Self-Cultivation. 'Bildung' from Humboldt to Thomas Mann* (Cambridge: Cambridge University Press, 1975); Friedrich Paulsen, *Geschichte des gelehrten Unterrichts auf den deutschen Schulen und Universitäten vom Ausgang des Mittelalters bis zur Gegenwart. Mit besonderer Rücksicht auf den klassischen Unterricht*, vol. 2 (Leipzig: Gruyter, 1921) is still a seminal guide to the nineteenth century German Geistesgeschichte; Rudolf Vierhaus, "Bildung," in *Geschichtliche Grundbegriffe*, vol. 1, ed. Otto Brunner, Werner Conze, and Reinhart Koselleck (Stuttgart: Klett-Cotta, 1972), 508–51. Louis Dumont's synoptic *German Ideology. From France to Germany and Back* (Chicago: University of Chicago Press, 1993) partly belongs to this tradition, especially in its analysis of Wilhelm von Humboldt, who according to the author established *Bildung* as a value, Dumont, *German Ideology*, 87. More detailed and instructive is Suzanne L. Marchand's, *Down from Olympus. Archaelogy and Philhellenism in Germany, 1750–1970* (Princeton: Princeton University Press, 1996), because it is one of the few and first efforts in English to probe how *Bildung* shaped the intellectual and political boundaries of an institution—in this case the profession of philology. See also the compelling study by David Gramit, *Cultivating Music. The Aspirations, Interests, and Limits of German Musical Culture, 1770–1848* (Berkeley: University of California Press, 2002), esp. 2, 93–124. Gramit demonstrates how music became one of the central practices of *Bildung* after it has been established as an autonomous field of aesthetics in the beginning of the nineteenth century.

16. Christoph Wilhelm Hufeland, *Makrobiotik oder die Kunst, das menschliche Leben zu verlängern* (Baden-Baden: Insel Taschenbuch, 1984), esp. 46–52.

17. Johann Christoph Friedrich GutsMuths, *Gymnastik für die Jugend enthaltend eine praktische Anweisung zu Leibesübungen. Ein Beytrag zur nöthigsten Verbesserung der körperlichen Erziehung* (1804) (Frankfurt am Main: Limpert, 1970), 39, 69; Friedrich Ludwig Jahn, *Deutsches Volksthum* (Leipzig: Philipp Reclam, 1813), 184.

18. Theodor Hentschke, *Allgemeine Tanzkunst. Theorie und Geschichte, antike und moderne (gesellschaftliche und theatralische) Tanzkunst und Schilderung der meisten National- und Charaktertänze* (Stralsund: Hausschildt, 1836), 2. Cf. also Rudolf Braun and David Gugerli, *Macht des Tanzes—Tanz der Mächtigen. Hoffeste und Herrschaftszeremoniell 1550–1914* (Munich: Beck, 1993), 232, and the literature given in the bibliography.

19. Cf. the literature given in Ulrich Engelhardt, *"Bildungsbürgertum." Begriffs- und Dogmengeschichte eines Etiketts* (Stuttgart: Klett & Cotta, 1986).

20. Assmann, *Arbeit*, 9–10; cf. Bollenbeck, *Bildung*, 160–64.

21. Another strategy would have been to adopt Hegel's definition of *Bildung*, especially the one elaborated in the *Phenomenology of Spirit*. It comes close to what Goethe understood as the design of life. Georg Wilhelm Friedrich Hegel, *Phänomenologie des Geistes* (Frankfurt am Main: Suhrkamp, 1973), 145–55, 384–87; cf. Georg Wilhelm Friedrich Hegel, "Rechts-, Pflichten- und Religionslehre für die Unterklasse (1810 ff.)," in *Werke in zwanzig Bänden*, vol. 4 (Frankfurt am Main: Suhrkamp, 1969), 259–62. Hegel's notion of self-formation is mediated through labor, either physical or intellectual. Goethe describes his dialectical notion of self-formation as following: "when in the exercise of his powers of observation man undertakes to confront the world of nature, he will at first experience a tremendous compulsion to bring what he finds there under his control. Before long, however, . . . he . . . must acknowledge their (forces of nature) power and pay homage to their effects. When this mutual interaction becomes evident he will make a discovery which, in a double sense, is limitless; among the objects he will find many different forms of existence and modes of change, a variety of relationships livingly interwoven; in himself, on the other hand, a potential for infinite growth through constant adaptation of his sensibilities and judgment to new ways of acquiring knowledge and responding with action," Johann Wolfgang von Goethe, *Scientific Studies* (New York: Suhrkamp, 1988), 61. Cf. Franco Moretti, *The Way of the World. The Bildungsroman in European Culture* (London: Verso, 1987), 50–51. Moretti maintains that the Goethean *Bildungsroman* created a trajectory of eternal youth that served as a philosophy of concreteness for the educated middle class. Not abstract thinking but concrete patterns of everyday life constituted its genuine realm.

22. *The Bible*, Genesis 1:27. Revised Standard Version.

23. The German version is as follows: "Und Gott schuf den Menschen zu seinem Bilde, zum Bilde Gottes schuf er ihn; und schuf sie als Mann und Weib," *Der Bibel*, Die Schöpfung 1:27. On the roots of the word "Bildung" see Ilse Schaarschmidt, "Die Bedeutungswandel der Worte 'bilden' und 'Bildung' in der Literaturperiode von Gottsched bis Herder," in Franz Rauhut and Ilse Schaarschmidt, *Beiträge zur Geschichte des Bildungsbegriffs* (Weinheim: Beltz, 1965), 28–36.

24. "Der Mensch in eine andere Form, Bildnis, Gestalt und Substanz geordnet und geschaffen ist [than the macrocosm] . . ." Paracelsus, *Vom Licht der Natur und des Geistes.* (Stuttgart: Reclam, 1984), 144. On the physical meaning of words "bilidon" and "bildunga" see Ernst Lichtenstein, *Zur Entwicklung des Bildungsbegriffs vom Meister Eckart bis Hegel*

(Heidelberg: Quelle & Meyer, 1966), 5. On the notion of *Bildung* in the seventeenth-century German mysticism see Günther Dohmen, *Bildung und Schule. Die Entstehung des deutschen Bildungsbegriffs und die Entwicklung seines Verhältnisses zur Schule*, vol. 1 (Weinheim: Beltz, 1964/65), 88–111.

25. Johann Gottlob Krüger, *Gedancken von der Erziehung der Kinder*, vol. 2, *Von der Bildung der Seele* (Halle: Hemmerde, 1752), 76. See also the strikingly similar view of Johann Peter Miller, a professor at the Lateinschule of Helmstedt and sympathetic toward the Moravian Brothers: "The reason why there are schools is so that those who recently came into this world would learn how they can lead a most enjoyable life now and in the future. In short, the whole school education is a constant instruction in enjoyment (*Vergnügen*). See Johann Peter Miller, "Die Schule des Vergnügens," *Altes und Neues von Schulsachen*, 2 (1753): 206.

26. Carl Friedrich Bahrdt, *Philanthropinischer Erziehungsplan oder vollständige Nachricht von dem ersten wirklichen Philanthropin zu Marschlins* (Frankfurt am Main: Eisenberg, 1776), 49.

27. "Alle kommen wir zur Vernunft nur durch Sprache und zur Sprache durch Tradition, durch Glauben an Wort der Väter," Johann Gottfried Herder, *Ideen zur Philosophie der Geschichte der Menschheit*, vol. 1 (Leipzig: Hartknoch, 1821), 340, 353.

28. Joachim Heinrich Campe, *Wörterbuch der Deutschen Sprache*, vol. 1. (Braunschweig: Schulbuchhandlung, 1807–9), 534.

29. According to Ulrich Herrmann, there has been a wide gap in research on what he calls the mentalities of education. Ulrich Herrmann, "Familie, Kindheit, Jugend," in *Handbuch der deutschen Bildungsgegschichte*, vol. 3, *1800–1870. Von der Neuordnung Deutschlands bis zur Gründung des Deutschen Reiches*, eds. Karl-Ernst Jeismann and Peter Lundgreen (Munich: Beck, 1987), 54; cf. also Karl-Ernst Jeismann, "Schulpolitik, Schulverwaltung, Schulgesetzgebung," in *Handbuch der deutschen Bildungsgegschichte*, vol. 3, *1800–1870. Von der Neuordnung Deutschlands bis zur Gründung des Deutschen Reiches*, eds. Karl-Ernst Jeismann and Peter Lundgreen (Munich: Beck, 1987), 109. One of the most ambitious ventures to study the educational mentalities of the German burghers between 1680 and 1815, Michael Maurer's *Die Biographie des Bürgers. Lebensformen und Denkweisen in der formativen Phase des deutschen Bürgertums (1680–1815)* (Göttingen: Vandenhoeck & Ruprecht, 1996), esp. 443–44, brings surprisingly little to the cultivation of the body. In the long chapter on "Bildung," this concept is understood in a narrow sense as an exercise of will and labor to earn a certificate for the future career as civil servant. Karl-Ernst Jeismann, in his recently reworked, *Das preußische Gymnasium in Staat und Gesellschaft*, has inserted the bodily aspect into the analysis on school politics.

30. Reinhart Koselleck, "Einleitung—Zur anthropologischen und semantischen Struktur der Bildung," in *Bildungsbürgertum im 19. Jahrhundert*, vol. 2, *Bildungsgüter und Bildungswissen*, ed. Reinhart Koselleck (Stuttgart: Klett-Cotta, 1990), 21. "Vielmehr gehörten Leib und Herz, Gemüt, alle Sinne und der Geist zum psychologisch stets aufs neue durchdachten Spannungsfeld, in dem sich Bildung zu vollziehen hätte."

31. Waltraud Heindl, *Gehorsame Rebellen. Bürokratie und Beamte in Österreich 1780 bis 1848* (Vienna: Böhlau, 1991), esp. 225–98; Ute Frevert, *Ehrenmänner. Das Duell in der bürgerlichen Gesellschaft* (Munich: Beck, 1991), esp. 198–214. McMillan has in mind an expansion of the traditional notion of *Bildung* when he sets out to show how "the ideal of self-cultivation (*Bildung*) was appropriated by groups who lacked extensive formal education; I also argue that diverse elements of the *Bürgertum*—ranging from academics to

artisanal journeymen—shared a distinctive work ethic, a specific orientation toward individual achievement as a promise and pitfall of the modern economy and meritocractic society," Daniel Alexander McMillan, "Germany Incarnate: Politics, Gender, and Sociability in the Gymnastics Movement, 1811–1871" (PhD diss., Columbia University, 1997), 14–15.

32. Wolfgang Hardtwig, "Auf dem Weg zum Bildungsbürgertum: die Lebensführungsart der jugendlichen Bildungsschicht 1750–1819," in *Bildungsbürgertum im 19. Jahrhundert*, vol. 3, *Lebensführung und ständische Vergesellschaftung*, ed., M. Rainer Lepsius (Stuttgart: Klett-Cotta, 1992), esp. 22–29. Also Manuel Frey, *Der reinliche Bürger. Entstehung und Verbreitung bürgerlicher Tugenden in Deutschland, 1760–1860* (Göttingen: Vandenhoeck & Ruprecht, 1997), esp. 50–53, interprets the hygienic movement in terms of disciplining or, in fact, as dual disciplining of the soul and body.

33. Henning Eichberg, *Leistung, Spannung, Geschwindigkeit. Sport und Tanz im gesellschaftlichen Wandel des 18./19. Jahrhunderts* (Stuttgart: Klett-Cotta, 1978), 168–201. cf. also Henning Eichberg, "Sport im 19. Jahrhundert—Genese einer industriellen Verhaltensform," in *Geschichte der Leibesübungen*, vol. 3/1, ed. Horst Ueberhorst (Berlin: Bartels & Wernitz, 1980), 385–401.

34. This is clearly spelled out in his conception of genealogy, which for Foucault does not constitute continuities of old or new traditions. On the contrary, he maintains that to "follow the complex course of descent is to maintain passing events in their proper dispersion; it is to identify the accidents, the minute deviations—or conversely, the complete reversals—the errors, the false appraisals, and the faulty calculations that gave birth to those things that continue to exist and have value for us," Michel Foucault, "Nietzsche, Genealogy, History," in *The Foucault Reader. An Introduction to Foucault's Thought, with Major New Unpublished Material*, ed. Paul Rabinow (London: Peregrine Books, 1984), 81.

35. A common assumption is that the body is roughly identical with sexuality in its different variations. This approach has been chosen, for instance, in an anthology by Catherine Gallagher and Thomas Laqueur in *The Making of the Modern Body. Sexuality and Society in the Nineteenth Century* (Berkeley: University of California Press, 1987). See the editors' "Introduction," esp. vii–viii, xv. Without refuting the essential meaning of sexuality organizing bodies, I have misgivings about this strategy. It is based on an anachronistic agenda—the concept of sexuality was introduced only in the 1850s—and fails to come to terms with the early nineteenth-century conception of the body. On the notion of sexuality see, for instance, Michelle Perrot, ed., *A History of Private Life. From the Fires of Revolution to the Great War* (Cambridge, Mass.: Harvard University Press, 1990), 578. See also Isabel V. Hull, *Sexuality, State, and Civil Society in Germany, 1700–1815* (Ithaca: Cornell University Press, 1996), 6–7, who systematically avoids applying the generic term "sexuality" to the period before 1815 and uses instead specific and contextual terms.

36. On the meanings attached to "bourgeoisie" (*Bürgertum*) in Germany around 1800, see Jürgen Kocka, "Bürgertum und Bürgerlichkeit als Probleme der deutschen Geschichte vom späten 18. Bis zum frühen 20. Jahrhundert," in *Bürger und Bürgerlichkeit im 19. Jahrhundert*, ed. Jürgen Kocka (Göttingen: Vandenhoeck & Ruprecht, 1987), esp. 23–30, 33–38. Kocka distinguishes four different meanings of *Bürger*: burgher, citizen, bourgeois, and the educated middle class. Hull, realizing the complex and deceptive meanings of *Bürgertum*, recurs to such lower-level terms as state and city officials as the carriers of civil society (*bürgerliche Gesellschaft*) see Hull, *Sexuality, State*, 201. Yet one should not exclude, as Hull does, the educated nobility from the *Bildungsbürgertum* because this class was, above all, the class of those who were educated and defined their social position through personal development.

37. On the program of bourgeois virtues see Rudolf Vierhaus, "Der Aufstieg des Bürgertums vom späten 18. Jahrhundert bis 1848/49," in *Bürger und Bürgerlichkeit*, 65–69. Cf. Frey, *Der reinliche Bürger*, 14–15.

38. On the utopia of a classless *bürgerliche Gesellschaft* as the driving force of the German bourgeoisie in the Vormärz see especially Lothar Gall, "Liberalismus und 'bürgerliche Gesellschaft.' Zu Charakter und Entwicklung der liberalen Bewegung in Deutschland," in *Historische Zeitschrift* 220 (1975): 324–56.

39. See especially the comprehensive book of Elisabeth Fehrenbach (ed.), *Adel und Bürgertum in Deutschland 1770–1848* (Munich: R. Oldenbourg Verlag, 1994), esp. her stimulating "Einführung," VII–XV. Fehrenbach shows both strong tendencies toward an increasing assimilation of the bourgeois bureaucracy and the aristocracy around 1800 and the resurgence of feudal consciousness in the Revolution of 1848.

40. Wolfgang Kaschuba, "Deutsche Bürgerlichkeit nach 1800. Kultur als symbolische Praxis," in *Bürgertum im 19. Jahrhundert*, vol. 2, *Wirtschaftsbürger und Bildungsbürger*, ed. Jürgen Kocka (Göttingen: Vandenhoeck & Ruprecht, 1995), 93.

41. Thomas Nipperdey understood in his, "Verein als soziale Struktur in Deutschland im späten 18 und frühen 19. Jahrhundert," in *Gesellschaft, Kultur, Theorie. Gesammelte Aufsätze zur neueren Geschichte* (Göttingen: Vandenhoeck & Ruprecht, 1976), see esp. 182–83, associations as the sign and vehicle of modernization. Yet his analysis is not sensitive to the questions that arise from "below." The intricate social networking of women in Hamburg, which Anne-Charlott Trepp has depicted in a most elaborate manner, indicates a new approach. The social clubs imitated and formalized many of the practices that had been established on a more informal level by a variety of reading circles, dinners, family circles, and private balls. See Anne-Charlott Trepp, *Sanfte Männlichkeit und selbständige Weiblichkeit. Frauen und Männer im Hamburger Bürgertum zwischen 1770 und 1840* (Göttingen: Vandenhoeck & Ruprecht, 1996), esp. 370–98. Cf. also Rebekka Habermas's studies on Merkels in Nuremberg, Rebekka Habermas, *Frauen und Männer des Bürgertums. Eine Familiengeschichte (1750–1850)* (Göttingen: Vandenhoeck & Ruprecht, 2000), esp. 137–71.

42. For my research I have consulted more than 25 journals, mainly of ephemeral and literary nature. Of these the most useful were *Journal des Luxus und Moden* and *Zeitung für die elegante Welt*. In particular, the regular reports in the *Journal des Luxus* on social life in spas and German capitals provided a systematic basis for research. These reports, however, virtually disappeared around 1820. Journals for women, such as the *Toiletten-Geschenk* were occasionally useful. Less useful were several of the most influential and respected journals, such as *Morgenblatt für die gebildeten Stände* (Tübingen, 1807–1865), *Freimüthige oder Berlinische Zeitung für Gebildete, unbefangene Leser* (Berlin, 1803–1840) or even such local journals as *Eos. Zeitschrift aus Baiern* and *Schwäbischer Merkur*. This sample suggests the increasing trivialization of the body after the 1820s: It became a self-evident issue.

*Part One*

# Quest for Bodily Autonomy

# Chapter Two

# Dietetics

In summer 1849, Prussian troops were restoring the old regime in Baden by attacking the last, desperate revolutionary troops. Karl Friedrich Straß, a high officer at the Prussian judicial administration, had other concerns. He was restoring his shattered health by conquering the shaded promenades of Pyrmont spa. Although the environment was pleasant indeed, Straß's life was no less systematic than that of Prussian soldiers in Baden. He was supposed to stay in fresh air, eat simple food, pay special attention to moderate physical exercise, sleep enough, and, above all, restore and retain the tranquility of his mind.[1] To successfully fulfill this mission Straß followed a detailed daily schedule. He woke up at six, strolled to the spring, drank 6 to 8 glasses of water, and took a short walk after each glass. After the last glass, he took, again, a walk, and, after an hour, had a light breakfast. Then was the time for a walk in fresh air or, if the doctor so wished, a bath. Before lunch Straß engaged in reading, socializing, music, and drawing. Lunch in company was at 1 pm. Between lunch and afternoon program, he enjoyed a relaxing cup of coffee. At 2 o'clock, Straß usually took an excursion to surrounding villages and hilltops. The light supper was served at 8 pm and at 10 o'clock Straß was in bed.[2] Karl Friedrich Straß's cure was successful and complete. Out of gratitude he wrote a detailed report of his visit to Pyrmont spa and made his experience public in a book in the following year.

During its formative years between 1790 and 1850, the German educated middle class subordinated its bodies to regimens like the one that Straß had experienced in Pyrmont spa. By doing so it reinvigorated a medical regimen and a method of lifestyle whose roots were at least as old as the roots of the political regime whose contours were threatened in 1848. This medical regimen was called dietetics.[3] Dietetics was the foundation of nineteenth-century lifestyle. It was not only a concern of medical doctors but also that of educated lay persons.

In the recent scholarship on eighteenth- and nineteenth-century medicine, the dietetic tradition has produced an academic anomaly. The increasing number of studies has not produced a systematic discussion of one of its most popular discourses and practices. It is understandable that for modern scholarship, dietetics in its traditional meaning is a chimera or, at best, a nice detail. It did not contribute to the rise of modern scientific medicine but was, rather, its old-fashioned nemesis.[4] Since the beginning of the 1980s, the new social history of medicine, inspired by Michel Foucault and Gerhard Oestreich, has contested and corrected the findings of this modernist success story. The price of the new knowledge and scientific progress, argued in the works of Ute Frevert and Claudia Huerkamp among others, could also be measured as professionalization, medicalization (Foucault), and disciplining (Oestreich) of the population.[5] The wealth of dietetic literature from the latter part of the eighteenth and the early nineteenth century was now analyzed and contextualized as medical enlightenment, as a means of implementing and promoting the medical policies of the state. This interpretation has remained unquestioned in recent studies that take a critical stand to what they perceive as Foucault's and Oestreich's modernist and anachronistic remnants.[6] Mary Lindemann's massive *Health and Healing in Eighteenth-Century Germany* is a case in point. By probing healing, lay medicine, and quacks in the eighteenth century, Lindemann challenges the traditional interpretations of professionalization and effective "medicalization."[7] She takes a new look at dietetics and discovers that it was used not only by doctors and authorities to implement their hygienic policies but also by laymen who simply wanted to enlighten themselves. Dietetics was one of the conceptual tools that lay and academic medicine shared.[8] This is an important finding. Yet we needed an account of dietetics not only as a medium of medical enlightenment and hygienic policies but also as a discipline, as a field of knowledge.

Thomas Broman has made important observations on the disciplinary nature of dietetics by the turn of the nineteenth century. In tracing the transformation of German academic medicine Broman has shown how, in the 1790s, the new Brunonian theory, enforced a simple and effective link between medical theory and its practical application at the bedside.[9] Although the Brunonians soon lost their influence, the old humoral link between theory and practice was irrevocably lost. Furthermore, after the decline of the Brunonian movement, according to Broman, theoretical and practical medicine started to separate. Whereas new natural sciences transformed theoretical medicine, the advocates of practical medicine continued to understand their field as art. This separation, though threatening the unity of the medical profession, was vital for the subsequent take-off of experimental medical research during the 1830s.[10] And the separation had fundamental consequences for dietetics as well. Through the Brunonian *coup d'état*, dietetics was dislocated from theoretical medicine to the art of healing, away from the center of medical discourse. It became, according to Broman, the medium of middle-class moralizing and medical enlightenment.[11]

To understand more fully the trajectory and social function of dietetics we have to proceed beyond Lindemann's and Broman's findings. Dietetics was not only socially applicable but also socially sensitive. By the end of the eighteenth century, manuals of general dietetics were accompanied by a host of literature that addressed dietetic problems of particular social classes. We need to ask what was included under "medical enlightenment?" Who was actually addressed, and how, by middle-class moralizing? Moreover, the academic status of dietetics was more complicated than what Broman suggests. Dietetics was a discipline with a carefully thought, though controversial, locus within the body of medical knowledge. Moreover, there is ample evidence that dietetics persisted much longer in academic education than what its Brunonian dislocation by 1800 implies. During the 1830s, it even regained some of its lost status as medical therapy. It seems that dietetics created a controversial but still functioning mediation between lay and professional medicine until the mid-nineteenth century. From the perspective of this productive tension between the lay adherence and professional rejection of dietetics we can also understand its social implications.

One of the difficulties in tracing the transformation of dietetics is embedded in its long tradition. Yet it was not the only science to carry this characteristic. Dietetics showed important parallels to other sciences of the late eighteenth century. The course of Cameralism between 1750 and 1830 provides a good point of reference.[12] Although Cameralism was not exactly "an old science," that is, it did not belong to the classical canon of sciences but found a permanent seat at German universities only after the mid-eighteenth century, it was traditional.[13] It was traditional because one of its conceptual sources was in the Aristotelic system of sciences. In the first book of his *Politics*, Aristotle discussed a doctrine called *oikonomos*, i.e., a description of the good order of a private household. *Oikonomos* located the conceptual basis of the "economy" in the private sphere. This privatized notion of economy was transported into the German husbandry writings (*Hausvaterliteratur*) which flourished during the latter half of the seventeenth century.[14] It included recommendations for the education, household, and moral conduct of household members of every social rank, from noble and princely families to peasant homes. Most importantly, it articulated the interests of German princes in promoting their power through economic and social policies. The discourse of the princely household, although under a clearly utilitarian influence, found its way into academia. In 1727, the universities of Halle and Frankfurt an der Oder established chairs in this field which soon adopted the name Cameralism.[15]

The basic problem of Cameralism was its heterogeneity. In their efforts to respond to administrational needs of princely courts, the first Cameralists were constantly at odds with the disciplinary and pedagogical nature of their field. The curriculum of Cameralism which F.X. Moshammer, a professor at Ingolstadt, offered during the 1780s in his lectures is characteristic. He embraced a huge variety of fields, such as philosophy, natural history (*Naturlehre*), law, mining, history, and technology.[16] Given the state's priority in organizing the economy, this combination could hardly be changed. It changed only when the economic priorities and constellations started to shift in the 1790s. The new generation of Cameralists replaced the state as the *modus vivendi* of economy with the concept of individual needs and calculation of interests. Yet the old Cameralism was taught alongside the new theories of national economy until the late 1820s.[17] The most intriguing feature in this disciplinary transformation is not only the radical change of social and political perspectives from state to civil society but also the new sense of philosophical and disciplinary unity within economics. By the emergence of national economics, economics had been reduced to economics proper, so to say, liberated from the immediate needs of governmental planning.[18] We can find a similar trajectory from a rich and multilayered aggregate of disciplines to a unified and reduced field of knowledge in the history of dietetics.

The peculiar role of dietetics was defined by its status as an old science on one hand, and by its social significance on the other hand. To clarify this, we have to follow how dietetics as an old science was carried down to the educated milieu of the early nineteenth century, second, how this milieu changed it into a new type of discipline, and, finally how this reconstituted science of dietetics served the needs of a particular class, the educated middle class. By fleshing out the two aspects of dietetics—scientific and social—we will be able to understand the role of dietetic ideology and the tensions of middle class lifestyle, in which very few practices were actually what they appeared to be to us, in which walking was not only walking, dancing only dancing, and drinking only drinking but also exercises in moral conduct.

## Classical Dietetics

In the classical medicine of the Hippocratic and Galenic tradition, which was canonized during the Middle Ages, health was understood as depending on the seven naturals, the six non-naturals, and the three contra-naturals. Although these categories overlapped at some important points, we can say, following the presentation of Antoinette Emch-Dériaz, that they roughly defined the scope of medical science.[19]

Physiology: the seven naturals:
- Elements (fire, air, water, earth)
- Qualities (hot, cold, dry, moist)
- Humors (blood, phlegm, yellow bile, black bile)
- Members of the Body
- Faculties
- Spirits (natural, vital, animal)
- Operations (hunger, digestion, retention, expulsion)

Dietetics: the six non-naturals:
- Air
- Food and Drink
- Motion and Rest
- Sleep and Waking
- Evacuations
- Passions[20]

Pathology: the three contra-naturals:
- Diseases
- The Causes of Diseases
- The Sequels of Diseases

The seven naturals were given by the constitution of the body; they were human nature and the basis of health. The pathological contra-naturals neither belonged to human nature nor contributed to its health but tried to destroy it. Finally, the six non-naturals did not belong to the human nature but still profoundly influenced its balance and health. Thus dietetics emerged as a science and art of directing the contingencies of the human body and its environment.

Dietetics was instituted within the theory of humors, the physiological theory of classical, Galenic medicine. The regulation of the human body, its metabolism, and contingent relationship with the environment was understood in Galenic medicine as an important tool in restoring and retaining health. Although the arguments against Galen and his legacy mounted after the late fifteenth century, the theory of humors persisted in medical curriculums and particularly in the basic assumptions of pathology and physiology so that, in the early nineteenth century, it was still the common currency of medical theorizing.[21] There was no lack of competition against the theory of humors. The leading medical institution in Germany, the University of Halle, was a case in point. In Friedrich Hoffmann it had a superior advocate of new mechanistic theories, i.e., iatromechanism, which explained human physiology and its pathological malfunctioning in terms of mechanical laws of nature. Georg Ernst Stahl, Hoffmann's colleague, disputed iatromechanism and advocated the doctrine of vitalism, according to which the human being was, above all, a living being whose specific characteristics were irreducible to any mechanical law. Vitalism, became, along with iatromechanism, the main contenders of the theory of humors in European medical thinking. But none of them succeeded in replacing the Galenic system. The result was not a paradigm change but, rather, the mushrooming of new and competing medical theories. The end of the eighteenth century witnessed a variety of different versions of iatromechanism, magnetism, and vitalism which all laid claim to the unified theory of health or human constitution. The reaction was to be expected. The profession and the educated clientele responded with scepticism and ridicule toward any medical theories. Hence there was space for a new practical emphasis within medicine.

By the turn of the nineteenth century, Hippocrates had replaced Galen as the symbol of sound medical practice. In 1805, a commentator expressed the nature of the new critique by claiming that Galen's medical thinking was too metaphysical. He was simply far too careless in adding "unfounded statements of elementary qualities and hidden forces" to physiological and pathological observations.[22] According to the same observer, Hippocrates was quite the opposite, making "extremely accurate observations on external factors, such as air, water, and climate."[23] Hippocrates now appeared as the true progenitor of an empirical and reliable medical practice, in contrast to Galenic medical theory.

In an interesting but confusing way the turn toward practical medicine of Hippocrates opened the venue to the revival of dietetics whose origins were in the theoretical medicine of Galen. How was this possible? The reasons are partly theoretical. As a discipline and a body of knowledge dietetics was flexible. Regardless of its close and convenient affiliation with the theory of humors, the pattern of six non-naturals flourished while the corresponding physiological theory was in decline. Both Stahl and, especially, Hoffmann were famous for their teaching and textbooks in dietetics. Like the increasing number of their colleagues and followers, they never abandoned the six non-naturals.[24] Until the 1770s, it is difficult to find a textbook that challenged or even essentially corrected the traditional conceptualization of dietetics. Nothing seems to suggest that dietetics had essentially changed since its formation during the Middle Ages.

Yet the status of dietetics in the body of medical knowledge was changing. In classical medicine, dietetics was a part of pathology, especially diagnostics, and a constitutive part of therapy. It provided an instrument of healing but unlike the other two instruments of therapy, surgery and medication, dietetics always had a special role in preventing diseases. Until the eighteenth century, the mutual balance between the therapeutic tools varied greatly—mainly because of the perpetual reliance on medication. This internal twisting continued until effective medicine and sophisticated methods of surgery were invented during the latter half of the nineteenth century. When the criticism against Galen's principles and influence increased and Hippocratic medicine went through a revival, the status of dietetics was expanded from a therapeutical tool to a broad prophylactic science. This prophylactic aspect of dietetic knowledge is important in understanding the revival of dietetics as a part of practical medicine. During the eighteenth century, German textbooks increasingly abandoned dietetics as a necessary part of medical therapy. Hermann Boerhaave's *Institutiones Medicæ* (1710) separated between the art of healing (*Curatoria*) and dietetics which was dealing with preventing diseases and prolonging life.[25] Johann Juncker, an influential student of Stahl and clinician at the University of Halle, saw dietetics as an insignificant, auxiliary method to secure the necessary nutrition, peace, and tranquility of mind for the patient to recover effectively.[26] Samuel Schaarschmidt's *Therapia Generalis*, which was posthumously published in 1749, was fully in line with this established systematization that ushered dietetics into the outskirts of medical therapy.[27] Towards the close of the century the exclusion of dietetics from mainstream medical textbooks was so profound, as the young medical doctor from Halle, August Friedrich Hecker, observed, that "there is hardly any writer whose texts on general therapy would deal with the diet of the patient, and those who do that focus only on nutrition and air."[28]

The six non-naturals had been separated from physiology and from therapy. Was classical dietetics, then, slipping outside academic medicine? There is evidence which supports this idea. There is also evidence that testifies to the opposite. The Hippocratic renaissance of the eighteenth century led, as James Riley has shown, to an increasing concern for environmental medicine and this concern endowed dietetics with a new flair.[29] Since the 1750s, medical doctors started to raise their voice for the reintroduction of the six non-naturals in the medical therapy. Christian Gottlieb Ludwig, a professor of physiology and therapy at the University of Leipzig, argued in his 1754 compendium, *Institutiones Therapiae generalis*, for a dietetic therapy.[30] Hecker was even more straightforward in his *Therapia Generalis* of 1789: not only food and air, but all the six non-naturals should have a permanent role in medical therapy. "I cannot understand," asked Hecker, "why the passions, sleep, waking, and evacuation should be omitted?"[31] Yet his voice for the dietetic revitalization of medical therapy conveyed not much more than the nostalgia for old medicine.

The genuine revival of dietetics took place in the grey zone of prophylaxis. As a part of medical therapy, dietetics was supposed to help restore the equilibrium of bodily fluids, i.e., health. As a prophylaxis, it was only indirectly contributing to this process, by preventing the outbreak of diseases. Hence it was only natural that the productive and positive possibilities of classical dietetics were to be discovered. During the second half of the eighteenth century, movement that Lindemann and Porter have called "popular medical enlightenment" or "medical popularization" started to spread.[32] To enlighten the population, its masses and elites, popular medical elightenment used dietetics. Its vocabulary was well known, not because it was natural and easy but because it was made natural and easy. Texts on the six non-naturals had been circulating in Europe since the thirteenth century, when the first versions of the famous dietetic poem, *Regimen Sanitatis Salernitanum*, saw the light. Dietetics was part of the constructed folklore and to reach the masses an enlightener had few choices but to accept and use this folklore.[33] Yet dietetics was more than a necessary evil in propagating health. It had important benefits in rationalizing human behavior in the way that combined physiological and pathological understanding of metabolism with a broad vision of moral conduct and lifestyle. In no other area this juncture of medical and moral conduct came clearer to fruition than education. John Locke was evidently inspired by dietetics in his *Some Thoughts Concerning Education* which, in fact, was constructed along the lines of a dietetic treatise. Johann Gottlob Krüger, Professor of Medicine at the University of Halle, was one of the first German scholars to notice this seeing "the famous English physician and philosopher, Locke," and "his book on the education of young noblemen" as model for his *Diät oder Lebensordnung* (Diet or the Order of Life) (1751). This book and the two-volume manual on education that Krüger published a year later effectively laid bare the foundations of an educational theory that rested on dietetics, on the

Table 2.1. Pediatric-Dietetic Literature in Germany, 1750–1830. Based on Kunze, *Die physische*, 187–99.

| *Years* | *N* | % |
|---|---|---|
| 1750–1770 | 12 | 8 |
| 1770–1790 | 41 | 27 |
| 1790–1810 | 77 | 51 |
| 1810–1830 | 21 | 14 |
| *Total* | 151 | 100 |

principle of hardening and endurance as the ideals of child rearing.[34] From Krüger to Johann Friedrich Zückert, and to the educational philanthropy of Johann Bernhard Basedow and Campe, we can follow, as Lydia Kunze and Christa Kersting recently have shown, the dietetic discourse of German education.[35] Dietetic writers, as Table 2.1. shows, readily turned their attention to education. While the eclipse in publication of pediatric-dietetic literature was reached between the French Revolution and the Wars of 1813–15, dietetic writing on children continued at a considerably high level until the 1830s. The educational practices of the late eighteenth and early nineteenth centuries, especially the ones with a penchant for physical exercise, were arguably lay extensions of dietetics. Education graphically displayed the strength of classical dietetics. Rather than separating the discourses of professionals and laymen, classical dietetics celebrated their mutual understanding. Yet mutuality could be a problem. It was shallow, arbitrary, and could prevent, as an increasing number of doctors and philosophers started to argue, the systematic understanding of both lifestyle and dietetics.

## Dietetics Revised: The Quest for Bodily Autonomy

In the introduction to his lectures on the vocation of scholars which he gave during the academic year 1794–95, Johann Gottlieb Fichte, a young professor of philosophy at the University of Jena, made clear in an acrimonious outburst what his lecture would not include:

> Now those [who find Fichte's book useless], who want to drag everything down to their level, cannot elevate themselves. They require for instance that all

printed text must be available as a cookbook, as a calculation book or as a statute. They denounce everything which does not comply with this requirement. But by doing all this they make a great injustice.[36]

Fichte's criticism was not a merely categorical rejection of a self-help philosophy. It was a precise departure from a rich tradition of writing on the vocation of scholars with which the eighteenth century was so familiar. Even more visionary texts could not escape this accusation. Christian Thomasius's lectures a hundred years earlier in Halle had launched a challenging program to combine genteel and scholarly lifestyles. Yet, looking from Fichte's perspective, Thomasius's solution was nothing but pedestrian, a technique, "how one can instruct young people in morality and in the art governing one's passions in a good manner."[37] Thomasius spent the rest of his life in elaborating a special science of decorum to implement his idea.[38] Much less ambitious but still in the same tradition was Jakob Sigmund Apinus's manual on *Vernünftiges Studenten Leben* (On Reasonable Student Life), published anonymously in 1726. Instead of a new vision Apinus described in detail what a student should eat—not too bad, not too delicious[39]—or "whether one should study sitting or lying down, walking or standing."[40] If anything, this was the kind of cookbook which Fichte wanted to scrap.

Fichte wanted something more than to scrap cookbooks. He wanted to leave behind the detailed realm of the body, conduct, and lifestyle, and this was the realm of dietetics. For those who would not follow him, Fichte promised a disgraceful future:

> Given that you cannot convince yourself [of the usefulness of Fichte's project] you will lose very little because, anyway, you are what you are. And humankind will not lose anything. It will just become clear by your actions that you will not have a share in the plan of the ennoblement of humankind. Whereas the ennoblement of humankind inevitably continues your ennoblement will be guided by good nature. It provides you rain and sunshine at the appropriate time, gives you decent food and free circulation of humors. And it might also give you some clever thoughts.[41]

Nature and the body could not prescribe the vocation of a scholar. This radical exclusion of dietetics from the reflection on the scholar's vocation was followed in the idealistic and classical literature of the nineteenth century. For instance, Friedrich Wilhelm Joseph von Schelling's *Vorlesungen über die Methode des academischen Studium* in Jena in 1802 and Friedrich Wilhelm Tittmann's *Ueber die Bestimmung des Gelehrten* (1833) followed this non-dietetic path.[42] We can say that, by 1800, classical dietetics was contested by a new kind of conception of lifestyle that emerged from the specific needs of scholars.

Although the dieticians wrote for the general public and not only for the scholars, Fichte's outburst included an important remark on the basic problem of classical dietetics as discipline: it was too heterogeneous to be scientifically convincing and too arbitrary to be useful as practical knowledge. During the final decade of the eighteenth century this had become a compelling argument among the German intellectuals. Within a few years, several efforts were made to reshape dietetics. The driving force behind this transformation was the logic of medical knowledge itself and the prospect for social application of new dietetic concepts.

A crucial year for a new conception of dietetics was the year 1796. It was the year when Christoph Wilhelm Hufeland, a young professor of medicine from Jena, published his *Über die Kunst, das menschliche Leben zu verlängern*.[43] Born in 1762 to the family of the physician-in-ordinary to the Duke of Weimar, Hufeland's social destiny combined two important parameters. He was to follow his father as a doctor and a court physician. After the premature death of his father in 1787, however, Hufeland found that this calling was not to be fulfilled. He remained a "public physician" (*Hofmedicus*). But due to his family background and obvious talent, Hufeland was soon priviledged to socialize with the most important names of Weimar court society. In 1792, he had the opportunity to give a series of lectures on the notion of vital power to Johann Wolfgang von Goethe's private club, *Freitagsgesellschaft*, in front of a renowned audience—Goethe, Herder, and the Duke himself were among the audience.[44] This event, more than anything else, defined the course of Hufeland's life. The Duke was so impressed by the young doctor's performance that he decided to nominate him to a chair at the University of Jena. Whether it was the lecture alone that made the Duke decide for Hufeland might be doubted, although the autobiography readily maintains so. Hufeland was not only a permanent member of the *Freitagsgesellschaft* but obviously a regular visitor, host, and friend to Goethe and his circle.[45] This opened paths for him, first to Jena, where Hufeland became a successful and popular professor, and, in 1801, to Berlin as the head of the famous hospital Charité and the director of the *Collegium medico-chirurgicum*, the leading committee on medical issues in Prussia. He also automatically became a permanent member of the Prussian academy of science. Besides his increasing political power—he was, for instance, one of the founding members of the new medical faculty of the University of Berlin in 1810—Hufeland had an almost overwhelming literary and academic influence. Already in Jena he started the *Journal der practischen Heilkunde*, the leading forum of medical discourse in Germany during the first half of the nineteenth century. Until the end of his life he continued to publish handbooks, treatises, and articles. Among his publications none could match the popularity of *Über die Kunst, das menschliche Leben zu verlängern*.

To be sure, Hufeland was not completely original in his venture on longevity. A few years earlier Hecker had advocated a theory of healing quite similar to Hufeland's art of longevity. They both were based on the notion of vital power (*Lebenskraft*).[46] The difference between them was their popularity: whereas Hecker's book was in its third and final edition in 1796, Hufeland's work became one of the most celebrated in the nineteenth century. The last non-historical re-edition is from 1860.

Can Hufeland's book be treated as a dietetic work? In fact, we do not find the word "dietetics" in the title of the book. It was also rarely used in the text.[47]

Furthermore, Hufeland understood his book as the foundation of a new independent science which was based on dietetics but whose goal was different. This new science was not designed to re-establish the health of the human body but to prolong its existence.[48] That is to say, Hufeland did not want to subsume his new science under medical therapy. This was nothing new, however. Since the beginning of the eighteenth century dietetics was set apart from medical therapy and assigned a prophylactic role. What was new appears in the bond between longevity and dietetics. Hufeland's book did contain a dietetics. We find in it the model of the non-naturals to which Hufeland had added education, marriage, and the culture of cleanliness.[49] And the purpose of this dietetics was longevity. The new science was not only set apart from therapy but also from pathology. Its role was not defined in a negative sense as protection against or cure from diseases but, rather, as something positive, the ennobling and perfection of human nature.[50]

More problematic than the relationship between dietetics and medicine was the question of whether this new science was a science, *Wissenschaft*. Thomas Broman has argued that an important component in the transformation of academic medicine, and hence in the rise of modern medicine, by the turn of the nineteenth century was the dislocation of history from the body of medical knowledge.[51] Hufeland's book was right in the center of this change. In fact, it contained a wealth of medical case histories from the ancient times. Hufeland was also pronouncedly historical in justifying his new science by carefully depicting the main stages of his field from the Greek world down to contemporary medicine. Yet as much as he was conscious of this tradition, he was convinced that the art of prolonging life should be established as a scientific discipline.[52] From the very outset this was an ambiguous idea, because dietetics only enumerated certain contingencies related to the body. In some of the classical works of eighteenth-century dietetics this inconvenience was solved by claiming physiology and pathology as antecedents of dietetic conduct of life. For instance, in his *Diät oder Lebensordnung* (1751) Krüger took for granted that the reader was well enough informed of his physiological and pathological theories in order to follow his exposition of dietetics.[53] Christian Jahn was more explicit in his *Norma Diatetica* (1757), by providing a physiological introduction to his topic.[54] Also, in Franz Anton May's famous, *Medicinische Fastenpredigten* (1793) we can find a similar physiological introduction as a brief account "of the necessary knowledge of the well organized human body and the physical and mental powers of the ancient Germans." This was neither enough nor adequate for Hufeland, who devoted half of his book to an analysis of the theoretical foundations of human nature. Hufeland placed them in what he called vital power (*Lebenskraft*).[55]

The origins of Hufeland's notion of a vital power were in vitalism. Although its progenitor Stahl had influential students in Germany, such as Juncker, Daniel Gohl, and Michael Alberti, his later influence would spread largely through France, especially Montpellier. Yet by the time French vitalism started to find resonance in Germany, by the middle of the century, Albrecht von Haller, the eminent physiologist at the University of Göttingen reduced the question of vital powers to a series of carefully planned physiological experiments. They convinced von Haller and an increasing number of his contemporaries of something which he called excitability.[56] This evidence gave a boost to a broader theory of a vital power that, until the 1770s, established its place in the medical and anthropological vocabulary. We find it in the physiological theory of Paul-Joseph Barthez, a leading figure at the Montpellier, as *Principe de Vie*; in Germany it was captured by Casimir Medicus as *Lebenskraft*. Finally, Johann Friedrich Blumenbach, a professor of medicine at the University of Göttingen and a towering figure among German natural scientists, became its most influential protagonist in 1781. Through his book *Über den Bildungstrieb und Zeugungsgeschäft* (On the Formative Drive and Procreation), inspired by von Haller, Blumenbach established the notion of vital power as a fundamental law of physiology that incited the subsequent physiological and anthropological discourse well into the nineteenth century.[57]

By the end of the eighteenth century, the legacy of Stahl, von Haller, and Blumenbach also affected the renewed debate on medicine from another angle. Von Haller's findings had reinvigorated an old theory of excitability as the basis of vital functions. John Brown, an obscure Scottish physician, recast this concept as a universal theory of medicine through his book *Elementa Medicinae* (1780). While Brown's influence in Scotland and England was modest indeed, in German-speaking Europe he captured many minds between the French Revolution and the Congress of Vienna. The followers of Brown, the Brunonian movement, was one of the main actors in the debates over the future of medicine.

How did Hufeland navigate among these rapidly changing theories? It is obvious that the young Hufeland was attracted by the vitalism of a Blumenbachian brand. As early as 1792, in his lectures to Goethe's *Freitagsgesellschaft*, he saw the essence of human life, i.e., the vital and active power, as irreducible to any set of mechanical laws of nature.[58] In the *Ideen über Pathogenie* of 1795 and two years later, in *Die Kunst*, Hufeland expanded the theory of vital power to pathology and prophylaxis or rather, the art of prolonging life. Although he increasingly felt challenged by Brunonian arguments after 1797, so that the *System der practischen Heilkunde* was almost completely in line with the Brunonian terminology of excitability and irritability, it is also important to notice his lingering commitment to Blumenbach and the classical brand of vitalism. Hufeland's Brunonianism was superficial and pragmatic.[59] In the Introduction he made his position clear.

> Instead of using the customary notion of vital power (*Lebenskraft*) I have used the word excitability (*Erregbarkeit*). Yet I have not used it to explicate a new idea but to avoid a misinterpretation in the philosophical grammar. Although I must admit that in signifying the generic category, . . . the notion "vital power" will remain useful and necessary.[60]

The notion of vital power articulated Hufeland's weltanschauung which can be discovered even in his posthumous *Enchiridion medicum.*[61] The premise of an irreducible and inexplicable vital power implied two theorems of major significance for the notion of dietetics. Hufeland maintained that vital power was only available in a limited amount.[62] Moreover, its automatic and constant externalization led to its weakening. Only through rest it could be regenerated.[63] Nevertheless, this externalization was essential for active human life, not as a mere function of external stimuli.

> The most immediate functions of the vital power are not only to receive impressions, such as irritation, and to react upon them, but also to change into organized nature the component parts which are added to the body; that is to unite them according to the laws of organization, and also to give them that structure and form which the end of organization requires, i.e., formative power, power of reproduction, and formative instinct (*Bildungstrieb*).[64]

Given the finite amount of vital power—it could be only strengthened or weakened, not increased—the science of correct, dietetic life was based upon the art of balancing the externalization and regeneration of vital power.

Hufeland's idea of a balanced consumption and reproduction of vital power reinforced the doctrine of moderation, a central part of classical dietetics. To avoid harmful effects of the non-naturals, one was advised to adopt a moral rule of the golden mean. Moderation was a convenient maxim for the art of mastering the contingencies of human life. But for Hufeland the purpose of human nature could not be mere moderation, which strongly connoted mediocrity in late eighteenth-century German and was only a moral maxim without any material content. Instead, one should strive for what he called "human nature ennobled and raised to perfection."[65] Since the externalization of vital power was the formative element of perfection, the emphasis of dietetics shifted toward a theory of human nature. Naturally, the attributes "ennobled" and "perfection," also belonged to the Neohumanistic vocabulary of *Bildung* and they were widely used in contemporary anthropology. With these parameters in mind, we can see that Hufeland made the dietetic discourse into the (utopian) theory of human nature.

This shift had important consequences for the practical part of Hufeland's book. It was divided into two sections: The first one recorded the pathological effects, which prevented the prolongation of life, and the second one prescribed the positive rules of longevity. The pathology, following Rousseau's arguments against the corrupting effects of civilization, was hardly original. In fact, it duplicated the ideas of such educators as Basedow, Campe, and Peter Villaume, who were acting in concert with physicians in promoting Rousseau's call for natural life in the 1770s and 1780s. What we find in this part of the book is a standard account of how this period was permeated by pampering education, sexual debauchery, overburdening of mental powers through excessive studies, unclean air of study-rooms and urban environment, excessive eating and drinking, overrefined and agitated passions and phantasy.[66] It is, however, important to notice the discrepancy of this pathology of culture with the rules of conduct, with the positive dietetics of macrobiotics, which the second section addressed. One could have expected that the criticism of the corrupted civilization would have justified or even demanded a program of eradicating the aberrations of contemporary civilization. At least, this was common in the moral discourse of the late eighteenth century. Physicians and pedagogues prescribed vigorous physical exercise, resistance against weather, and strengthening of one's body as means of overcoming the culture of overrefinement.[67] It was the program of hardening. Hufeland advised differently. He carefully pointed out how, in physical exercise, "attention must be always paid to the uniform distribution of vital power: for harmony and equality in the motions are the foundation of health and life."[68] Or, for that matter, how one should avoid overly warm baths,[69] and watch one's sleeping time, which should be optimized between six and eight hours.[70] This advice found a natural justification in the economy of vital power, in the balance of its externalization and regeneration.

Hufeland sought to establish a scientific dietetics. The discipline was no longer a random collection of prophylactic and therapeutic prescriptions but had become a unified body of knowledge, a science (*Wissenschaft*) in the rigorous sense which Fichte could also have accepted. It was anything but clear whether Hufeland had convinced his audience. We do not know whether Fichte rejected his revised dietetics. Yet an equally qualified authority investigated the epistemological status of scientific dietetics immediately after *Die Kunst* was published. Hufeland had sent his work to Immanuel Kant, waiting for a friendly gesture. Kant, increasingly obsessed with his health, illnesses, and the functioning of his aging body, spent one long month with Hufeland's book, producing an extensive answer which contained a dietetic treatise, "On the Power of Human Mind to Direct Pathological Emotions Through Firm Intention."[71] Wiesing has recently labeled Kant's comments on Hufeland's book as a harmless compilation in which Kant "in addition to a few theoretical remarks also depicted his personal experiences."[72] The private character of Kant's remarks is noticeable, but rather than letting it provide an excuse to dismiss the text, we should pay attention to its important epistemological implications.

From the very outset, Hufeland's book clearly did not provide the kind of general and objective rules which, for instance, Johann Peter Frank had constructed in the six volumes of his *System einer vollständigen medicinischen Polizey* (A System of Perfect Medical Policy) (1779–1819). Frank had linked his project to the absolutistic state that aspired to increase and conserve its population.[73] But, as Kant remarked, Hufeland's subject field was related to private experiences. This approach had quite a peculiar problem. One was

> compelled to use "I" which in a dogmatic presentation shows presumptuousness. If it is not a shared experience but an inward experiment or observation the use of "I" deserves our forgiveness. To provide material for judgement "I" has to

> undertake this experiment because something which is not already liked by everyone through oneself or through guidance must be presented for judgement only after "I" has used this observation for oneself.[74]

Therefore, dietetics could not provide the necessary objectivity of publicly shared experiences: it was not science. Dietetics was, rather, a narrative, as Kant called it, in which the six non-naturals yielded only rhetorical cohesion, not the logical and apodictic unity of a theory or scientific experience. Closely connected to the epistemological question was the pragmatic problem of how, to whom, and by whom dietetic knowledge should and could be applied. Kant suggested that dietetics could be applied only personally, through one's own deliberation to one's own life.[75] Given the narrative form of private experiences this seemed to follow from the epistemic nature of dietetic knowledge.

In effect, Kant's comments on Hufeland's enterprise were quite damaging. Hufeland could not, according to Kant's criteria, redeem his promise to establish a science. Yet contrary to Kant's suggestion, even a private narrative could have uses beyond private introspection. It not only provided material for a future (scientific) judgement but could also be used publicly. By 1800, we can distinguish two forms which, in fact, employed this strategy: the dietetic narrative of Germanic tribalism and the discourse of health education.[76]

After Rousseau, anthropological narratives of a lost natural state had become increasingly popular. A variation on this narrative was the story of Germanic tribalism. Franz Anton May, the Mannheim physician and Heidelberg professor of midwifery, was among the first to employ it for dietetic purposes in his public lectures that he gave in Mannheim in 1793 and 1794. May was a local figure with a strong following in his home town of Mannheim. A political monarchist, he rejected the French Revolution and attacked against those Germans who sympathized with "the French mutiny" and especially the capture and execution of the King and his family in 1793 and 1794.[77] His political concern was combined, however, with a concern about the dietetic enlightenment of the population.[78] To expand the scope of the audience May developed in his Mannheim-lectures a specific dietetic narrative in which the "archetypal health and uprightness of the ancient Germans" served as the beginning and model.[79] It was contrasted with the ending, the present, in which the corruption of the youth displayed a lack of knowledge of nature and the creation, a lack of pure religion, and a lack of dietetic knowledge.[80] The dietetic regulations—in the standard format of the six non-naturals—which now followed prescribed the conditions for restoration, had two coinciding objectives: physical and political. The ideal type of a healthy man

> is anyone whose parents are healthy, strong, and mature, who is proportionately built, not spoiled as child, nourished by simple food, raised in fresh country air, and protected from debauchery. He can move his body and use the powers of his soul with ease, delightfully, cheerfully and without exhaustion. He can also endure the change of weather without any harm. It is also important that he does not need any prophylactic bloodletting nor laxatives. He passionately engages

> into his work with all powers of his soul and body and begets healthy children. He overcomes the attacks of any disease with the old Germanic temperament.[81]

For May dietetics was a means of cultural and political restoration of the tribal conditions which the Germans had lost due to corrupting culture—and particularly through French influence.

Though never a dominant topic in the dietetic literature, the tribal narrative persisted throughout the early nineteenth century. In 1828, Johann Michael Leupoldt was convinced that dietetic rules could be prescribed only according to national distinctions and, furthermore, that those that applied to the German *Volk* necessarily had the highest validity because the life of humankind culminated in this very people.[82] Also Carl Wilhelm Ideler, who envisioned a system of dietetics in 1846, was equally convinced that dietetics was possible only on the basis of a national conception of history.[83]

Besides the dietetics of tribal narrative, the six non-naturals served medical enlightenment and health education. Frank, Simon André Tissot, and Bernhard Christian Faust were among those who most actively and successfully popularized and disseminated medical knowledge.[84] Although dietetics was an important tool in medical enlightenment, a second look at the used dietetic literature and in particular their audiences and narrative strategies is needed. Unlike Kant's philosophical introspection, the tone of the dietetic enlighteners was not introspective, but observing and prescriptive. Tissot's *Avis au peuple sur sa santé* (1761), one of the most influential works of medical enlightenment during the eighteenth century, set the standards in Germany as well, when Hirzel translated the book in 1768. The massive work of 736 pages was not meant to be read by the people itself but by the ministers who would then instruct their communities.[85] Senff's *Gesundheitskatechismus* (1781) followed Tissot in tone and size—despite its title, the book went 514 pages and assumed the help of ministers.[86] A step further in the medical instruction for commoners was Faust's *Gesundheits-Katechismus* (1794), which was meant to be used in home and school education. The book was thin, handy, and used uncomplicated language, mainly in dialogue form. Faust also made a crucial conceptual change in adopting religious language, which suppressed the dietetic tone.[87] This tendency was encouraged by another development whose seeds already can be seen in Tissot's book. Hundreds of pages of Tissot's work were filled with detailed descriptions of diseases and respective therapies adequate for commoners. The dietetic elements which were hidden in individual descriptions were thus effectively overshadowed by nosological and therapeutical discourse. Senff still incorporated a short description of dietetics and therapy in his book, sandwiched between physiology and long descriptions of diseases and medication. Faust's *Gesundheits-Katechismus* followed the same structure. The book was divided in two parts: the first one dealt with health extensively, considering among other things education, nursing, nutrition, and fresh air, and to a lesser extent physical exercise and sleep; the other part discussed diseases and had no dietetic elements.[88] That this tone was not unknown to May show lectures on

"The Art to Preserve Good Health," which he started in Heidelberg around 1800. They addressed the same audience as Faust's catechism and emulated the same religious tone by emphasizing how the human being was more than an animal, how he should use his free will and reason, "how he should be religious and moral in his thinking and action. He should defend himself against the wild passions with reason and religion."[89] May's favorite topic was the sixth non-natural, passions, whose control and regulation provided a convenient excuse to discuss moral issues.

These examples show crucial features of dietetics for commoners. It was designed in view of the specific needs of people living in the countryside or in the crowded dwellings of urban centers. Its point of departure was mostly in specific problems and diseases, rather than in the promotion and perfection of good life. The voice from above which enunciated these prescriptions made regular use of religious language, which replaced traditional dietetics. It was a style quite different from the dietetic discourse that addressed the educated middle class.[90]

May was well aware of the social distinctions between dietetic audiences. When the cultivated audience of the Nationaltheater in Mannheim saw the premier of Schiller's *Räuber* in 1782, the effect was so overwhelming for both the audience and the actors that May became concerned. Several times he was seen behind the screen consulting and examining the actors, among them August Wilhelm Iffland, the genial interpreter of Schiller. In the same year he published an article, "On the Diseases of Actors and the Difficulties of Curing Them," providing detailed dietetic recommendations for performers, especially for their conduct of over-stimulated passions.[91] Although extraordinary in his intellectual vigor, May followed a long tradition of dietetic literature that dealt with the health and longevity of scholars.[92]

One of the most influential treatises on the dietetics of scholars in the eighteenth century was Georg Wolfgang Wedel's *Diæta Literatorum* (1674).[93] This book, a minor bestseller in its time, was re-edited for the fourth time in 1704, and as late as 1729 its eighth edition came out. In 1753, it was translated into German as, *Von der Diät der Gelehrten* (On the Dietetics of Scholars).[94] *Diaeta* displayed several topics that made the core of this genre. Above all, it followed quite carefully the order of the six non-naturals. After identifying scholars as sedentary bodies, Wedel then described the specific conditions of air in their studies, the appropriate, light food they needed, the problems of digestion and bowel movement, their need of moderate exercise (walking), adequate sleep, and avoidance of overburdening, and, finally, the beneficial influence of music, spa, and moderate exercise on the balance of mind.[95] The epicurean tone remained in the dietetics of scholars throughout the eighteenth century.[96] When Tissot in 1768 revitalized the discourse on scholarly dietetics,[97] his diagnosis of the scholarly lifestyle remained close to Wedel's. "The diseases of scholars have two main sources: the unruly motions of the mind and the constant immobility of the body. In order to accurately describe this state of affairs we need only to profoundly depict the harmful impacts of these two influences."[98] Tissot vigorously warned scholars of overburdening, which he discovered in several different activities. Not only intellectual labor but also religious enthusiasm could destroy the delicate balance of a scholar's body.[99] As a prophylaxis, he offered diet and also fresh air and exercise, especially gymnastics.[100] Yet everything should be moderate, appropriate to the feeble and sensitive body of a sedentary person.

Where did Hufeland stand? Was his dietetics a modification of the tribal narrative which May so eagerly offered? Was he, perhaps, a medical enlightener à la Faust? Or did he address the concerns of scholars? Hufeland's position appeared ambiguous. He did not explicitly exclude any social class from his dietetics. In the preface of his *Die Kunst*, Hufeland embraced the widest possible audience: medical doctors, lay persons, and school students.[101] Yet given its epistemic form as private experience, the restriction of Hufeland's dietetics to scholars or, rather to well-educated population at large, was, in fact, strongly suggested.[102] At least, this was how Kant, in his comment to Hufeland's book, wanted to see a dietetic program emerging. By seeing dietetics as an art of sustaining and abstaining (*sustine et abstine*), a modification of stoic ethics, Kant presupposed "a power which can be provided only by philosophy or its spirit, which has to be presupposed absolutely."[103] That is to say, only rigorously educated and philosophically cultivated minds were capable of conducting dietetics in this Kantian sense. It was an apotheosis of the dietetics for scholars and, at the same time, a new kind of justification for an old science. As a commentator noticed, Kant's emphasis on stoic self-control replaced the hitherto practice of dietetics that intimidated healthy persons with useless, frightening, and pedestrian prescriptions of lifestyle with a private experience that "invited to emulation."[104] This new style was neither for commoners who wanted to be taught nor for scholars who wanted to teach or to hear a convincing argument, but, rather, for individuals of the educated middle class who wanted self-regulation.

One of the most systematic readers of Kant's widely discussed article was Karl Friedrich Burdach, a young lecturer at the University of Leipzig. Born in Leipzig to the family of a medical doctor, Burdach attended the local university and defended his medical dissertation in 1798. Unlike Hufeland, who was promoted early, Burdach confronted severe obstacles during his early career. He desperately looked for a professorship at the University of Leipzig but to no avail. In 1811, he finally gave in and accepted a nomination to the University of Tartu.[105] After three years, Burdach, seemingly unhappy at the Estonian university, left for the University of Königsberg. During his early years in Leipzig, Burdach had written on a variety of philosophical, propedeutical, and dietetic topics, but after 1808, he turned to pathology and especially physiology.[106] In Königsberg, he became a leading figure in pathological and physiological studies, along with his colleague Karl Ernst von Baer.

In 1805, Burdach published *Die Diätetik für Gesunde* (Dietetics for Healthy), a work that appeared unrelated to his physiological studies and definitely remote to what became his expertise and the source of his reputation. Yet the book was important. It was important for Burdach himself who forty years later thought about it with fondness and pride.[107] It was also important because it compellingly elaborated on the social implications of Kant's stoic understanding of dietetics. A program such as May's or Faust's, Burdach observed, could not pay attention to how the different classes could apply given knowledge, especially in relation to what he understood as their sense of intellectual autonomy.[108] Burdach wrote for the educated class, for cultivated minds, not immature ones, for those whose tasks were complicated, "not for those who are still in the state of nature and are occupied with the internal and external impulses from their limited environment."[109] Burdach was interested in the autonomy of his selected audience. In particular, he insisted that a person should have autonomy and the right to self-determination in relation to his own body. Furthermore, his maxim implied an opportunity to go beyond the mere preservation of health—dietetics—toward *Hygiastik*, i.e., perfecting one's own health.[110]

> The individual applies the rules and principles of *Hygiastik* in order to preserve and perfect his own health. It is therefore different from other disciplines; . . . it is different from public hygiene or the study of measures which the state has to take to protect the health of its citizens; . . . it is also different from dietetic education or the art of directing, promoting and supporting the powers of man so that he reaches his most perfect health.[111]

Burdach spelled out the requirement for dietetic self-help in a most radical way, but not as a compilation of technical advice. Instead he formulated a maxim, a request for the self-determination and bodily autonomy of the individual.

Burdach's program excluded not only the lower classes but also women. His book was dedicated especially for "the young man whose vocation is to become a useful member of the society through academic education."[112] Women were not addressed. They were not expected to be active users of Burdach's dietetics, although several dietetic writers had addressed women's special concerns as mothers.[113] In general, classical dietetics was ambivalent in relation to female bodies. Rousseau and his German followers had adopted hardening as a universal medicine against the degeneration of the human civilization. During the 1790s, this program developed into a cult of masculinity, boosted by the wars of the French Revolution and the subsequent Napoleonic Wars. Since Hufeland had serious caveats against excessive hardening and training of muscles, his idea of a balanced consumption of vital power actually provided arguments against masculinization.[114] Yet the position of women in the general dietetic discourse was only indirect, unless specific prescriptions were given for the preservation of their beauty and skin or for pregnancy, child rearing and giving birth.

The requirement of autonomy and freedom for the educated man found ample support among dietetic writers. Their manner was often exclusive, sometimes even truculent, as in the case of Gustav Groß, who in the 1820s did not want to reach out to "those who are poor, have no right to self-formation (*feinere Bildung*), and therefore belong to the despicable part of the population."[115] What we find in these examples of dietetic reflection was an argument for bodily autonomy of the educated man, whom the dieticians expected to be able to conduct his body and its environment and thus have the right of shaping mutual relationships. Ideler was correct in observing the self-limiting, subservient, and discriminatory character of this type of dietetics and offered in his handbook, *Die allgemeine Diätetik für Gebildete* (1846), dietetics in which the human being, not a member of a particular class, though still a man, " . . . would himself determine his conduct of life (*Lebensgesetz*)."[116] It was, however, debatable whether Ideler's own project, that "the only true foundation of dietetics was the idea of moral freedom," had any chance to materialize.[117] Was this, one could ask, only a postulate which pretended to universalize specific lifestyles of educated middle class men by forgetting their specific characters as members of a social group and individuals from specific localities?

In the early nineteenth century, a number of specific circumstances and institutions shaped the ideal of bodily autonomy and, in fact, showed its remarkable force as a strategy of lifestyle. We can discover traces of its influence in areas as distant as education and the prevention of epidemics, above all the horrendous attacks of cholera which, after creating an enormous intensity in South-Asia, attacked Europe, reached Moscow in 1830, a year later took over first Poland, then Austria, Prussia, Hamburg, England, and France, and, by 1838, had conquered the whole continent, then suddenly retreated, in order to return with more or less devastating power at regular intervals. In reality the dietetics of bodily autonomy came closest to its ideal in a social environment that became popular during the early nineteenth century: the spa, the site of "cultivated and conversational life."[118]

## Notes

1. Karl Friedrich Heinrich Straß, *Pyrmont und dessen Umgebungen. Ein Taschenbuch für Curgäste und Reisende. Aus Dankbarkeit gegen die kräftigenden Quellen des herrlichen Bades* (Pyrmont: Georg Uslar, 1850), 39–41.

2. Straß, *Pyrmont*, 42–45.

3. On the current scholarship see Antoinette Emch-Dériaz's "The Non-Naturals Made Easy," in *The Popularization of Medicine, 1650–1850*, ed. Roy Porter (London: Routledge, 1992), 134–59. Emch-Dériaz concentrates mainly on Tissot but provides an excellent conceptualization of classical dietetics. See also J. Rather, "The 'Six Things Non-Natural': A Note on the Origins and Fate of a Doctrine and a Phrase," *Clio Medica* 3 (1968): 337–47; Fredrik Berg, "Hygienens omfattning i äldre tider. Sex res non naturales" *Lychnos* (1962): 91–127. A detailed account of the academic teaching of the classical dietetics can be found in Hans-Heinz Eulner, "Die Lehre von der Ernährung im Universitätsunterricht," in *Ernährung und Ernährungslehre im 19. Jahrhundert*, ed. Edith Heischkel-Artelt (Göttingen: Vandenhoeck & Ruprecht, 1976), 76–98. Gerd Göckenjan, *Kurieren und Staat machen. Gesundheit und Medizin in der bürgerlichen Welt* (Frankfurt am Main: Suhrkamp, 1985), 74–94, and Jens Lachmund and Gunnar Stollberg, *Patientenwelten. Krankheit und Medizin*

*vom späten 18. bis zum frühen 20. Jahrhundet im Spiegel vom Autobiographien* (Opladen: Leske + Budrich, 1995), 37–41, 60–66, concentrate on the social and political implications of dietetics.

4. Erwin Ackerknecht's dismissive statement on classical dietetics is characteristic: "The relatively late change from a sacred to a hygienic and therapeutic diet was apparently the work of the Greeks, who also gave the practice its name. They used the term often in a larger sense: diet as health-directed regulation not only of the food intake, but also of air, sleep, exercise, excretion, and sensations. But very early they used the word diet in the more limited sense in which it is used today and in which I use it in this article," Erwin H. Ackerknecht, "The End of Greek Diet," *Bulletin of the History of Medicine* 45 (1971): 242.

5. See Claudia Huerkamp, *Der Aufstieg der Ärzte im 19. Jahrhundert. Vom gelehrten Stand zum professionellen Experten: Das Beispiel Preußens* (Göttingen: Vandenhoeck & Ruprecht, 1985), esp. 131–39, 164–66. Ute Frevert concentrates in her study on the lower class and their medicalization and submission to state control, Ute Frevert, *Krankheit als politisches Problem 1770–1880. Soziale Unterschichten in Preußen zwischen meidizinischer Polizei und staatlicher Sozialversicherung* (Göttingen: Vandenhoeck & Ruprecht, 1984), esp. 84–148.

6. The studies in Roy Porter, ed., *Patients and practitioners. Lay perceptions of medicine in pre-industrial society* (Cambridge: Cambridge University Press, 1985) provide good examples of the rising sensitivity toward ventures from below, i.e., lay medicine. In Germany, Francisca Loetz has criticized anachronistic and modernist approaches, taking a more subtle look at the concrete conditions in which social medicalization (*medizinische Vergesellschaftung*) took place, Franzisca Loetz, *Vom Kranken zum Patienten. "Medikalisierung" und medizinische Vergesellschaftung am Beispiel Badens 1750–1850* (Stuttgart: Franz Steiner, 1993), 86. Thomas Broman has more specifically criticized the traditional modernist conception of professionalization. He suggests that we can distinguish certain specific forms which belong to a pre-modern form of professionalization. See Thomas S. Broman, *The Transformation of German Academic Medicine 1750–1820* (New York: Cambridge University Press, 1996), 2.

7. Mary Lindemann, *Health & Healing in Eighteenth-Century Germany* (Baltimore: Johns Hopkins University Press, 1996), 372.

8. Lindemann, *Health and Healing*, 262–65. See also Loetz's instructive account of the uses of dietetics as medical utopia around 1800, Loetz, *Vom Kranken*, 74–78.

9. The term "Brunonian" refers to the late eighteenth-century physician from Scotland, John Brown, and his simplistic but powerful theory of pathology. In Germany, Brown and the Brunonians found a short but intensive reception. On the reception of Brunonianism in Germany see Urban Wiesing, *Kunst oder Wissenschaft? Konzeptionen der Medizin in der deutschen Romantik* (Stuttgart: Fromman-Holzboog, 1995), 70–75. See also Broman, *Transformation*, chapters 3–5.

10. Broman, *Transformation*, 184–92.

11. Broman, *Transformation*, 111.

12. My account of Cameralism is based on Keith Tribe's *Governing Economy. The Reformation of German Economic Discourse 1750–1840* (Cambridge: Cambridge University Press, 1988), Angela Raupach's "Zum Verhältnis von Politik und Ökonomie im Kameralismus. Ein Beitrag zur sozialen Theoriebildung in Deutschland in ihrer Genese als Polizei" (PhD diss., Hamburg, 1982), and Jutta Brückner's *Staatswissenschaften, Kameralismus und Naturrecht. Ein Beitrag zur Geschichte der Politischen Wissenschaft im*

*Deutschland des späten 17. und frühen 18. Jahrhunderts* (Munich: Beck, 1977).

13. By "old sciences," I mean the heterogenous group of disciplines the roots of which were in the Aristotelian notion of knowledge. In addition to dietetics and dancing, the doctrine of temperaments and affects, combinatorics, cameralism, and physiognomy can be subsumed under this category. They all shared the stigma of being "old-fashioned," of preceding modern social sciences.

14. See for instance, Norbert Waszek's paper *The Teaching of Cameralism, "Staatswissenschaften," and Economics in Early Nineteenth-Century Germany. A Case Study (University of Berlin) In Its National Context*. Fachbereich Wirtschaftswissenschaften Universität Hannover. Diskussionspapier 103 (Hannover, 1987), 5 and the references given. See also Tribe, *Governing Economy*, 22–29. Raupach, *Zum Verhältnis*, 17–19, emphasizes the practical needs of princely economies, especially the development of taxation as the cornerstone of Cameralism.

15. Waszek, *The Teaching*, 6. I am thankful for André Wakefield for his comments on my interpretation of Cameralism and especially his remarks on the difference between the old, Aristotelian notion of oikonomos, which operated on moral categories, and the new, utilitarian concept of "Oeconomie," launched in the 1720s. There is, however, a difference between these private economies and the notion of economic systems, applied by the later theories of national and political economy.

16. Tribe, *Governing Economy*, 95–96. Cf. Raupach, *Zum Verhältnis*, 20. See also Brückner, *Staatswissenschaften*, 292, on the composition of agricultural science (*Landwirtschaft*).

17. Tribe, *Governing Economy*, 149–82.

18. This does not mean that the transformation from Cameralism to modern theories of political economy was lineal but new standards of scientific knowledge (*Wissenschaft*) were needed. Yet the old and new model of economy shared the goal of increasing one's (prince's, state's or individual's) wealth.

19. On the dietetic conceptualization see Emch-Dériaz's "The Non-Naturals," 134–35.

20. Emch-Dériaz uses the term hygienic instead of dietetics, following the French nomenclature. Furthermore she speaks only of the passions of the soul. But, obviously, the notion of passion was flexible and did not demarcate between bodily and mental passions.

21. On the theory of humors and its influence in general, see Karl Edward Rotschuh, *Konzepte der Medizin in Vergangenheit und Gegenwart* (Stuttgart: Hippokrates-Verlag, 1978), 219–23.

22. Carl Friedrich Burdach, *Die Diätetik für Gesunde*, vol. 1 (Leipzig: Wichmann, 1805), 80.

23. Burdach, *Die Diätetik für Gesunde*, 79. On Hippocratism in the Eighteenth Century, see Jackie Pigeaud, "La Renaissance hippocratique au XVIIIème siècle," in *Hippokratische Medizin und antike Philosophie*, eds. Renate Wittern and Pierre Pellegrin (Hildesheim: Olms, 1996), 583–610.

24. See Friedrich Hoffmann, *Gründliche Unterweisung, wie ein Mensch vor dem frühzeitigen Tod und allerhand Arten Kranckheiten durch ordentliche Lebens-Art sich verwehren könne* (Halle, 1715) and the encyclopedic *Kurzgefaßte Diätetic oder hinlänglicher Unterricht* (Jena: Goller, 1744). Johann Storch translated Stahl's major work on dietetics, *Theoretische und practische Abhandlung von der Diaet* in 1739.

25. Hermann Boerhaave, *Institutiones Medicæ, in usus annuæ exercitationis domesticos digestæ. Cum præfatione nova de studio medico difficili, sed jucundo, Johannis Philippi Burggravii* (Francofurti ad Moenum: Georgii Heinrici Oehrlingii, 1710).

26. Johann Juncker, *Conspectus Therapiae Generalis, cum Notis in Materiam Medicam Tabulis XX. Methodo Stahliana Conscriptus*. 2nd ed. (Halle: Impensis Orphanotrophei, 1736), 11.

27. Samuel Schaarschmidt, *Therapia Generalis oder Abhandlung von denen üblichen Artzneien, nach ihren wahren Eigenschaften und Würckungen, Nebst der Anweisung zu deren gehörigen Gebrauch, auf Verlangen seiner Zuhörer* (Berlin: Verlag Joh. Jacob Schützens, 1749), 3.

28. August Friedrich Hecker, *Therapia Generalis oder Handbuch der allgemeinen Heilkunde* (Berlin: Christian Friedrich Himburg, 1789), XVIII.

29. Of German authors Riley mentions Friedrich Hoffmann in particular, see James C. Riley, *The Eighteenth-Century Campaign to Avoid Disease* (London: MacMillan, 1987), 34–44.

30. Christian Gottlieb Ludwig, *Institutiones Therapiae generalis praelectionibus academicis accommodatae* (Lipsiae: Gleditschiana, 1754), 28–32.

31. Hecker, *Therapia Generalis*, XVIII. We can find almost exactly the same argument in Carl Wilhelm Ideler's *Die allgemeine Diätetik für Gebildete* (Halle: C.A. Schwetschke und Sohn, 1846), XIV.

32. Lindemann, *Health and Healing*, 65–71. See also Roy Porter, "Introduction," in *The Popularization of Medicine 1650–1850*, ed. Roy Porter (London: Routledge, 1992), especially 6–10 and in the same volume Emch-Dériaz's "The Non-Naturals," 136–39.

33. On the tradition of popular dietetic literature and its transmission through the Sanitatis Salernitanum in Latin and vernacular until the nineteenth century see Melitta Weiss Adamson, *Medieval Dietetics. Food and Drink in Regimen Sanitatis Literature from 800 to 1400* (Frankfurt am Main: Lang, 1995), 97–102.

34. Krüger's notion of educational dietetics was based on an idea of moderate hardening: "I wish to say only that one ought to learn to endure everything but not to be enslaved by anything. How happy one would be, if one could follow this rule in educating children," Johann Gottlieb Krüger, *Diät oder Lebensordnung* (Halle: Hemmerde, 1751), 26–27. His *Gedancken von der Erziehung der Kinder*, vol. 1, *Von der Bildung des Leibes* (Halle: Carl Hermann Hemmerde, 1752), 3–4, and *Gedancken von der Erziehung der Kinder*, vol. 2, *Von der Bildung der Seele* (Halle: Carl Hermann Hemmerde, 1752), 2–3, 49 followed Locke in combining physical and intellectual education into an educational vision of a unified personality through dietetic hardening. On Krüger see John Hufert's remarks in, *Bewegungsdiätetik. Ein Paradigma auf der Grundlage von Krüger, Feuchtersleben und Zdarsky* (Ahrensburg: Czwalina, 1987), esp. 20–43.

35. Christa Kersting, *Die Genese der Pädagogik im 18. Jahrhundert. Campes "Allgemeine Revision" im Kontext der neuzeitlichen Wissenschaft* (Weinheim: Deutscher Studien Verlag, 1992), 195. Cf. Lydia Kunze, *Die physische Erziehung der Kinder* (Marburg: Diss., 1971), 108–10, and Heikki Lempa, *Bildung der Triebe. Der deutsche Philanthropismus (1768–1788)* (Turku: Turun yliopisto, 1993), 65–71.

36. Johann Gottlieb Fichte, "Einige Vorlesungen über die Bestimmung des Gelehrten (1794)," in *J.G. Fichte-Gesamtausgabe der Bayerischen Akademie der Wissenschaften*, vol. I, 3 (Stuttgart: Friedrich Frommann Verlag, 1966), 26.

37. Christian Thomasius, "Der Studierenden Jugend zu Leipzig in einem Discours, Von denen Mängeln der Aristotelischen Ethic, und von andern das Jus Publicum betreffenden Sachen. Zwey Collegia Über die Christliche Sitten-Lehre und über das Jus Publicum," in *Allerhand bißher publicirte Kleine Deutsche Schriften. Mit Fleiß colligiret und zusammen getragen. Nebst etlichen Beylagen und einer Vorrede* (Halle: Christoph Salfeld, 1701), 212.

38. A good overview of Thomasius's program is given in his *Summarischer Entwurf der Grundlehren, die einem Studioso Juris zu wissen und auf Universitäten zu lernen nötig sind* (1699).

39. Sigmund Jakob Apinus, *Vernünftiges Studenten Leben, welches zeiget, Was sowol ein Candidatus Academiae, als auch ein würcklicher Studiosus, bey dem Anfang, Fortgang und Ende seiner Academischen Fahrt zu thun und zu lassen hat* (Jena: Johann Matthäus Kaltenbrunner, 1726), 29–30.

40. Apinus, *Vernünftiges Studenten Leben*, 57.

41. Fichte, "Einige Vorlesungen," 26.

42. Friedrich Wilhelm Tittmann, *Ueber die Bestimmung des Gelehrten und seine Bildung durch Schule und Universität* (Berlin: Reimer, 1833).

43. Hufeland has been researched widely, though not in the context of classical dietetics. On Hufeland in general, see Walter Brednow, *Christoph Wilhelm Hufeland, Arzt und Erzieher im Lichte der Aufklärung* (Berlin: Akademie-Verlag, 1964); Klaus Pfeifer, *Christoph Wilhelm Hufeland. Mensch und Werk* (Halle: Niemeyer, 1968). More specific are Stefan Goldmann, *Christoph Wilhelm Hufeland im Goethekreis: eine psychoanalytische Studie zur Autobiographie und ihrer Topik* (Stuttgart: M & P, 1993) and Hans Joachim Schwanitz, *Die Theorie der praktischen Medizin zu Beginn des 19. Jahrhunderts: eine historische und wissenschaftstheoretische Untersuchung anhand des "Journals der practischen Arzneykunde und Wundarzneykunde" von Ch. W. Hufeland* (Cologne: Pahl-Rugenstein, 1979).

44. See the detailed account of Hufeland's encounters with Goethe and his circle in Weimar, Goldmann, *Hufeland im Goethekreis*, 121–34. The papers of the society show that Hufeland was giving a longer series of lectures rather than an occasional presentation, which is what he maintains in the autobiography, Christoph Wilhelm Hufeland, *Hufeland. Leibarzt und Volkserzieher. Selbstbiographie von Christoph Wilhelm Hufeland* (Stuttgart: Verlag Robert Lutz, 1937), 78. Goldmann, *Hufeland im Goethekreis*, 125, refers to Böttiger's account.

45. Hufeland was a man whose friendship was appreciated by Goethe, Schiller, von Humboldt, and Hegel, to name only the most prominent. In von Humboldt's personal diaries from the 1790s, when he spent much of his time in Jena and Weimar, Hufeland's name appears regularly among the agreeable guests and caring hosts. Based on von Humboldt's meticulous notes on names and chores, visits, meetings, and letters received and written from the year 1794 in Jena and Weimar, we can find that he met with Hufeland several times: March 30, "Abend mit Professor Hufeland auf dem Clubb" [in Jena], April 3, May 21, September 21, and October 27, in Wilhelm von Humboldt, *Gesammelte Schriften*, vol. 15, *Tagebücher I* (Berlin: B. Behr's Verlag, 1918), 242, 245, 251, 253. For Goethe, Hufeland was a trusted guest whose work was considered, though not actively discussed. In a letter to Christiane Vulpius, August 24, 1797, the poet asked Christiane to send a copy of Hufeland's "Book on longevity" to his mother, Johann Wolfgang von Goethe, *Goethes Briefe*, vol. 2 (Hamburg: Christian Wegener Verlag, 1964), 304. A certain sign of personal closeness can

be seen also in how the young professor Hufeland delivered a letter and a publication from Lichtenberg to Goethe 1795, Johann Wolfgang von Goethe, *Briefe an Goethe. Gesamtausgabe in Regestform*, vol 1 (Weimar: Hermann Böhlau, 1980), 426.

46. Hecker, *Therapia Generalis*, 20.

47. The only major conceptual change was the new term *Makrobiotik*, which Hufeland introduced in the third edition of 1805.

48. Hufeland, *Makrobiotik*, 11. An even clearer statement of this distinction between therapy and the art of prolonging life can be found in Hufeland's *System der practischen Heilkunde* (1800) in which *Makrobiotik*, as he now called the art of prolonging life, was assigned the preservation of health. See Christoph Wilhelm Hufeland, *System der practischen Heilkunde. Ein Handbuch für academische Vorlesungen und für den practischen Gebrauch*, vol. 1, *Allgemeine Therapeutic* (Jena und Leipzig: Friedrich Frommann, 1800), 1.

49. This can be located in the practical part of the book.

50. Hufeland, *Makrobiotik*, 14. Guenter Risse and Thomas Broman have argued that the increasing scepticism of late eighteenth-century physicians toward any philosophy of medicine amounted to an emphasis of medical practice over theory. According to them, Hufeland was one of the leaders of this movement. See Guenter Risse, "Kant, Schelling, and the search for a Philosophical 'Science' of Medicine in Germany," in *Journal of the History of Medicine* 27 (1972), 153 and Broman, *Transformation*, 119–27. Urban Wiesing takes a somewhat mediating position by depicting Hufeland as a promoter of a scientific art of medicine, Wiesing, *Kunst oder Wissenschaft?*, 88–89. This interpretation captures well the disputes over the medical education and professional status of physicians, but it is less adequate in describing the program of prolonging life which quite obviously challenged the separation of lay and professional medicine, on one hand, and the distinction between scientific theory and bedside practice on the other hand. Macrobiotics was a new science.

51. Broman, *Transformation*, 137, 148, shows how historical knowledge, historicizing cases or narratives of ancient events and diseases served to justify medicine until the end of the eighteenth century.

52. Hufeland, *Makrobiotik*, 33.

53. Krüger, *Diät oder Lebensordnung*, 9.

54. Christian Jahn, *Norma Diaetetica oder regelmäßige Abhandlung wie ein Mensch . . . sein Leben und Gesundheit nebst wenigen Arzeneyen lange erhalten* (Dresden: Johann Nicol. Gerlach, 1757), 14–22.

55. Hufeland, *Makrobiotik*, 34.

56. On von Haller see Rotschuh, *Konzepte der Medizin*, 343–44.

57. Blumenbach formulated his widely influential ideas in "Über den Bildungstrieb (Nisus formativus) und seinen Einfluß auf die Generation und Reproduction" *Göttingischem Magazin der Wissenschaft und Literatur* I/5 (1780): 247–66 and in his book *Über den Bildungstrieb und das Zeugunsgeschäfte* (Göttingen: Dieterich, 1781). On vitalism and its influence in Germany see Timothy Lenoir's important *The Strategy of Life. Teleology and Mechanics in Nineteenth Century German Biology* (Dordrecht: D. Reidel Publishing Company, 1982), esp. 17–24, gives an instructive account of Blumenbach's theory of *Bildungstrieb* and its repercussions especially in Kant's theory of teleology of nature. Cf. Rothschuh, *Konzepte der Medizin*, 291–98, 303–5, 323–30. A more limited account of the "science of life," especially in Goethe, can be found in Maike Arz, *Literatur und*

*Lebenskraft. Vitalistische Naturforschung um 1800* (Stuttgart: M&P, 1996), 24–35.

58. Goldmann, *Hufeland im Goethekreis*, 121–34; Hufeland, *Selbstbiographie*, 78.

59. Broman, *Transformation*, 156, sees Brunonianism substantial for Hufeland's medical theories.

60. Hufeland, *System der practischen Heilkunde 1*, XIV.

61. Christoph Wilhelm Hufeland, *Enchiridion medicum oder Anleitung zur medizinischen Praxis. Vermächtniss einer fünfzigjährigen Erfahrung*, 5th ed. (Berlin: Jonas Verlagsbuchhandlung, 1839), 53.

62. Hufeland, *Makrobiotik*, 47–49.

63. Hufeland, *Makrobiotik*, 45.

64. Hufeland, *Makrobiotik*, 46.

65. Hufeland, *Makrobiotik*, 14.

66. Hufeland, *Makrobiotik*, 119–45.

67. Johann Friedrich Zückert, *Von der diätetischen Erziehung der entwöhnten und erwachsenen Kinder bis in ihr mannbares Alter* (Berlin: August Mylius, 1765), 72–157. This was also a guideline for the educators of the *Philanthropismus*, Basedow, Campe, Villaume, and Trapp. On *the Philanthropismus* and dietetics, see Kersting, *Die Genese der Pädagogik*, esp. 42–95. On the movement in general see Auguste Pinloche's *Geschichte des Philanthropismus* (Leipzig: Brandstetter, 1896).

68. Hufeland, *Makrobiotik*, 160.

69. Hufeland, *Makrobiotik*, 164.

70. Hufeland, *Makrobiotik*, 175.

71. See the intriguing analysis of Hartmut and Gernot Böhme in their *Das Andere der Vernunft. Zur Entwicklung von Rationalitätsstrukturen am Beispiel Kants* (Frankfurt am Main: Suhrkamp, 1985), especially in Chapter 8: "Fin de Partie: Bruchstücke eines bezwungenen Lebens," 427–55, and also 389–97.

72. Although Kant influenced medical philosophy through his critical method, we cannot ignore his immediate involvement in the debates. Broman does not pay attention to Kant's review of Hufeland's writing. Wiesing takes Kant's statement as a misplaced narrative with a largely private concern, Wiesing, *Kunst oder Wissenschaft*, 51.

73. Erna Lesky, "Introduction," in Frank, Johann Peter, *A System of Complete Medical Police. Selections* (Baltimore: Johns Hopkins University Press, 1976), XV.

74. Immanuel Kant, *Werke*, vol. 7 (Berlin: Cassirer, 1912), 412. "genötigt, mein Ich laut werden zu lassen, was im dogmatischen Vortrage Unbescheidenheit verrät, aber Verzeihung verdient, wenn es nicht gemeine Erfahrung, sondern ein inneres Experiment oder Beobachtung betrifft, welche ich zuerst an mir selbst angestellt haben muß, um etwas, was nicht jedermann von selbst, und ohne darauf geführt zu sein, beifällt, zu seiner Beurteilung vorzulegen."

75. Kant, *Werke*, vol. 7, 412. This turn to personal and individual dietetics was warmly endorsed by the anonymous reviewer of Kant's *Macht des Gemüthes* (1798), in *Allgemeine Literatur-Zeitung* 184 (1799): 648.

76. Instead of "nationalism" and "nationalistic," the terms "tribalism" and "tribal" are much more appropriate for capturing the sources of German political and social unity which May and his companions attempted to enforce. I will discuss the sources of this notion more specifically in chapter four on gymnastics.

77. See the best modern biography of May, Eduard Seidler, *Lebensplan und Gesundheitsführung. Franz Anton Mai und die medizinische Aufklärung in Mannheim* (Mannheim: Boehringer, 1979), 117.

78. Franz Anton May, *Medicinische Fastenpredigten oder Vorlesungen über Körper und Seelen-Diätetik, zur Verbesserung der Gesundheit und Sitten*, vol. 1 (Mannheim: Schwan und Götz, 1793), Vorbericht.

79. May, *Fastenpredigten*, vol. 1, Vorbericht.

80. May, *Fastenpredigten*, vol. 1, 9.

81. May, *Fastenpredigten*, vol. 1, 50–51.

82. Johann Michael Leupoldt, *Eubiotik. Oder Grundzüge der Kunst als richtig, tüchtig, wohl und lang zu leben* (Berlin; Leipzig: Reimer, 1828), 16–17

83. Ideler, *Die allgemeine Diätetik für Gebildete*, IV.

84. See Lindemann, *Health and Healing*, esp. 65–71. Concerning Tissot, see Emch-Dériaz's "The Non-Naturals," passim. On Frank's and Faust's influence and the dissemination of dietetic-medical literature at the end of the eighteenth century, see Kunze, *Die physische Erziehung der Kinder*, passim.

85. I refer to the German edition, Samuel André Tissot, *Anleitung für das Landvolk in Absicht auf seine Gesundheit.* Aus dem Französischen übersetzt durch H.C. Hirzel (Zürich: Fueßlin, 1768).

86. Senff saw himself as a classic enlightener who helped the ignorant people: "But, how an earth can you even know it?," Adam Andreas Senff, *Gesundheitskatechismus für das Landvolk und den gemeinen Mann* (Berlin und Stettin: Friedrich Nicolai, 1781), Preface.

87. He was also criticized for the religious tone of his book. See Alfons Labisch, *Homo Hygienicus. Gesundheit und Medizin in der Neuzeit* (Frankfurt am Main: Campus Verlag, 1992), 96–97.

88. The breakdown of the first edition of Faust's book is telling: 1. On Health and One's Duties of Preserving Health (Chapters I, II), 2. Physiology (III), 3. On Nursing Infants (IV), 4. On Physical Education (V), 5. On Clothing (VI), 6. On Air (VII), 7. On Cleanliness, Washing, and Bathing (VIII), 8. On Nutrition (IX), 9. On Drinks (X, XI, XII), 10. On Tobacco (XIII), 11. On Motion and Rest (XIV), 12. On Sleep (XV), 13. On Housing (XVI), 14. On Fevers (*Erhitzungen*) and Chills (XVII), 15. On Preservation of Different Parts of the Human Body (XVIII), 16. On Beauty and the Perfection of the Human Body (XIX). See Bernhard Christian Faust, *Gesundheits-Katechismus zum Gebrauche in den Schulen und dem häuslichen Unterrichte* (Bückeburg: Althaus, 1794), passim.

89. Franz Anton May, *Die Kunst die blühende Gesundheit zu erhalten und die verlorne durch zweckmäßige Krankenpflege wieder herzustellen. Eine Einleitung zu Vorlesungen über die Gesundheit-Erhaltungs-Lehre und vernünftige Krankenpflege.* Dritte vermehrte und verbesserte Auflage des Gesundheits-Katechismus und Krankenwärter-Unterrichts, vol. 1 (Mannheim: Tobias Löffler, 1820), 6.

90. The current scholarship, mainly interested in the lower class, has not paid attention to the differences between dietetics for commoners and educated middle class (*Bildungsbürgertum*).

91. See Franz Anton May, "Von den Krankheiten der Schauspieler, und der Schwierigkeit, dieselbe zu behandeln," in *Vermischte Schriften* (Mannheim: Neue Hof- und akademische Buchhandlung, 1786), 310–38. Cf. Seidler, *Lebensplan*, 67–75.

92. On the origins of dietetics of scholars and its reception in the Humanism see Werner Friedrich Kümmel's instructive "Der Homo litteratus und die Kunst, gesund zu leben. Zur Entfaltung eines Zweiges der Diätetik im Humanismus," in *Mitteilungen. Kommission für Humanismusforschung* 11 (1984). Kümmel emphasizes the seminal impact of Marsilio Ficino's *De vita sana* (1482) and its several re-editions on the dissemination and transmission of the dietetics of scholars, Kümmel, "Der Homo litteratus," 74-75.

93. The book was a dissertation that Wedelius wrote for his student, Johannes Rottenberger at the University of Jena.

94. Erna Lesky, "Van Swietens Hypochondrie. Zur Berufskrankheit der Gelehrten und zur Musiktherapie," in *Clio Medica* 8 (1973), 190. Lesky's article gives a good introduction into the dietetics of scholars in the seventeenth and eighteenth centuries. Yet I disagree on her claim that Bernardino Ramazzini's and Ficino's ideas would have dominated the dietetic discourse on scholars, Lesky, "Van Swietens," 175, 180. Ramazzini's great book *De morbis artificum diatriba* was not published until 1700. By the time Wedel's small book had been reprinted at least three times.

95. Georg Wolfgang Wedel[ius], [Johannes Rottenberger] *Diæta Literatorum*. Editio Quarta cum Additamenta Paradoxis (Erfurt: Müller, 1704), 19–25.

96. See the dissertation of Christian August Kaysler, *Diaeta ad longaevitatem* (Lipsiae: Langenheim, 1752) and Andreas Rüdiger, [Ridigerus, Andreas], *Commentationes de diaeta Eruditorum* (Lipsiae, 1728). An active dietetic writer was Stahl's disciple, Michael Alberti, of whose dissertations several dealt with the topics of longevity but not necessarily in the classical spirit. See for instance, Michael Alberti, *De Aurora Musis amica et sana. Früh studirn dient zur Seelen- und Leibes-Gesundheit.* [Praes. Michael Alberti. Resp. Sigismundus Mauritius Schipalius.] Halle, Dissertatio (Halle: Hendel, 1746) and Michael Alberti, *De concionum mensura. Wie lange für Lehrer und Zuhörer zu predigen gesund sei.* [Präs. Michael Alberti. Resp. Johann Friedrich Otto.] Halle, Dissertatio (Halle: Hendel, 1739).

97. On the influence of ethics on the conduct of the body in the early eighteenth century, see especially Wolff's *Ethik*, the chapter on duties toward one's own body, Christian Wolff, *Vernünfftige Gedancken von den Menschen Thun und Lassen, zu Beförderung ihrer Glückseligkeit, den Liebhabern der Wahrheit* (Franckfurt und Leipzig, 1733), 260–349.

98. Simon André Tissot, *Von der Gesundheit der Gelehrten* (Zürich: Fueßlin, 1770), 11.

99. Tissot, *Gesundheit der Gelehrten*, 15–16, 31–32. Tissot mentions a case of a Moravian woman. "I knew a woman who lived quite reasonably until she was twenty-five years old. But after being unfortunately introduced to the sect of the Moravian Brothers, she was inspired and penetrated by the love of Jesus Christ—whom she called her lamb—to the extent that she was totally preoccupied with this sole idea. Because of this she became completely childish. She lived in this manner for six months and finally died of consumption."

100. Tissot, *Gesundheit der Gelehrten*, 99.

101. Hufeland, *Makrobiotik*, 14.

102. Goethe's mother was annoyed by Hufeland's aristocratic tone and the use of Latin type. Although she found the book interesting, she asked the son not to send same kind of products to her anymore, Johann Wolfgang von Goethe, *Briefe an Goethe*, vol. 1 (Hamburg: Christian Wegener Verlag, 1965), 214.

103. Kant, *Werke*, vol. 7, 230. "ein Vermögen, das nur Philosophie, oder der Geist derselben, den man schlechthin voraussetzen muß, geben kann."

104. Anonymous, "Review of Kant's *Macht des Gemüthes* (1798)" in *Allgemeine Literatur-Zeitung* 184 (1799): 648.

105. Karl Friedrich Burdach, *Rückblick auf mein Leben. Selbstbiographie* (Leipzig: Leopold Voß, 1848), 215.

106. Burdach, *Rückblick*, 154.

107. Burdach, *Rückblick*, 111.

108. Burdach, *Die Diätetik für Gesunde*, X–XI.

109. Burdach, *Die Diätetik für Gesunde*, XII, 53–54.

110. Burdach, *Die Diätetik für Gesunde*, 5, called his science "Hygiastik."

111. Burdach, *Die Diätetik für Gesunde*, 63.

112. Burdach, *Die Diätetik für Gesunde*, XIV.

113. See for instance, Johann Nepomuk Feiler, *Handbuch der Diätetik* (Landshut: Krull, 1821), 304; Leopold Fleckles, *Die Krankheiten der Reichen. Diätetische Grundlinien für das höhere und conversationelle Leben* (Wien: Carl Gerold, 1834), 199; Leupoldt, *Eubiotik*, 176. There was, however, a separate and rapidly increasing genre that emulated the dietetic tone—cosmetic literature *(Schönheitsliteratur)*.

114. Hufeland, *Makrobiotik*, 100.

115. Gustav W. Groß, *Diätetisches Handbuch für Gesunde und Kranke mit vorzüglicher Berücksichtigung der homöopathischen Heilkunst* (Leipzig: Reclam, 1824), VIII.

116. Ideler, *Die allgemeine Diätetik für Gebildete*, 3.

117. Ideler, *Die allgemeine Diätetik für Gebildete*, V.

118. See the section on "Der höhere Mensch" (the civilized man) in Fleckles, *Krankheiten der Reichen*, 176–95.

# Chapter Three

# Restoring the Balance

## Spa

In 1835, Ferdinand Gustav Kühne, a Saxonian writer and teacher, opined that the Germanic realm was inundated with spas, that nowhere else were there so many of them than in Central Europe.

> One has estimated that in France there are only ten health spas, eight in Italy, twelve in Hungary, three in Sweden, two in Spain, and also two in England, whereas Denmark and great Russia have each only one important spa. In German speaking countries, including also Bohemia and Switzerland, there are 149 establishments, in which the health sparkles.[1]

Although Kühne was misinformed about the number of English, French, and Italian spas—Osann had given much higher estimates—he might have been right in the ranking order.[2] Since the last third of the eighteenth century, spas became enormously popular summer resorts making the German-speaking area the realm of spas.[3]

The spas that Kühne observed, the leisurely summer resorts, had gone through a significant social and structural evolution since the end of the eighteenth century. Medieval and early modern cities were often surrounded by a network of bathing facilities and everybody used them. As we know for instance of Pyrmont in the early seventeenth century, peasants, artisans, city dwellers, as well as patricians, aristocrats, and scholars, found their ways to spas to clean and cure themselves. After the late seventeenth century, a noticeable change took place: in several spas, the lower class was separated to its own areas.[4] At the same time, spa administrations made their facilities more attractive to the upper echelons of society. The first ballroom in a German spa was built in Aachen at the end of the seventeenth century.[5] Also the shabby shopping stands that still crowded the main boulevards of spas like Pyrmont were replaced by permanent luxury boutiques by mid-eighteenth century.[6] As a further sign of increasing sense of distinction and luxury, major spas started to enhance their walkways from the 1770s on. Not only the main promenades and boulevards but also the walking paths to the surroundings were paved; the wealthiest, such as Pyrmont, Aachen, and Wiesbaden, built arcades (*Wandelhalle*) as indoors walking areas.[7] Around 1800, a standard spa consisted of one or several springs, a central promenade (*Allee*), dining room and ballrooms, lodgings, and a network of walkways leading to the nearby mountains, hilltops or to the seashore.

To discuss the structural changes that German spas went through between 1770 and 1840 and how these changes reflected the dietetic lifestyle I turn to Pyrmont spa. Pyrmont was the most important spa in Northern Germany until the early nineteenth century. Despite its decline against the competition of Carlsbad, Baden Baden, Wiesbaden, and Ems, Pyrmont still enjoyed high reputation among spa doctors and their patients throughout the nineteenth century. In many ways it was a classical German spa, with classical spa structures, organization of space, and activities.

A typical Central European city was round, surrounded by thick walls that compressed it into compactly organized, limited space around a market square, on which its most important buildings were located.[8] By these standards Pyrmont was an atypical city. It had neither a wall nor a market square. It was not round but, rather, oblong, a city that had evolved around a street. This street, *Hauptallee*, was a promenade. It was not a space for transportation and traffic, but one for strolling.[9] In the late eighteenth century, Pyrmont was still a rural village. During the summer months, its few streets were filled with thousands of spa-goers, but during the silent winter, the city became deserted. This seasonal fluctuation created the oscillation between cosmopolitan flair and rural parochialism typical for a spa town.

Historically, Pyrmont was cast around two centers: the castle and the spring, and the spring became dominant. In 1526, the count of Waldeck had started to build a castle by the river of Emmer, close to the villages of Oesdorf and Lügde near Hameln.[10] The area had a healing spring since ancient times, but the reputation of its miraculous powers started to spread after the mid-fourteenth century. In 1556, the count had almost finished the construction of his fort when thousands of crippled and ailing people from all walks of life and corners of Europe arrived in Pyrmont to use its springs.[11] The exodus started already in late April and within a month more than ten thousand diseased were camping around the spring, many of them in most miserable condition, hungry and cold, waiting for cure from the water that was supposed to heal all kind of illnesses and ailments. From now on diseased from all social classes frequently used the spring. Following the Thirty Years War, Pyrmont established itself as the gathering point of royal and high noble families. In 1668, the prince of Waldeck realizing the political and economic importance of the spring for his small principality, built a bathing house on the spring. The adjacent meadow was planted with lindens to line a boulevard for his guests to walk. During the summer 1681, forty royal and princely families came to Pyrmont.[12]

During the eighteenth century, the pinces of Waldeck made their facilities the most famous and attractive spa in German lands. While the spring itself was important, special attention was paid to buildings for social and convivial activities. Between 1724 and 1732, a ballroom was built, a scene of elevated balls, stage for plays, site for concerts, and a casino.[13] In the 1770s, it was accompanied by a public coffee house and a few years later a theater. All these facilities located on the main boulevard whose ambience was enhanced by an increasing number of lavish boutiques.[14] The first, temporary stands were erected soon after the boulevard but during the eighteenth century they became permanent small stores for luxury goods displaying items behind glass windows.[15] At the end of the eighteenth century, Pyrmont could boast with a vibrant and seductive social nexus for people to see and be seen. The enhanced social scene boded well with the improved bathing facilities. In 1777, an imposing new bathing house with lodgings in the upper floors was built next to the old spring.[16] Pyrmont was famous for its iron waters and springs. The new salt spring, *Solbad*, fifteen minutes away from the main boulevard in Oesdorf opened in 1809, and soon after a new bathing house on the main boulevard was built. In addition, on Hufeland's recommendation Pyrmont's administration opened a so-called gas spring with carbonate coming from the ground. The third step in improvements took place in the middle of the 1830s, when the administration shifted its attention to beautification and landscaping. The colonnades from the old bathing house to the boulevard, the park (*Kurpark*), a new bathing house next to the old spring, and the square around the old spring (*Brunnenplatz*) were developed.

By the 1860s, Pyrmont had reached its maturity as a spa. It now displayed a spatial hierarchy, vital for the everyday workings of an efficient and agreeable spa. The most regulated and observed space was the *Hauptallee*, the main boulevard. It was the center of Pyrmont, a center not only for sociability and leisure but also for the curative functions of the spa. All the facilities for convivial purposes, the coffee house, theater, ballroom, and walking colonnade, located on the *Hauptallee* or one of its side boulevards. Although the *Solbad* became quite popular, the *Hauptallee* retained its centrality. The constant complaints about the cumbersome and costly transportation to the *Solbad* underlined the popularity of the main boulevard.

Beyond the center opened the outskirts of the city. Unlike old cities, such as Aachen or Wiesbaden, Pyrmont lacked significant sites of interest in its wider urban area. For those who were looking for ones, spa guides could recommend only the churches and among them especially the temple of the Quaker community which had settled down in Pyrmont in 1797.[17] Its reputation was enhanced by the attention that Goethe and royal visitors paid to it. Far more important than the insignificant outskirts were the surroundings of the city. They were the magnets that occupied a permanent place in a spa-guest's daily schedule as destinations of excursions. The most popular was Königsberg, a hilltop with panoramic view over the valley of Emmer, where Frederick II had spent much of his time during his visits to Pyrmont in 1744–46. Royal flair and a pavilion for breakfast and dancing made it the favorite destination among spa-goers. After 1850, when the area around the main boulevard was renovated through a new extensive princely garden, the hill north of the center, Bomberg, was opened to walking excursions. It was conveniently within reach by following the Kloisterallee, the adjacent parallel street of the main boulevard. An exhilarating view opened to a walker over the city and Emmer two miles down to the village of Lügde. After 1850, a network of pathways to Bomberg were gradually built during the decades making it a popular place of walking tours. Those who were better off and were looking for more distant attractions found their ways to Hameln and Lügde.

What was the impetus of creating and enhancing spa facilities. Certainly, the ideology of beautification, to embellish physical environment, to shape nature aesthetically agreeable for human perception played an important role, as we shall see later when we discuss walking practices. But the environment was also a dietetic concern. The principle of Pyrmont's spatial structure, as in most of German spas, was the complementary nature of the center, the outskirts, and the distant destinations. This principle was carefully spelled out in spa guides which normally started with the description of the environment, proceeded to facilities, and finally outlined a number of walking tours.[18] Just because the center made moving from a spa facility to another so effortless the guests could find the effort of strolling to distant places pleasurable.[19] And this was fully in line with dietetics.

But the environment and facilities alone could not make a spa cure. As Heinrich Matthias Marcard, a leading spa doctor and the long-time physician of Pyrmont spa, pointed out in 1805, one has to follow the regimen of a daily schedule because: "He who always oscillates back and forth, between what satisfies his desires and what is useful for him, will never reach his goal."[20] Therefore any successful spa cure was contingent on how the dietetic factors, the six non-naturals, were balanced and, above all, how successfully they were translated into a daily schedule. By the end of the eighteenth century, German spa doctors had reached a rough consensus of a healthy daily schedule. The dispute about the correct time of taking waters and baths had been resolved in favor of early morning. Early in the morning, not later than 6 or 7 am, water, spa doctors argued, absorbed easier into the body because then the body had less fluid than during the day or in the evening. The coolness of morning air prevented excessive perspiration and thus preserved the balance of bodily fluids.[21] The balance and optimal absorption of fluids determined most of the daily schedule. For instance, breakfast was taken not sooner than an hour after the last glass of spring water had been consumed. This time was long enough to let the waters impact the body.[22] A bath, also prescribed in the morning hours, was carefully enveloped between resting times after breakfast and before lunch. If one took waters or baths in the afternoon, similar restrictions applied. Laws of humoral balance determined a spa guest's daily life, and these laws applied in most German spas, as Table 3.1. shows.

Table 3.1. Dietetic Schedules at German Spas.

| *Hours* | *Pyrmont*[23] | *Carlsbad*[24] | *Kissingen*[25] |
|---|---|---|---|
| 6–8 | Spring, Walking | Spring, Walking | Spring, Walking |
| 8–9 | Breakfast | Spring, Walking | Breakfast |
| 9–10 | Bath, Walking | Breakfast, Dance | Promenades, Socializing |
| 10–11 | Walking, Socializing, Newspaper, Music | Walking, Socializing, Correspondence | Bath |
| 11–12 | Walking, Socializing, Newspaper, Music, Drawing | Bathing or Walking, Socializing | Promenades, Socializing |
| 12–1 | Walking, Socializing, Newspaper, Music, Drawing | Walking, Socializing | Lunch |
| 1–2 | Lunch in Company | Lunch in Company | Lunch |
| 2–3 | Coffee | Walking, Excursions, Socializing | Coffee |
| 3–4 | Walking, Excursions | Walking, Excursions, Socializing | Walking, Excursions, Socializing, Theater, Concerts |
| 4–5 | Walking, Excursions | Walking, Excursions, Socializing | Walking, Excursions, Socializing, Theater, Concerts |
| 5–6 | Spring or Walking, Excursions | Walking, Excursions, Socializing, Theater | Walking, Excursions, Socializing, Theater, Concerts |
| 6–7 | Theater, Assemblies, Card Play | Spring, Bath | Spring, Walking, Socializing for Supper |
| 7–8 | Theater, Assemblies, Card Play | Walking | Walking, Socializing for Supper |
| 8–10 | Supper | Supper, Ball | Supper |
| 10–12 | Going to Bed, Ball, Card Play | Going to Bed, Ball | Going to Bed, Ball, Socializing |

A closer look at German spa schedules reveals an interesting structural variation. Whereas water-taking, baths, and meals furnished the backbone of daily routines, diversions of different sorts filled the rest of the time. The first drinking session was regularly accompanied and followed by walking sessions; breakfast and lunch were digested in socializing and promenading; and the evening was often completed by dancing. Yet only certain types of activities qualified for spa diversion. In no way an activity that caused excessive exhaustion and perspiration or was overly strenuous could find its way into a spa guest's daily program. Marcard reminded that even walking and promenading might be dangerous if practiced excessively.[26] The main purpose of all exercise was to produce motion and this motion could be active or passive. Passive motion, such as being carried in a carriage or sedan, was especially useful because it moved or, rather, shook the body and its fluids. And above all, passive motion was not strenuous. This was a good medical justification for spa doctors' recommendations to rent a carriage and take off to near-by towns and villages for an afternoon excursion.[27] It would certainly not harm the cure that horse cab owners made a nice profit of this therapy.

Spa doctors tried to ban exhaustion and exertion in all spa activities. For scholars who wanted to continue on their unfinished works or businessmen running extensive correspondence they firmly prescribed light reading, socializing, and conversation.[28] In 1836, the administration of the Kissingen spa opened the Conversation Lounge (*Conversationssaal*), if not first at least one of the most famous buildings of its kind providing facilities for easy conversation and peaceful corners for reading journals and newspapers.[29] Newspaper reading, literary circles, and consumption of light novels was a central diversion also in Pyrmont and Carlsbad.[30] Although spa guests recognized the entertaining function of spa diversions, one should not see them merely as entertainment. There was a ranking order among diversions: doctors and well-educated guests preferred amusements that enhanced healthy mind set and healthy passions, cheerfulness and joy of life. Light reading, amusing conversations, and peaceful strolling certainly met the requirements of healthy mind set.

Problematic were excessive and overly stimulating activities, such as flirting, dancing, and gambling. The leading physician at Carlsbad spa, Eduard Hlawaczek, spelled out an important addition to this list when he sternly warned that, "one should refrain, whenever possible, from sexual intercourse during the whole spa visit."[31] Yet much of the air of a spa depended on its status as an attractive marriage market. Heinrich Koenig's protagonist, Mrs. von Salisch, an impoverished lady, was a typical user of this market. To arrange her niece a good marriage she went to great lengths to capture the attention of two wealthy businessmen, Albert and Gottfried Elzheim. After having engaged them and their friend Dr. Lüdemann to a walk to Friedensthal, a Quaker colony close to Pyrmont, the relationship of Mrs. von Salisch's niece and Albert took a decisive turn, and a year later they were married.[32] Besides the marriage prospects, which still was contractual and controlled by families, erotic flair was enhanced by the presence of a tangible number of single men and women. By the mid-nineteenth century, the number of single men at the Pyrmont spa could occasionally exceed that of family men. Almost as distinguishable was the presence of single women who came from

Hannover and other nearby areas to spend a week or two at a major spa. In Wildbad spa in Württemberg women's visits to spas independently from their husbands or male relatives were also very common, as Gudrun König recently has discovered.[33] For a man who meticulously followed his doctor's prescriptions of celibacy an additional temptation were prostitutes. Although we do not know much about their activities and numbers—any respectable spa guide carefully avoided such topics—popular spa novels give enough evidence to conclude their presence. According to Schmidt-Lisber, Pyrmont's administrators had forbidden the prostitutes to "step on the *Hauptallee* during the day time. In the evening one could not prevent them to do that, because they were not distinguishable from several other ladies."[34] For the administration of Pyrmont the prostitutes were hardly a grave problem that needed detailed regulation, unlike smoking or the behavior of peasants.[35]

If the reality occasionally transgressed the dietetic vow of celibacy, even more so it did in dancing. Dancing was never completely banned, because doctors considered moderate dances, such as the minuet a good exercise, while discouraging the whirling and exhausting waltz. Balls were a regular part of a spa schedule. Depending on the style and clientele of a spa, assemblies could start in the morning, as in Carlsbad and Pyrmont, or they could be a part of the afternoon program, as the *dejeuners* and assemblies of Kissingen and Pyrmont.[36] Grandiose balls took place in the evening, after the dinner, and were organized once or twice a week. In Wiesbaden, for instance, great numbers of occasional visitors came in during the weekend with no other purpose than to attend the balls and see dignitaries.[37]

Gambling was one of the most widely-spread preoccupation at German spas and a most problematic diversion. It was a good example of how spa life was torn between dietetic regulations, transgressive patterns of behavior, and economic necessities. Spa doctors condemned gambling when it became an obsession and stirred the balance of a spa guest's emotional economy and they had good reasons for doing so.[38] Since the late eighteenth century, when spa reviews became regular, a common complaint was about widely spread gambling that caused havoc among spa guests, disrupted social life, and brought players to the brink of personal catastrophe.[39] Pyrmont's administrators were aware of these complaints and tried to contain the problem. Between 1820 and 1860, several regulations were issued that strictly prohibited gambling of lower classes and any person of moderate means. This ruling served two purposes. While seemingly protecting the lower classes against this ostentatiously upper class vice, it enforced gambling as an upper class diversion. Yet a total ban of gambling was not an option, not only because gambling was very popular but also because the small principality of Waldeck-Pyrmont became increasingly dependent on the revenues from gambling. Since the middle of the eighteenth century, the princes of Waldeck had lavishly invested in Pyrmont's facilities. By the turn of the century it became clear that these efforts had overwhelmed the limited resources of the small state. In a desperate search for additional resources gambling was one of the most lucrative. It did not need much investments and the flow of revenues was steady. After the casino was opened in a separate building in the 1830s, the casino became the main support for the overall maintenance of the spa. The entrepreneurs who run the business were obligated to pay for various public services, such as the cleaning of the *Hauptallee*, subsidize the trimming of trees, planting flowers, and caring for lighting.[40] When gambling was banned and the casino of Pyrmont spa closed in 1864, the principality had to find compensation for the loss of revenues to cover more than half of the maintenance of spa facilities.[41]

Although a major challenge for the dietetic lifestyle, gambling was an exception that confirmed the rule. The spa guests followed the daily schedule, because an individual rhythm of life was not only against doctors' prescriptions but also socially restrictive. The one who missed or avoided the drinking sessions in the morning, would have tremendous difficulties to navigate in the delicate social networks of a spa. It was most common to make the social arrangements for the day during the drinking session at the fountain or at the adjacent promenade in the morning.[42] For a short social endeavor, the first opportunity opened right after the drinking session and breakfast. Because of the imminent lunch some guests preferred the afternoon for social engagements. Then, between 2 and 5, the Pyrmontians could see groups of spa-goers in a variety of settings wandering toward nearby hilltops, caves, or villages. They could also see wealthier guests renting carriages for excursions to Hameln or other nearby cities.[43] All the spa-goers were entertaining themselves but also following the prescriptions of their dietetic therapy. Social pressure and physician's authority kept the control and put limits to spa guests' desires for strenuous and overly stimulating diversions.

What was the influence of spas on middle class lifestyle? Where they merely curiosities and expressions of upper class extravagance or did they have a more general bearing on everyday life? During the nineteenth century, spa attendance was steadily increasing. Whereas only 200 guests found their ways to Kissingen in the summer of 1800, fifty years later there were 3,828 and by the turn of the century 15,000 guests proper and over 20,000 visitors.[44] Pyrmont, a popular spa already in 1800, started with 1,424 guests proper (peasants were not included by name), reaching to 2,800 by the middle of the century, and, in 1900, the number of guests was solidly at 18,954.[45] In Carlsbad, there were 10,000 visitors in 1865. By the middle of the century, the number of guests of all German and Austrian spas easily reached 100,000.[46] Moreover, since several spas included only respectable persons with name and title in their statistics and yet still allowed peasants to use their facilities, the real number was even significantly higher than 100,000.

Besides the numbers one should also consider the intensity of a spa experience. A visit to a spa was most often a lengthy vacation. Although several spas attracted casual visitors who came on Sundays to enjoy assemblies and casinos, regular guests stayed several weeks. A cure was supposed to last from 4 to 6 weeks, a short cure from 2 to 3 weeks. When Goethe came to Pyrmont in 1801, he stayed six weeks from mid-June to mid-July.[47] Somewhat extreme in his enthusiasm for spas was Aron Hirsch Heymann, a long-standing leader of the Jewish community in Berlin. He was a spa enthusiast who made annual visits to Marienbad where he spent time with Gerson Bleichröder, the banker of Bismarck, and other Jewish notables from Berlin. In 1872, instead of going to Marienbad, Heymann headed on May 28 to Carlsbad where he met several Jewish businessmen and organized a well-attended civic gathering. After several weeks in Carlsbad, Heymann and his wife decided to visit their "home spa," Marienbad, as well as the Kissingen spa, where Bismarck used to spend his summers. On July 8, they continued their tour with a stint at Wiesbaden, and from there, on August 19, with a stop at Baden-Baden, the biggest and most international spa in Germany. No earlier than September 4 were the Heymanns back in Berlin.

In order to enhance the curative impact of a spa therapy, doctors encouraged their patients to follow a special "after-cure" (*Nachkur*), namely to continue to follow the diet, daily rhythm, and drinking waters at home as much as possible because the real effects of the cure were supposed to materialize several weeks after the visit. Theodor Valentiner, a long-term physician at Pyrmont spa recommended in 1859 that after a spa cure "should follow a certain time of peace. . . . A pleasant journey of several weeks and a visit to acquaintances in the country are a much better after-cure [than work]."[48] A lengthy spa visit combined with an after-cure of several weeks had an impact on one's lifestyle. The spas were an ideal environment that served as a dietetic model and, as we shall see, as a physical model for reshaping the urban landscape in Germany.

## Battle over Waters

In the summer of 1818, an obscure medical doctor and pharmacist in Dresden, Friedrich Adolph Struve, opened his small factory which produced mineral waters, almost identical copies of spa waters of Carlsbad, Marienbad, Pyrmont, and Ems. Sending bottled mineral water was not new. Most of the famous spas had for centuries made handsome profits on retailing their precious waters over long distances. Not even the production of artificial mineral waters was unprecedented. French and English chemists had started industrial production of mineral waters years before Struve's venture could start. What made Struve's factory and particularly his method so extraordinary in Europe was the level of scientific accuracy and the solid quality of his products. After detailed studies, visits to all famous spas in Germanic realm, and innovations in discovering new important minerals in waters, Struve set new standards. In fact, he claimed to have produced waters whose remedial qualities were identical with those of the original spa waters.[49]

Some spa administrators and doctors perceived Struve's facilities, which by 1823 were available in Dresden, Berlin, and Leipzig, as threat, although Struve carefully pointed out the complementing nature of his endeavor.[50] The fear of unfair competition persisted. In the early 1830s, Austria had forbidden soliciting artificial mineral waters.[51] As late as 1841, Adolf Pleischl, professor at the University of Vienna, launched a salvo of accusations against Struve's facilities and methods that he considered adversaries of natural springs in general, and in particular Bohemian springs, the crown jewelry of Austrian spas.[52] Nevertheless, Struve's facilities quickly spread over Northern, Eastern, and Central Europe. In the early 1840s, most major German cities had a *Trinkanstalt* and important European capitals and cities, such as Petersburg, Moscow, Warsaw, Königsberg, Kiev, and Birmingham boasted with a drinking facility in Struve's style. But the numbers were still quite modest. An estimate from 1843 gives the number of visitors to drinking institutes at 3,500 a year.[53] In Berlin, the breakdown shows 744 visitors to the local drinking facility in the season of 1840.[54] Compared to the major spas the figure was modest indeed. In Pyrmont, more than 2,805 visitors came during the season of 1840 and this figure did not include 946 peasants and other persons of humble means.[55] And Pyrmont was only the seventh in rank among German spas, far behind the numbers of Carlsbad which easily lured 10,000 spa-goers a year.[56]

If the material and economic threat of Struve's enterprise was so insignificant, why did critique, fear, and hesitance persist? An important fact was the image. In his statistical breakdown of the Drinking Institute (*Trinkanstalt*) in Berlin from the year 1840 August Vetter detailed all the waters that the customers had used:

> The total number of drinkers was 744. Most of them turned to, as usual, the incredibly curative springs of Carlsbad. Also this year their success completely met all the realistic expectations that one could raise. 279 persons used that water. The springs of Ems were used by 45 persons of which more than two thirds drank Kesselbrunnen. Vichy (quelle grand grille) was drunken with excellent effect by nine patients.[57]

These were warm waters. The statistics tells that those who used cold waters preferred Kreuzbrunnen of Marienbad (225 drinkers) whereas such a famous water as Pyrmont's Heilwasser could attract only 12 users.[58] It was the image of spas which was solicited in the form of water. This had become possible because the nature of water had been transformed. It was no more a natural water but a replica of a natural water, a replica that a scientific method had made possible. This was the very reason for a debate that started after Struve had expanded his facilities in 1823 and soon divided spa doctors and administrators.

The question was about water and its chemical analysis. Although a Swedish scientist, Torbern Bergman (1735–84), had discovered the chemical analysis of waters and their mineral components, the results were only rarely paired with efforts to produce or recombine waters. Struve's endeavor changed the constellation by enhancing chemical analysis so that the "copying" of particular mineral waters became possible. Leading chemists, Michael Faraday and Jöns Berzelius, quickly lend their authority to support Struve's findings. But those who saw the medical consequences of Struve's invention, were as quick to reject it. Hufeland, who became Struve's major adversary, though approving the remedial benefits of artificial waters, draw the line between the original and its copy. Whereas Struve's product included all the detectable components of spa waters, it did not include all components because, Hufeland argued, chemistry was constantly advancing and especially because

> should one not assume that there was to us completely unknown Third and that this Third was exactly the best, spiritual, and animating force. And as long as I will live, I will remain a representative and an advocate of this spiritual and animating force in nature, and also in mineral springs. In fact, I have made this animating force the basis of my entire medical theory.[59]

Although Struve's discovery was influential indeed and gained substantially in support during the following two decades, those who sided with Hufeland did not loose their grip of discourse and, especially, of medical teaching until the 1840s, as Valentiner with certain bitterness noticed in 1873.[60] But the main and immediate importance of Struve's discovery was its bearing on the framing of discussion. Water became a key concern of therapy and also of spa therapy.

Almost simultaneously with Struve's enterprise, a peasant from Silesia, Vincenz Prießnitz, started to experiment with physical water therapy. Regardless of his lack of education or, perhaps, because of that, he was able to direct medical attention to physical impact of waters by using cold showers and baths in healing a variety of ailments. His institute at Gräfenberg attracted hundreds of curious customers and doctors.[61] After 1848, Sebastian Kneipp, a Bavarian priest, created a similar kind of hydrotherapy, *Kneippsche Kur*, that became popular in Germany, France, and Holland.[62] Although Kneipp wrote extensively and constantly talked about his "method," neither he nor Prießnitz could create a new conceptual basis for water therapy. Yet they shook the traditional dietetic understanding of water's curative power and helped Struve's scientific analysis gain influence. In 1841, Bernhard Preiss discussed a new field that he, presumably for the first time in German language, called balneotherapy (*Balneotherapie*).[63] Few years later, August Vetter, a disciple of Struve, published the second edition of his *Theoretisch-praktisches Handbuch der allgemeinen und speciellen Heilquellenlehre* which introduced the standards of discussing spas in the context of Struve's water analysis. In 1851, we can read in Brockhaus's *Allgemeine deutsche Real-Encyclopädie* that "the doctrine of baths in general, the doctrine of their types and uses is called balneology."[64] In 1854, came out the first extensive manual on balneology, Hermann Helfft's *Handbuch der Balneotherapie* which as early as 1873 had reached its eighth edition. A new discipline on spas was established and this discipline was becoming increasingly influential also in public discussion on spas.

In Pyrmont, Theodor Menke and his colleague and successor Valentiner were keenly interested in chemical analysis of waters. Menke was the host of the conference of German natural scientists which took place in Pyrmont in 1839. Much of his scientific work focused on the chemical analysis of waters. Even more so it was with Valentiner who considered himself a natural scientist, highly rejective of any natural philosophy that would obstruct the clear vision of scientific observation.[65] Given this development we could expect a boost of medicalization of spa facilities in Pyrmont. But it did not take place: the guides, personal testimonies, and administrational regulations do not reveal any significant change in spa life between 1780 and 1870. At the same time, as Douglas MacKaman has shown, the French spas were almost completely medicalized, torturing customers in a variety of different showers, curbing social interaction, and changing the rules of conduct.[66] But in Pyrmont, and in several other German spas as well, we can see a curious combination of increasing medicalization of discourse and persisting cultivation of sociability. The scientific transformation, it seems, changed only the theoretical justifications of therapies, whereas the traditional dietetic arrangements of these therapies were left intact.

## Notes

1. Ferdinand Gustav Kühne, "Bade-Leiden und Freuden. Ein Capriccio" in *Zeitung für die elegante Welt* 251 (1835): 1002.

2. See Emil Osann, *Physikalisch-medicinische Darstellung der bekannten Heilquellen der vorzüglichsten Länder Europa's* (Berlin: Dümmler, 1829), passim.

3. See, for instance, Christoph Wilhelm Hufeland and Friedrich Justin Bertuch, "Nöthige Erinnerung an die Bäder und ihre Wiedereinführung in Teutschland; nebst einer Einweisung zu ihrem Gebrauch und bequemer Einrichtung derselben in den Wohnhäusern," *Journal des Luxus und der Moden* (May 1801): 237–50. In fact, we do not have the exact figures.

4. Reinhold Kuhnert, *Urbanität auf dem Lande. Badereisen nach Pyrmont im 18. Jahrhundert* (Göttingen: Vandenhoeck & Ruprecht, 1984), 33–34.

5. Burkhard Fuhs, *Mondäne Orte einer vornehmen Gesellschaft. Kultur und Geschichte der Kurstädte 1700–1900* (Hildesheim: Georg Olms Verlag, 1992), 67.

6. Fuhs, *Mondäne Orte*, 55. In Wiesbaden, the luxury boutiques were in place around 1800, Fuhs, *Mondäne Orte*, 208.

7. In Carlsbad, the enhancement of walkways took place in the first decade of the nineteenth century, see "Neue Anlagen in Karlsbad," in *Journal des Luxus und der Moden* (Januar 1801): 11–12. For Pyrmont see Ilona Schäfer-Schmidt, "Die Entwicklung der Kuranlagen in Bad Pyrmont," in *Kurstädte in Deutschland. Zur Geschichte einer Baugattung*, ed. Rolf Bothe (Berlin: Frölich & Kaufmann, 1984), 430–31. An arcade was created in Pyrmont fairly late, only in 1843, Schäfer-Schmidt, "Die Entwicklung," 443. On colonnades and arcades in spas, see Rolf Bothe, ed., *Kurstädte in Deutschland. Zur Geschichte einer Baugattung* (Berlin: Frölich & Kaufmann, 1984), esp. 17–25 and the picture of the arcades in Wiesbaden, 25. In Driburg, a competitor of Pyrmont, the arcades were already built in 1822. According to Bothe, "Bad Driburg," in *Kurstädte in Deutschland. Zur Geschichte einer Baugattung*, ed. Rolf Bothe (Berlin: Frölich & Kaufmann, 1984), 307–8, it also contained boutiques and became a model for spa arcades in the first half of the nineteenth century.

8. The research on city walls and their impact on urban culture in Central Europe is still sparse. On Germany, the best study is Peter Grobe, *Die Entfestigung Münchens* (Munich: Stadtarchiv, 1970). Helmut Friedmann, *Alt-Mannheim im Wandel seiner Physiognomie, Struktur und Funktionen (1606–1965)* (Bad Codesberg: Budensanstalt für Landeskunde und Raumordnung, 1968), outlines the leveling of city walls in Mannheim. On Hamburg, see Bocklitz's detailed but insufficiently documented study, "Hamburgische Festungsanlagen," in Armin Clasen Klaus Bocklitz, *Studien zur Topographie Hamburgs*, vol. 14, *Beiträge zur Geschichte Hamburgs* (Hamburg: Christians, 1979), 94–154.

9. Also in Aachen, the *Promenade* was a central place, but it was not exclusively for pedestrians. A picture from 1727 shows strollers intermingling with riders and carriages, Ernst Kasper and Klaus Klever, *Das Kaiserbad. Der Neubau und sein historischer Hintergrund* (Bratislava, 1995), 20.

10. Karl Theodor Menke, *Pyrmont und seine Umgebungen mit besonderer Hinsicht auf seine Mineralquellen; historisch, geographisch, physikalisch und medicinisch dargestellt* (Pyrmont: Georg Uslar, 1840), 129.

11. Menke, *Pyrmont 1840*, 320–21.

12. My account of Pyrmont follows mainly Wilhelm Mehrdorf's "Geschichte des Bades Pyrmont" in *Chronik von Bad Pyrmont* (Bad Pyrmont, 1985).

13. Mehrdorf, "Geschichte des Bades Pyrmont," 70.

14. Mehrdorf, "Geschichte des Bades Pyrmont," 72.

15. Mehrdorf, "Geschichte des Bades Pyrmont," 72.

16. Menke, *Pyrmont 1840*, 138.

17. Herbert Fritsche, *Pyrmont. Aus der Gnadengeschichte einer Stätte* (Bad Pyrmont: Verlag Leonhard Friedrich, 1946), 24–25.

18. See, for instance, Straß, *Pyrmont*, 69; Gottfried Käppel, *Pyrmont's Merkwürdigkeiten. Eine Skizze für Reisende und Kurgäste.* (Pyrmont: Helwingsche Buchhandlung, 1810), 38–93.; Henrich Matthias Marcard, *Beschreibung von Pyrmont*, vol. 1 (Leipzig: Weidmanns Erben und Reich., 1784), 3–113; Menke, *Pyrmont 1840*, 139–259.

19. On the spas as sites of pleasure see Karin Wurst, *Fabricating Pleasure. Fashion Entertainment, and Cultural Consumption in Germany, 1780–1830* (Detroit: Wayne State University Press, 2005), esp. 255–61.

20. "Wer immer hin und her schwankt, zwischen dem was seinen Begierden schmeichelt, und ziwschen dem was ihm nützlich ist, der kommt nicht zum Ziele." Henrich Matthias Marcard, *Kleines Pyrmonter Brunnenbuch für Curgäste zu Hause und an der Quelle* (Pyrmont: Helwingsche Buchhandlung, 1805), 96.

21. Henrich Matthias Marcard, *Beschreibung von Pyrmont*, vol. 2 (Leipzig: Weidmanns Erben und Reich, 1785), 276. Christoph Wilhelm Hufeland,, *Praktische Uebersicht des vorzüglichsten Heilquellen Deutschlands nach eignen Erfarungen.* (Berlin: Reimer, 1820), 28, explains the preference of morning drinking by the highest level of sensitivity of the stomach nerves in the morning and, therefore, the enhanced impact of waters on the body. Friedrich Steinmetz, *Pyrmont und seine Mineralquellen. Anleitung zu Trink- und Badecuren, in Bezug auf die neueste Analyse* (Pyrmont: G. Uslar, 1825), makes the same argument.

22. Marcard, *Beschreibung von Pyrmont*, vol. 2, 296. Cf. Friedrich August von Ammon, *Brunnendiätetik. Anweisungen zum zweckmässigen Gebrauche der Gesundbrunnen und Mineralbäder Deutschlands.* (Leipzig: Weidmann'sche Buchhandlung, 1841), 64.

23. Menke, *Pyrmont 1840*, 445–48. Cf. Marcard, *Kleines*, 95–107 and Straß, *Pyrmont*, 42–45. In Pyrmont, the peasants could use the spring from 4 to 6 am.

24. Eduard Hlawaczek, *Karlsbad in medicinischer, pitoresker und geselliger Beziehung. Für Kurgäste* (Prag: Kronbergers Wittwe und Weber, 1838), 119. Cf. Joseph Carl Eduard Hoser, *Beschreibung von Karlsbad* (Prag: Calve, 1797), 129–31, gives, in 1797, a more flexible account that does not detail the afternoon program but mentions a host of mainly convivial activities between 3 pm and midnight.

25. Franz Anton Balling, *Die Heilquellen und Bäder zu Kissingen. Für Kurgäste.* (Frankfurt a.M. und Kissingen: Carl Jügel, 1855), 329–32. Cf. Gottfried Eisenmann, *Die Heilquellen des Kissinger Saalthales. Physisch, chemisch und therapeutisch* (Erlangen: Palm und Enke, 1837), 77–98, provides a similar account of the daily routines of Kissingen. And even the travel guide from 1900, *Kissingen Spa: the International Health-resort, in its Medical and Social Aspects* (Munich: Kurverein Bad Kissingen, 1900), 47–57 relies on this tested schedule.

26. Marcard, *Pyrmont.* Vol. 2, 305 and Marcard, *Kleines*, 84.

27. See, for instance, Menke, *Pyrmont 1840*, 349–50. Also Marcard, *Pyrmont.* Vol. 2, 298, describes passive motion, riding, as a recommendable option. The distinction between passive and active motion as physical exercise was common in the old medicine. A more detailed description of this distinction can be found for instance in Gerhard Ulrich Anton Vieth, *Versuch einer Encyklopädie der Leibesübungen*, vol. 2, *System der Leibesübungen* (Berlin: Carl Ludwig Hartmann, 1795), 14–15.

28. Straß, *Pyrmont*, 41; Menke, *Pyrmont 1840*, 444. Theodor Valentiner, *Pyrmont für Kurgäste und Fremde* (Kiel: Carl Schröder & Comp., 1859), 39, saw, besides professional exertion, especially dangerous women's obsession with correspondence. Also Marcard, *Pyrmont.* Vol. 2, 311, made clear that both professional and leisurely, passionate reading and intellectual exertion were harmful for the cure. Eisenmann, *Heilquellen*, 97–98, particularly warned businessman against continuing their correspondence at a spa.

29. Balling, *Heilquellen*, 330.

30. Käppel, *Pyrmont's Merkwürdigkeiten*, 152. In the eighteenth century, Pyrmont was known for its reading circles, Kuhnert, *Urbanität*, 19. On Carlsbad see, Hlawaczek, *Karlsbad*, 115.

31. "Eben so enthalte man sich wo möglich während der ganzen Kurzeit des Beischlafes," Hlawaczek, *Karlsbad*, 43. Cf. Käppel, *Pyrmont's Merkwürdigkeiten*, 152; Wilhelm Ferdinand Chaßot von Florencourt, *Sittliche Schilderungen entworfen auf einer Reise von Braunschweig, über Pyrmont, Rinteln etc. nach Cassel in Briefen an einen Freund* (Berlin: Felischische Buchhandlung, 1801), 206; Straß, *Pyrmont*, 39; Johann Wendt, *Die Heilquellen zu Kissingen im Königreiche Baiern* (Breslau: Gosohorsky, 1837), 158. Hufeland, *Heilquellen*, 50, considered any kind of love life harmful for a spa cure.

32. Heinrich Koenig, *Eine Pyrmonter Nachcur. Roman* (Leipzig: Brockhaus, 1869), 41–45.

33. Gudrun M. König, *Eine Kulturgeschichte des Spazierganges. Spuren einer bürgerlichen Praktik 1780–1850* (Vienna: Böhlau, 1996), 192. The gender relationships at Pyrmont spa are analyzed more detailed in Heikki Lempa, "The Spa: Emotional Economy and Social Classes in Nineteenth-Century Pyrmont" *Central European History* 1 (2002): 51–52, 64–66.

34. H. Schmidt-Lisber, *Die Reise nach Pyrmont. Wahrheit und Dichtung* (Braunschweig: Waisenhaus, 1828), 48. According to Käppel, *Pyrmont's Merkwürdigkeiten*, 42, prostitutes used mainly the side streets and alleys.

35. In the regulations for the city police and the guards of the Main Boulevard, prostitutes were not mentioned. See *Staatsbad Pyrmont Archiv*, Einzelabhandlungen, Nr. 7: "Instruktionen II 1823–1892."

36. On Pyrmont, see Käppel, *Pyrmont's Merkwürdigkeiten*, 89. On Carlsbad, see Hlawaczek, *Karlsbad*, 44.

37. "Bruchstück einer Reise von Frankfurt nach Wisbaden, Langenschwalbach, Schlangenbad und Brückenau, nebst Nachrichten von diesen Bädern im Monat August 1808," *Journal des Luxus und der Moden* (September 1808): 629.

38. Marcard, *Pyrmont*. Vol. 2, 299; Ammon, *Brunnendiaetetik*, 76; Steinmetz, *Pyrmont*, 64–65.

39. Käppel, *Pyrmont's Merkwürdigkeiten*, 77; "Ueber die Hazard-Spiele im Bade zu Flinsberg in Schlesien," *Journal des Luxus und der Moden* (May 1798): 289–94; "Pyrmont," *Journal des Luxus und der Moden* (September 1801): 493; "Neue Beschreibung von Eger und Schwalbach," *Journal des Luxus und der Moden* (February 1800): 74.

40. *Staatsbad Pyrmont Archiv*, Einzelabhandlungen, Nr. 31: "Spielbank I, 1812–1866," 2. "Concept zu einem neuen Pacht Contract über die Spiel Bank zu Pyrmont während der Brunnen Cur-Zeit" esp. §§ 7, 13. The contract was to cover the years 1835–46. See also the casino contract from 1855, *Staatsbad Pyrmont Archiv*, Einzelabhandlungen, Nr. 31: "Spielbank I, 1812–1866," 11. "Vertrag über die Verpachtung des Spiels und des Badelogirhauses zu Pyrmont" June 12, 1855, J.v. Wellens.

41. Staatsarchiv Marburg, Best. 121, Nr. 2081: "Aufhebung der Spielbank zu *Pyrmont*." 1862–1864. Cf. Mehrdorf, "Geschichte des Bades Pyrmont," 105–10.

42. Adolph Bühren in his *Vier Wochen in Pyrmont, oder Wer's Glück hat, führt die Braut heim. Erzählung in Briefen* (Braunschweig: G.C.E. Meyer, 1824), 165, has his main character find the company for a walk to the caves of Dunsthöhle during the morning promenade. We have similar reports from Carlsbad: "In the morning people socialize there [by the spring] without any consideration for rank and order. There one can already make arrangements for the afternoon recreation as happened often during my visit. Here, by the spring, the lover of beautiful, wild nature, the indefatigable walker can already make appointments with kindred spirits," "Carlsbad und Töplitz," *Journal des Luxus und der Moden* (November 1798): 628.

43. Bühren, *Vier Wochen*, 46, 50–51, 125; Käppel, *Pyrmont's Merkwürdigkeiten*, 88, 93; Straß, *Pyrmont*, 45.

44. Anonymous, *Kissingen*, 55; Hermann Welsch, *The Springs and Baths of Kissingen* (Kissingen: Author, 1888), 5–6.

45. As known, spa statistics was notoriously unreliable because different criteria were applied to count a guest as a guest proper. Some spas, such as Kissingen distinguished carefully between visitors (*Passanten*) and guests proper (*Kurgäste*), whereas others inflated their statistics by including both as guests proper. Pyrmont was one of these "generous" spas, see Sibylle Lehmann, *Das fürstliche Schauspielhaus in Bad Pyrmont. Die Funktion eines Kurtheaters im 19. Jahrhundert* (Göttingen: Hubert & Co, 1994), 110.

46. Mehrdorf, "Geschichte des Bades Pyrmont," 91, lists the leading German spas in 1865 as following: Pyrmont with 6,537 guests proper was the 7th most visited spa in Germany after Baden-Baden (45,000), Wiesbaden (29,000), Carlsbad (10,000), Ems (8,000), Teplitz (7,000), Kissingen (7,000). The eighth most popular spa, Schwalbach, had 4,800 visitors. Only these eight most popular spas had more than 110,000 guests. Considering the great differences in spa statistics, overlapping visits by same guests to different spas, varying lengths of stay, and the lack or unreliability of statistics of peasant guests, these figures are hardly accurate. Yet they clearly show the range, because the smaller spas, and there were hundreds of them in Germany, quickly added the numbers of visitors.

47. Johann Wolfgang Goethe, *Sämtliche Werke nach Epochen des Schaffens. Münchner Ausgabe*, vol. 14, *Autobiographische Schriften* (München: Carl Hanser Verlag, 1986), 70–75.

48. "Eine Zeit der Ruhe folge auf die Kur, . . . Eine mehrwöchentliche behagliche Reise, ein Aufenthalt bei Verwandten auf dem Lande sind eine ungleich bessere Nachkur," Valentiner, *Pyrmont*, 51.

49. There is no modern study on Struve and his facilities. Some of the basic information can be gathered from Julius Minding, "Geschichtliche Bemerkungen über die Struveschen Nachbildungen, nebst Nachrichten über das Leben des Erfinders," in *Annalen der Struveschen Brunnenanstalten*, vol. 1 (Berlin: August Hirschwald, 1841), 1–45. Cf. August Vetter, "Vorrede," in *Annalen der Struveschen Brunnenanstalten*, vol. 1 (Berlin: August Hirschwald, 1841), III–X. According to Vetter the factory was opened already in 1817. Also Theodor Valentiner, "Vorwort" in Theodor Valentiner, ed., *Handbuch der allgemeinen und speciellen Balneotherapie* (Berlin: G. Reimer, 1873), III–VIII provides important details of Struve and his followers.

50. Hlawaczek, *Karlsbad*, 14, saw the manufactured water of Carlsbad only as an artificial copy that never could reach the "secret forces of nature" veiled in the original waters of Carlsbad.

51. Conrath [Brunnenarzt in Franzensbad], "Heilquellen zu K. Franzensbad bei Eger. Mit einer Nachschrift von Osann und Hufeland," *Journal der practischen Arzneykunde und Wundarzneykunst* 78, no. 3 (1834): 120.

52. August Vetter, "Beantwortung der gegen den Ersatz natürlicher durch künstliche Mineralwasser von Hrn Prof. A. Pleischl in Wien erhobenen Einwände," in *Annalen der Struveschen Brunnenanstalten*, vol. 3 (Berlin: August Hirschwald, 1843), 138–39.

53. Vetter, "Beantwortung," 143.

54. August Vetter, "Die Saison von 1840 in der Berliner Brunnenanstalt," in *Annalen der Struveschen Brunnenanstalten*, vol. 1 (Berlin: August Hirschwald, 1841), 171–72.

55. Valentiner, *Pyrmont*, 135.

56. Mehrdorf, "Geschichte des Bades Pyrmont," 91. See also Johannes Steudel, "Therapeutische und soziologische Funktion der Mineralbäder im 19. Jahrhundert" in *Der Arzt und der Kranke in der Gesellschaft des 19. Jahrhunderts*, ed. Walter Artelt and Walter Ruegg (Stuttgart: Ferdinand Enke Verlag, 1967), 89.

57. Vetter, "Saison," 171–72.

58. Vetter, "Saison," 172.

59. Hufeland's comment in Johann Evangelist Wetzler, "Bemerkungen über einige versandete Struve'sche Mineralwasser. Nebst einer Nachschrift von Hufeland," *Journal der practischen Arzneykunde und Wundarzneykunst* 65, no. 3 (1827): 123. This "metaphysical"

difference between Struve and Hufeland was paralleled by an important cognitive difference. Whereas Struve's discoveries implied and, in fact, were followed by a series of manipulations of waters toward their medical and technological utilization Hufeland's discoveries were directed to "neue Kräfte, neue Wunder, . . . , bis ans Ende der Tage." The nature was unlimited but our powers were limited, Friedrich Adolf August Struve, "Bemerkungen über einige gegen seine künstlichen Mineralwässer gemachten Einwendungen," *Journal der practischen Arzneykunde und Wundarzneykunst* 68, no. 4 (1829): 101. Rather than being technological categories "Kraft" and "Wunder" were aesthetic notions. Hufeland did not understand himself as one who manipulated nature but as a representative (*Vertreter*) and an advocate (*Sachwalter*) of the spiritual and living aspect of nature, Wetzler, "Struvesche," 123. In other words, he expressed nature, formulated in words its physical expressions but did not manipulate it.

60. Theodor Valentiner, "Allgemeine Balneotherapie," in *Handbuch der allgemeinen und speciellen Balneotherapie*, ed. Valentiner, Theodor (Berlin: G. Reimer, 1873), 11–12. Valentiner, a leading spa doctor from Pyrmont, mentioned Hufeland, his disciple Osann, and especially Sobernheim as the main adversaries of the new theory.

61. On Proessnitz there is no adequate research. I have used Valentiner, "Allgemeine Balneotherapie," 11.

62. Jean M. Irion, "Historical Overview of Aquatic Rehabilitation" in *Aquatic Rehabilitation*, ed. Richard G. Ruoti, David M. Morris, and Andrew J. Cole (Philadelphia: Lippincott, 1997), 5.

63. Bernhard Preiss, *Beobachtungen über die Heilkraft der Bäder zu Warmbrunn als Beiträge zur Pathologie und Balneotherapie* (Breslau, 1841).

64. "Die Lehre von Bädern überhaupt, ihren Arten und deren therapeutischen Anwendung heißt Balneologie," *Allgemeine deutsche Real-Encyclopädie* 1851, 224.

65. Valentiner, "Allgemeine Balneotherapie," 12.

66. Douglas Peter MacKaman, *Leisure Settings. Bourgeois Culture, Medicine, and the Spa in Modern France* (Chicago: University of Chicago Press, 1998), 96–100.

*Part Two*

# Practices of Bodily Education

# Chapter Four

# Gymnastics

"The history of medicine," claimed Karl Friedrich Koch, director of the gymnastic institute in Magdeburg, in 1830, "shows us the time when gymnastics and the art of healing were identical, instructed and exercised by same persons."[1] In a sentence, Koch captured the transformation of physical education during the first decades of the nineteenth century. In 1831, he would see the first students enroll in Ernst Eiselen's program for gymnastic teachers in Berlin.[2]

What was gymnastics? How did it become more than healing and exercise? For German gymnasts the answer was: It became an autonomous field with rules of its own. In 1816, Friedrich Ludwig Jahn saw in gymnastics a discipline that reestablished "the lost harmony of humanity," while Christian Friedrich Geisler celebrated it "as an essential component of the perfect education of young men."[3] Gymnastics had become (or so it claimed) the substitute for the old orders and regimens of the body. But by thirty years later, Koch noted, "gymnastics teachers" were still dependent on medicine, or more precisely, dietetics. And that wasn't all. When Koch opened his institute in 1828, the 170 new students, though well-trained in gymnastics, were plagued by bad posture. To correct this malformation and educational failure, Koch suggested that their curriculum "reinvigorate the old art of dancing."[4] In the 1830s, gymnastics, despite claims to independency and disciplinary maturity, was a fragile construct that carried an historical burden. When such masters of gymnastics as Koch reflected upon the possibilities and problems of their field, they were haunted by the remembrance of a time when physical education was in the hands of other specialties. Koch enumerated two of them: dietetics and dancing. Johann Heinrich Krause, a philologist, and Otto Heinrich Jaeger, a Swabian gymnastics leader, remembered a third: the old Greek pentathlon, which provided a different goal for physical training.[5] All these prove that modern German gymnastics, as much as it wished to stand as its own creature, was the heir of premodern traditions of physical education.

Rather than looking to tradition, scholarship on German gymnastics rests on the assumption of a rupture. It was, first of all, political. Historians have explored the (proto)political nature of German gymnastics seeing it either as the godfather of German liberalism or the origin of the Germanic movement. In its German incarnation, they argue, gymnastics was an incubator of modern political nationalism and an instrument for mobilizing the rising bourgeoisie in the aftermath of the Napoleonic Wars.[6] Sports historians also have supported the idea of a rupture, charting a host of innovations in gymnastics and physical education after the late eighteenth century.[7] While social and sports history have shared the assumption of historical discontinuity in German gymnastics, they have remained largely separate fields of research. Only recently have studies of gymnastics and its social uses found each other. Henning Eichberg's broad historical and anthropological explorations into German and English sports, dancing, and gymnastics have revealed a wholesale transformation of bodily configurations between 1770 and 1820: static and geometric motions replaced by dynamic motions, the minuet replaced by the waltz, regulated fencing replaced with intensive boxing.[8] Besides symbolizing the modernization of German society, the transformation of gymnastic movement revealed a number of social innovations. As Christiane Eisenberg has shown, German gymnastics was organized in a network of male organizations (*Männerbund*) that carefully guarded their masculine and martial culture by concentrating on the exercise most appropriate to it—javelin, wrestling, and climbing, for instance, while dancing was weeded out as effeminate or feeble.[9] But why were javelin, wrestling, and climbing more manly than dancing?

To answer this question we have to follow the slow rise of gymnastics as an independent field of practice and knowledge between the 1770s and 1820, and focus on Johann Christoph Friedrich GutsMuths's innovations; and we must navigate through the Napoleonic Wars that so profoundly influenced the work of Jahn, the founding father of the German gymnastics movement (*Turnbewegung*). Finally, we must consider the limits of experiences set by stubborn old traditions, provincial resistance, and competing ideas of what good and useful gymnastics was supposed to be.

## The Classical Canon of Physical Exercise

The history of German or any national gymnastics starts with the so-called old exercise. Among the various sports and physical diversions that occupied European life from the late Middle Ages onward, two possessed special cohesion, marked by rules and repertories of their own: aristocratic and academic *Exercitien*.[10] Although city dwellers and peasants regularly engaged in wrestling, fencing, shooting competitions, and dancing, only aristocrats and students organized and preserved a systematic cultivation of physical exercise canonized in the ritual triad of dancing, riding, and fencing. After the sixteenth century, the popular versions of fencing and riding began to disappear and the flourishing literature on dancing, riding, and fencing, and support of professional instructors in these fields helped the nobility appropriate these common forms of physical exercise and mold them to its own needs. Besides the martial skills they maintained, aristocratic exercises served the self-representation of a gentleman. Dancing, riding, and fencing masters, as Eichberg has shown, restructured their fields in accordance with the hierarchical order of court society.[11] Not surprisingly, they soon occupied the major part of an aristocratic education. In prominent knights' academies (*Ritterakademien*), such as Kassel, Lüneburg, Tübingen, and Soroe, a young nobleman could spend almost as many hours with physical exercise as with sciences and languages together.[12] By the early seventeenth century, *Exercitien* had become the *modus vivendi* of genteel education and an aristocratic privilege, sanctioned and supported by the princes.

By the end of the seventeenth century, physical exercise found its way into academic curricula. The reasons for this are not quite clear. Advocates of Humanism and Reformation stressed classical learning and were critical of physical exercise. The incentives for its incorporation into academic and social life came from increasing state intervention after the Thirty Years' War.[13] Physical exercise became one of the more important ways of attracting students from the nobility and even strongly humanistic universities, such as Jena, hired dancing, riding, and fencing masters. In Göttingen, the leading university of the eighteenth century, the academic cultivation of the gentleman reached its high point. A predominantly aristocratic university, Göttingen was proud of the dancing, riding, and fencing opportunities, which as disciplines equaled the natural sciences and classical languages.[14]

Though the classical canon of physical exercise comprised riding, fencing, and dancing, vaulting (*Voltigieren*), acrobatics on a pommel horse or a table, often was included. In Göttingen in particular, vaulting was very popular. Although all these exercises shared a high level of complexity and sophisticated rules, they developed in quite different directions. Dancing, the most inexpensive and accessible of them, began to lose its social exclusiveness by the middle of the eighteenth century when non-academic burghers and city dwellers adopted social dancing (and its instruction) for themselves. With riding, the opposite happened.

An exclusive and expensive exercise, it took an abrupt decline after the turn of the nineteenth century. Its gymnastic variation, vaulting on the pommel horse, which traditionally provided technical practice for riding, was incorporated in the new gymnastics, *Turnen*.

The most distinguished exercise was fencing. In aristocratic dueling and the ritualized student dueling of *Mensur*, fencing remained an important but culturally ambivalent form of exercise well into the twentieth century. The classic French art of rapier, introduced in Germany around the middle of the seventeenth century by Wilhelm Kreußler, reached a high level of sophistication during the eighteenth century.[15] Rather than an art of self-defense, rapier fencing was considered part of practical mathematics because of its geometrical forms.[16] But as fencing was increasingly formalized as a sport, traditional dueling took an alternative path. While aristocrats and bourgeois duelists, sanctioned by the code of honor, replaced the rapier with the pistol as their weapon of choice, students continued to duel with the sword. In the 1790s, an increasing aversion to French culture, including the rapier, brought about the reincarnation of old German fencing as practiced by commoners. Student fraternities resumed fencing by saber (*Hiebfechten*), the common weapon of the sixteenth and seventeenth centuries. Although institutionally sanctioned, fencing lost the level of sophistication that it had reached during the eighteenth century. In *Mensur*, for instance, the rules of fraternities seriously limited effective defense, which had been central to rapier fencing. The best student duelist was regarded as he who could show his nerve and calmly wait for a painful blow.[17]

Why did the genteel version of this exercise decline after the middle of the eighteenth century? We know that the aristocratic way of life was going through profound change. Increasing requirements for civil servants imposed obligations of formal education on impoverished aristocrats who were dependent on salaried income. This, in turn, was reflected in the educational institutions that aristocrats used for the education of their sons, the military academies and genteel universities such as Göttingen and Frankfurt an der Oder. They started to put more emphasis on subjects useful for administrative careers. Moreover, during the last decades of the eighteenth century, medical and dietetic writers began to challenge the traditional genteel and academic cultivation of the body.

It was no accident that certain key principles of dietetics were reinvented as traditional aristocratic and academic exercise was on the decline. The traditional dietetics of the six non-naturals provided a convenient framework to discuss gymnastics as an application of the third non-natural, motion and rest.[18] Even more influential was new dietetics that treated life as a well-balanced system of human nature in its environment. In this new dietetics, physical exercise, in order to restore or preserve the balance, had to be moderate. A good dietetics doctor prescribed exercise, as Krüger and Tissot argued, to establish and maintain harmony between sensation and motion. Although physicians acknowledged the benefit of muscular strength and dexterity, they did not recognize them as goals of physical exercise. Fencing and vaulting on the pommel horse, for instance, were considered too aggressive and vigorous. But riding in a sedan or a carriage was appropriate and beneficial, and most recommended walking and dancing the minuet and other moderate dances.[19]

The indirect critique or, at best, lukewarm endorsement of traditional genteel sports by physicians was taken to a new level when dietetic ideas were transplanted into educational programs. After the initial reception of Locke's *Some Thoughts Concerning Education* in the 1740s, dietetics became an important theme in German pedagogical discourse. Krüger, Zückert, and the members of the dominant pedagogical movement of the late eighteenth century, *Philanthropismus*, framed their ideas in dietetics.[20] With such influence on the rise of pedagogy and establishment of educational practices, dietetics implanted a deep concern for physical exercise, albeit its own limited version, within German education. Peter Villaume, a member of *Philanthropismus* from Halberstadt, argued that diet, medicine, and exercise should be the primary tools of physical education. For Villaume, the rationale of diet and medicine for physical education was obvious. They provided instruments for ethical moderation, for strengthening and stabilization (which he called "hardening") of the body to resist "the storms of passions."[21] But Villaume's was not exactly the traditional idea of moderation, which prescribed an agreeable, even soothing regimen of physical motion to benefit the human body. By emphasizing hardening as the best means of preserving the balance between the body and its environment, he removed the constraints against vigorous exercise.

Rather than preserving the balance of the body with its environment, Villaume's idea of exercise increased the physical powers of the body and supported its natural instinct for movement.[22] In consequence, Villaume was now confronted by a new and important question: How far could human beings develop in terms of physical performance, "at what point must we say that a human being cannot develop any further?"[23] Besides the classical, aristocratic exercises, a host of new exercises were developed and used at the educational institutions of *Philanthropismus* during the 1770s and 1780s. Unlike traditional dancing, fencing, and riding, whose purpose was aesthetic perfection and mastery of the body, these new exercises were not evaluated according to rules of perfection—many of them did not have established sets of rules. In part, they went back to popular physical culture, such as stone (shot) putting, but *Philanthropismus* also borrowed from Greek athletics, adopting running and jumping into its curriculum.[24] Unlike the aristocratic examples, the new exercises were measurable. Yet Villaume, not fully aware of the extent to which the new exercises might jeopardize the dietetic order of physical motion, chose not to introduce an objective scale of assessment. He repeatedly underscored that the goal of physical exercise was, first, "the development and perfection of powers," including strength, dexterity, and endurance, and, second, creation and preservation of the aesthetic proportions of the body.[25] Running and jumping were "useful," because they increased endurance, strengthened muscles, and helped to save one's life in emergency situations, such as fires.[26] But Villaume appreciated exercise that cultivated the symmetry and harmony of the body, such as dancing and fencing.[27] And as much as exercise fostered the development of human powers and the aesthetic cultivation of the body, it remained confined within the limits of moderation, which was the primary purpose of any physical education.

In his *Von der Bildung des Körpers*, published in 1787 as the eighth volume of Joachim Heinrich Campe's pedagogical encyclopedia, Villaume successfully amalgamated the aristocratic arguments and dietetics with the reinvention of ancient exercise. His achievement was unmistakable, yet the price was just as unmistakable. Both kinds of exercise, aristocratic and ancient, now were subordinated to a dietetic regimen in which moral utility outranked physical perfection. One could ask whether this was legitimate, whether something essential to physical exercise had been sacrificed to "moral conduct."[28] For those who preached aristocratic and academic exercise for its own sake, it would have been legitimate to ask whether Villaume's version of physical exercise actually caused a decline in the cultivation of the body or, in extreme cases, the disappearance of aesthetic excellence of the body. But besides Gerhard Ulrich Anton Vieth, a teacher of mathematics and gymnastics in Dessau, there were very few to raise this objection.

Originally from Jever, Vieth's formative education was at the University of Göttingen.[29] Besides his studies in mathematics and natural sciences, he was an enthusiastic gymnast, actively taking advantage of opportunities for riding, fencing, dancing, and vaulting on the pommel horse, for which Göttingen was famous. Although he was hired as a teacher at the grammar school in Dessau in 1786, his contacts to the advocates of *Philanthropismus* remained desultory.[30] Vieth, who became the headmaster of the school in 1799, was, above all, a dutiful director and conscientious teacher of mathematics.[31] He never taught gymnastics or other physical exercise in any systematic way. Yet he continued his own regimen of physical exercise, and it was this hobby that brought him his reputation, through the publication of an encyclopedic manual of physical exercise in 1794. The book, *Versuch einer Encyklopädie der Leibesübungen*, comprised two volumes: an historical inventory of all possible forms of physical exercise from ancient peoples down to contemporary European, Asian, and American sports, and a systematic presentation of physical exercise.

Vieth had a zeal for systematization.[32] The second volume of his encyclopedia was entitled *System der Leibesübungen* (System of the Exercise of the Body), which included a meticulous taxonomy of contemporary physical exercise. Its basis was kinetic. In any exercise, as he defined it, motion was either active or passive. Passive exercise comprised, among others, swinging, riding in a carriage, bathing, and massage. They were exercises in which the body was subjected to motion, whereas in active exercise the body itself brought about movement.[33] After this distinction, Vieth then denied place to elementary exercise, such as jumping, bending, and stretching. The exercises he included were complex, those that incorporated their own configurations, geometrically defined movements that were applicable to the body as a whole. His analysis of skating, for example, was based on careful geometric calculations of possible curves, angles, and figurations.[34] Within this mathematical definition of physical motion, illustrated by a list of all possible movements of different parts of the body, the academic and aristocratic exercise not only were emphasized but also preserved in their traditional configurations. And, as a former student at the University of Göttingen, Vieth valued dancing, riding, fencing, and vaulting on the pommel horse above all other exercises.

Was Vieth's system an anachronism, as has been implied by recent scholarship?[35] Vieth insisted that physical exercise was for "well-being and amusement."[36] Although he included physical motion in the cultivation of the body, he did not consider it as part of education. Rather, we can see him as an advocate of physical exercise or, if passive exercises were included, of a system of bodily culture that flourished outside the schoolyard, in city promenades and social clubs where it assumed an aesthetic function, based on the perfection of performance. Within the schoolyard physical exercise was assessed not by the perfection of performance but by the measure of accomplishment, in other words, by improvement and increase of skill.

## GutsMuths

In 1788, Christian Gotthilf Salzmann, the director of the *Philanthropinum* in Schnepfenthal in the duchy of Sachsen-Coburg und Gotha, reported that a new teacher trained the students in running, vaulting, and jumping over a ditch and crossbar. Everything was strictly regulated. Salzmann tells us that "Mr. GutsMuths carefully compiles a table on all these forms of exercise. By doing so, as accurately as possible, he can evaluate how much each disciple's abilities develop and what their weekly progress is."[37]

Born in Quedlinburg in 1759, Johann Christoph Friedrich GutsMuths went to the University of Halle, where he attended Ernst Christian Trapp's lectures on pedagogical seminary (1778–82), the first of its kind in Germany and famous for its advocacy of *Philanthropismus*. In 1785, his career as a private tutor took an unexpected turn when he was asked to take his pupil to Schnepfenthal, where Salzmann had founded an educational institution in 1784. Salzmann was so impressed by the young tutor that he hired him as a teacher. GutsMuths accepted the offer and never left Schnepfenthal again; he taught at the *Philanthropinum* until his death in 1839. At first, GutsMuths was in charge of geography and French but he soon discovered physical education to be his real interest.[38] The publication of *Gymnastik* in 1793 made him the leading authority on physical education in Germany. During the following twenty-five years, he continued to write on physical and moral education. He published a book on games in 1796 and on swimming in 1798. Three years later, we find him occupied with handicrafts.[39] After 1800, he expanded his sphere of influence by founding the *Bibliothek der Pädagogischen Litteratur*, the leading pedagogical journal in Germany until 1820.

The breadth of his influence and the spread of his writings made GutsMuths the leading figure in physical education in Germany.[40]

The centerpiece of GutsMuths's program was the *Gymnastik* of which originality he was deeply convinced. As he correctly noticed, the extant patterns of physical exercise either were connected to functions of a particular social class, such as fencing for self-defense or dueling, or they had a moral function. Yet he claimed that there was physical exercise that was self-reflexive serving the perfectibility of the body: "Although all manual work trains the body, that does not make it gymnastics. The purpose of manual work is to produce an object outside the exercising person. The purpose of gymnastics, however, is embedded in the exercising person himself."[41] Furthermore, the only practice that concerned itself only with the perfection of the practicing subject was pedagogy. That is to say, the physical exercise had to adopt pedagogical goals in order to reach conceptual autonomy, to become a practice with rules of its own.[42]

GutsMuths created gymnastics largely from ancient exercise. Villaume had noticed their usefulness and he also had witnessed their application in a number of *Philanthropinums*. But unlike Villaume, who had emphasized their moral and dietetic utility and resisted the temptation to make them conducive to meritocratic evaluation, GutsMuths had no inhibitions about these steps. As a teacher of gymnastics in Schnepfenthal, he collected materials and classified different forms of exercise into a coherent and formal system of motion. Classifying physical exercises was neither unique nor unprecedented. As Vieth in the first volume of his encyclopedia of physical exercise had demonstrated, the occidental civilizations had a rich tradition of manuals and studies on dancing, riding, fencing, and swimming. In reflection of their respective fields, European masters of genteel exercise had reached a high level of sophistication and cohesion. GutsMuths' singular contribution was a new kind of approach for formalizing physical exercise and distilling it to the elementary motions of the body.[43]

A surprising feature in GutsMuths' and Villaume's books is their endless number of exercises. This seems to place them at a distance from genteel activities and closer to dietetic prescriptions, which traditionally listed a number of exercises by virtue of their therapeutic usefulness. Villaume described fifty-two different physical exercises, including for the first time such activities as games, running, jumping, manual work, the Greek pentathlon, climbing, carrying loads, dancing, fencing, walking, shooting, riding, military drill, and exercise for the senses.[44] The list comprised three major traditions: aristocratic and pedagogical games, Greek exercise, and the aristocratic and academic traditions of dancing, fencing, and riding. In GutsMuths' *Gymnastik,* we find not only a considerable reduction in the number of exercises—GutsMuths listed only twenty-nine—but also a qualitative change. He rejected genteel exercise, excluding aristocratic fencing and riding as inappropriate, and including dancing only with caveats. Moreover, the games were separated from physical exercise proper and described in *Spiele zur Übung und Erholung* that appeared two years after the *Gymnastik.*

The core of GutsMuths' curriculum consisted of the Greek pentathlon and several new exercises that he invented in Schnepfenthal.[45]

For an example of an old exercise fused into a new system, consider jumping. The long jump, especially, was an important part of the ancient pentathlon. It was also a practical exercise that Basedow had introduced in the *Philanthropinum* of Dessau during the 1770s. Villaume had witnessed its students making "ten to twelve-foot-long jumps," and he observed that "all forms of exercise are organized to proceed gradually from easier to more exerting ones. For these exercises there is a special ditch in Dessau, narrow at both ends and in the middle about eight feet wide."[46] But this account was hardly more than a detailed description of what he saw. There is no sign of the formal approach that characterized GutsMuths' concept of jumping. The exact evaluation and measurement of each individual performance presupposed a careful taxonomy of different types and degrees of jumping.[47] GutsMuths distinguished five different types: 1. high jump without a vault, 2. high jump with a vault, 3. "deep" jump without and with a vault, 4. long jump without and with a vault, 5. combined high and long jump and "deep" and long jump. Each of these categories was arranged according to the degree of complexity of the corresponding exercise. For instance, the high jump without a vault, by far the most extensive category, consisted of elementary exercise, such as plain jumping in place and jumping on one foot and genuine exercise. The difference between elementary and genuine exercise was clear. The former were preparatory in nature whereas the genuine could be measured. They resulted in real performance.[48]

Measurability was the first criterion of GutsMuths' gymnastics, and it was closely related to, in fact dependent on, simplicity.[49] Although the forms of genuine exercise, such as the high-long and deep-long jump, were complicated, their complexity was manageable because the performance of them could be divided into their component parts. In aristocratic exercise, vaulting on the pommel horse had been the classical mode of jump. For GutsMuths, it was not manageable because it contained non-generic features: It was not a pure jump but belonged to a category that he called balancing.[50] His new gymnastics simply could not absorb this aristocratic exercise because its taxonomic principles were different. Taxonomic incompatibility was a significant problem for GutsMuths and he tried to solve it in the second edition of *Gymnastik* (1804) by including both dancing and fencing.

GutsMuths did not know enough about fencing, so he entrusted its discussion to the fencing master of the University of Erlangen, Johann Adam Karl Roux, a descendant of a famous old family of fencing instructors, who had published a manual on fencing as physical exercise in 1798.[51] Roux was convinced that "all rules that the art of fencing follows, as long as it remains within the boundaries of reason, correspond exactly with the constitution of our body and the sword. Its first principles are derived from general mathematics."[52] With the classical rapier, especially, the geometrical structuring of space determined the configurations of the exercise. The elements of fencing were derived from the weapon, and the fixed number of possible positions it might take in relation to the adversary.[53] The anatomy of the body did not play a dominant role in the classical configurations of fencing because it was designed to serve self-defense. Roux could not solve the problem of how to transform fencing into a pure exercise, as GutsMuths had required. His chapter on fencing in the 1804 edition of *Gymnastik* remained faithful to the classical tradition, full of technical details on different attacks and defenses, but without instruction in the elementary forms of movements and their effects on the body.[54]

With dancing, GutsMuths was more successful. He believed that "our common dances do not deserve to be recommended unconditionally as gymnastic exercise, . . . because their main content derives from love."[55] Contemporary dancing was "pretentious," "feeble" and "artificial," whereas GutsMuths' gymnastics were supposed to express true "powerful" and "flexible" manliness, i.e., the principles of morality and strong-mindedness.[56] To overcome what he considered the hopelessly effeminate features of social dancing, GutsMuths accidentally found a solution. He discovered that by attaching a rope to a small sandbag, he had an educational instrument for use in dancing. By spinning the rope in a circle at a specified height, the teacher could make the pupils jump at a certain tempo.[57] The arrangement was most convenient for single "dancers." Simple, unified, and pure movement replaced the inconvenient complexities of social dancing. GutsMuths's device had reduced educational dancing to a variation of jumping. This was exactly the opposite of what was actually happening in social dancing, where jumps were being replaced by sweeping steps that never lost contact with the floor. GutsMuths, however, was interested in silencing the erotic connotations of dancing and celebrating its manly, purely physical benefits. This does not mean that GutsMuths rejected the idea of exercise for women.[58] But he rejected what he considered the feminization of physical conduct in favor of manliness, which he held up as a moral ideal. The rules of simplicity, measurability, and anatomical utility that defined jumping in GutsMuths's new gymnastics were also applied to running, climbing, and lifting, creating a true taxonomy of physical exercise, a "system."[59] The influence of this system was significant and broad. By 1846, more than twenty new editions and translations of GutsMuths's *Gymnastik* had been published in German, English, Danish, Italian, Greek, and Dutch.[60]

During the first decade of the nineteenth century, formalization of physical exercise continued. Its most radical and consequent solution can be found in Johann Heinrich Pestalozzi's methodical gymnastics. Influenced by a disciple of Fichte, Pestalozzi created a purely formal system of exercise that consisted of simple movements of all the joints and the combinations of these into elementary motions.[61] Although Pestalozzi was much criticized, he influenced the shaping of educational gymnastics. His work was much relied upon by the Swedish gymnast and educator Per Henrik Ling and the gymnastic reformer of Hesse, Adolf Spieß.[62] Their works perfected the formalization of gymnastics, making possible its mass application to public-school education after the revolution of 1848.

We have followed three efforts to reshape physical exercise as educational or cultural activity: Villaume's dietetic gymnastics, Vieth's genteel gymnastics, and GutsMuths's pure gymnastics. All endorsed physical exercise as a method of human perfection. By 1809, the time of educational naivete had passed. It was in this year that a young teacher at Plamann's academy in Berlin decided to take his students to the surrounding meadows to play games and perform exercises in the open air. Attendance increased to several dozen during 1810, and the meetings became more regular. In July 1811, the first public gymnastics field was opened in the Hasenhaide, not far from the city center. What history books have dubbed the German gymnastics movement was born. The terms of physical exercise and its social appropriation went through a dramatic change. Overnight gymnastics was no longer an educational question alone but a vehicle for military mobilization and, finally, a community. These were to be the parameters of German gymnastics. But many of the controversies between dietetics, genteel exercise, and gymnastics continued after 1811.

## Jahn: Shaping a Tribal Body

The young teacher at Plamann's institute who in 1809 took his students outdoors to exercise was Friedrich Ludwig Jahn. Christiane Eisenberg has characterized Jahn as a charismatic leader.[63] A man who grew up in a rural community in an impoverished part of Prussia, a man who against many odds went to university, a man whose eccentric lifestyle was as notorious as it was celebrated and who did not fail to use his considerable physical strength when needed, already display features of a character beyond the ordinary. In his professional life, as well, he faced more than the usual number of obstacles. Having failed in the qualifying exam (*Staatsexamen*) needed for a position at a *Gymnasium*, he never achieved academic recognition. He yearned to be military leader but never became more than a subordinate commander of a volunteer detachment during the war of 1813–15. But despite these failures and despite the fragile political recognition of his gymnastics, he still succeeded in mobilizing a sizeable movement. One could ask, however, whether his charisma is enough to understand Jahn, his movement, and the configuration of physical exercise that he established during the eight years of his activities. Instead of concentrating on Jahn's person and career, I will focus on the formative influence of GutsMuths on Jahn's work, his unique experience of the war of 1813–15, and his historical and political ideas, especially that of tribal Germanness.

When Jahn embarked on his gymnastic venture in 1809, he did not hesitate to borrow from the repertory of physical exercises systematized by Villaume and GutsMuths over the past two decades. By 1816, when Jahn felt he had reached the status of a national educator, he still used the same exercises. In Hasenhaide and dozens of other sports fields, the curriculum was filled with hiking, running, pulling, carrying, pushing, climbing, throwing, wrestling, exercise on the vaulting-horse, and games. The horizontal bar and parallel bars were Jahn's own contribution.[64] He also shared some of GutsMuths's aversion to aristocratic exercises, which he decried as the expressions of charm—"the first thing to be rejected in an overly overindulged time."[65] But Jahn saw the benefits in some of these genteel exercises and adopted them, albeit with new vocabulary and purpose. For instance, he decided that the vaulting-horse deserved to be included in his program. But instead of the "foreign" *Voltigieren* his gymnasts used the German term *Schwingen* (swinging). The same Germanization occurred in fencing. While neither Eiselen nor Jahn included fencing in their manual of gymnastics, *Deutsche Turnkunst* (1816), the increasing popularity of fencing during the 1820s convinced Eiselen to create a Germanic style and vocabulary for fencing.[66] As for dancing, Jahn excluded it from his program.[67]

While the programs of Jahn and GutsMuths embraced, by and large, the same exercises, their views of the social organization for exercise differed greatly. Jahn's *Deutsche Turnkunst* paid close attention to the location, arrangements, and clubs (*Turnverein*), which were more than mere stages for gymnastic exercise. It was important, said the manual, that the sports fields (*Turnplätze*) be encircled by a fence and a moat because the arena was supposed to hold 200 to 400 gymnasts and convey the symbols of their community to the crowds that regularly gathered—and were expected to gather—to follow the physical performance of Jahn's students. Jahn had calculated that this number was large enough to be visually impressive but not too large to prevent the gymnasts from being fully visible to the observers.[68] Each activity had its volunteer trainer (*Turnwart*), himself well-trained in gymnastics, and a number of leaders (*Vorturner*) nominated from among the best gymnasts but the differences in status demonstrated a system less of a teacher and pupils than of *primus inter pares*. This equality of effort was enhanced by the casual and friendly use of "thou," not the formal *Sie* (You), and by simple uniforms, prescribed by the rules that Jahn and Eiselen stipulated for the community of gymnasts.

The spread of Jahn's gymnastics after 1811 was spectacular so much so that by 1813 his missionary zeal encouraged several communities in Prussia and North Germany to open sports fields of their own. Berlin and Breslau became centers of the movement. From there, Jahn's young emissaries—Hans Ferdinand Maßmann, Eduard Dürre, Wilhelm Beneke, and Wolfgang Harnisch, to name the most influential—spread the word and example, so that in Prussia alone some 100 gymnastics clubs had been founded by 1818 and enrolled about 6,000 members. The network of sports fields included also Hamburg, Mecklenburg, Thuringia, Hesse, Württemberg (Stuttgart and Tübingen), Baden (Heidelberg, Mannheim, Wertheim) and Bavaria (Bayreuth and Erlangen) by 1817. Dieter Düding has estimated the number of active gymnasts in Germany by 1818 at 12,000, organized in 150 clubs.[69] The center of gravity was in Northern Germany, especially Prussia. Only nine clubs existed south of the Main, and none was located in the major Upper Bavarian cities, Munich and Augsburg. The lands of Hapsburg and

Saxony also were important gaps in the network. Students at the University of Leipzig were inspired by Hasenhaide but obviously had no direct connections to Jahn or his emissaries.[70]

The rapid expansion of gymnastics clubs came to an abrupt halt in October 1819, when the German princes agreed to measures against subversive activities. In addition to the student fraternities (*Burschenschaften*), they indicted the gymnastics movement as a principal source of social unrest. Jahn himself was imprisoned, then released on a probation that lasted until 1825. *Turnen* was prohibited on Prussian soil. Most of the German princes followed Prussia's lead and either abolished Jahn's gymnastics or put it under more or less strict surveillance. In most German communities, with some exceptions such as Tübingen and Hamburg, the movement went underground. Not until 1842 did Prussia rescind the ban and open the doors to the second revival of the gymnastics movement.

Who were the gymnasts, those who followed Jahn's call for physical exercise and whose activities seemed to threaten the authorities? Historians have seen the early gymnastics movement as the first modern mass movement in Germany.[71] Yet "the masses" were hardly involved. The starting point of the movement were the advocates of gymnastics whom Jahn sent from Berlin to spread the word. These gymnastics missionaries were recruited from among Jahn's personal disciples in Berlin, students who supported the *Burschenschaften*, and the volunteer detachment under Major von Lützow, the so-called *Lützowsches Freikorps*, in the war of 1813–15. The beginnings of gymnastics in Hamburg show how this missionary work proceeded. In 1815, Wilhelm Beneke, one of Jahn's favorites, arrived in Hamburg from Berlin to finish his education as merchant.[72] He soon organized a circle of friends who started gymnastics exercises in Jahn's style. The members of this group mostly were students from local *Gymnasiums* and seminars, but after 1817 some young merchants and tradesmen joined them.[73] At the high point of this early gymnastic club, in 1819, the membership peaked at 166, hardly a mass attendance. By the following year, after the ban on gymnastics clubs had been issued in Prussia, only twenty members dared to continue their training. For the next twenty-five years, membership remained at the low level of a few dozen.[74] In active and enthusiastic student chapters, such as Breslau, membership occasionally reached several hundred.[75] But in Berlin, birthplace of the movement, attendance rarely exceeded 200.[76] Not until the 1840s did gymnastics clubs start to attract the members en masse. By the middle of the 1840s, membership in the *Hamburgische Turnanstalt* began to rise, reaching 433 in 1850 and 699 in 1861. According to Düding, the number of active gymnasts in Germany in 1847 was between 40,000 and 50,000, and the clubs also held a large number of young men who did not participate in exercise.[77]

The moderate size of the early gymnastics movement, even considering its heavy recruitment among high school students, does not evidence a political mass movement. More crucial than size was the organization of the movement. Did it follow the explicitly political agitation of the French Revolution, or was it more like peasant and journeyman revolts, well-known in Saxony and areas west of

Rhine in the early 1790s? Neither seems completely true of Jahn's movement. Jahn, in fact, was not a democratic Jacobin but a keen supporter of constitutional monarchy. Yet, paired with his personal and charismatic style, his constitutionalism aimed at transforming society, rather than restoring it to its former state, as so many peasant and journeyman revolts did. The gymnastics clubs were social and political models of equality and camaraderie—admirable qualities but not necessarily conducive to democracy, especially liberal, constitutional democracy. Rather than a modern liberal democrat, Jahn was an intellectual heir of the Reformation and the Pietist awakening of the late seventeenth century.[78] Many of the forms of social and ideological mobilization that Jahn so efficiently exploited to spread the message all over Germany and beyond its borders, including personal contacts and persuasion, correspondence, and emissaries, had been used by the Reformation and the Pietist movements. Like Jahn, they shaped public opinion by developing an extensive popular literature and a wealth of popular songs to support and disseminate their cause.[79] But Jahn substituted Germanness for religion. Although Luther himself had a concept of Germanness, which he marshaled against the papal forces, the Pietistic movements were either provincially attached to a local prince, such as Spener and Francke to the Prussian princes, or developed a cosmopolitan agenda as with Zinzendorf and his Moravian followers.[80] Jahn's starting point was different. He had inherited a half century of intellectual development that had endowed the German language with a special ability to express the social unity of its speakers.[81] Moreover, the language of Germanness and Jahn's often obscure and vaguely formulated political and ideological opinions were substantially shaped by the war of 1813–15, not in response to but as an experience of that war.

Jahn had felt deeply the devastating collapse of the Prussian forces against Napoleon in 1806, and he was excited by the approaching opportunity for revenge. When war finally broke out in 1813, Jahn became an organizer of *Lützowsches Freikorps* enticing several of his disciples from Berlin to join the unit. The enlistment of gymnasts from Berlin was so great that exercises were mostly canceled for the years 1813–14. The close connection between Lützow's militia troops and the gymnastics movement raises a question. Were Jahn's gymnastics used in preparation for war or was it the battlefield that militarized the movement? The gymnasts were only a small group of a few hundred among 3,847 troops of the *Lützowsches Freikorps* and not more than a drop among the 22,119 volunteers of the whole Prussian army.[82] But Jahn's position as recruiter and civil adviser for Major von Lützow gave the gymnasts special status within the unit. The most important deeds of Lützow's militia were brought about its (partly unintentional) strategy to operate behind the enemy lines. They mostly engaged in guerilla attacks, ambushes, espionage, and sabotage against French troops and German collaborators.[83] Guerrilla maneuvers did have their advantages: minor loss of manpower, opportunities for private initiative, and especially, places for heroism—real or construed. Despite the complaints of Jahn and other members of Lützow's troops, and later historical writing about the lack of "real battles" in the history of the detachment, it was in the environment of guerrilla war that the unique experience of a gymnast could make its mark.

> What gleams there in the forest, in the sunshine?
> Listen, it comes closer and closer.
> It wanders down to us, in gloomy rows,
> and the trumpets are shrilling
> and filling the soul with dread.
> And when you ask the black fellows
> They answer: It is Lützow's wild and bold hunt!
>
> What sweeps through the gloomy forest
> and roams from hill to hill?
> It lies in nightly wait;
> you hear them shout and the gun fires,
> the French henchmen drop down.
> And when you ask the black hunters,
> They answer: It is Lützow's wild and bold hunt![84]

This dark, poetic savagery, recorded by Theodor Körner, the poet of Lützow's troops and himself a guerrilla, wrapped a strange mixture of mysticism and a "cheerful" spirit of violence in the vivid imagery of nature. The raw material of such images would not have occurred on an ordinary battlefield of mass maneuvers and casualties, such as the battle of Leipzig in 1813, noted for the brutal fate of those killed in action and the huge suffering of thousands of wounded soldiers.[85] Johann Christian Reil, a leading medical doctor from Berlin, described in his letter to vom Stein, that after the battle of Leipzig "in the yard of the grammar school I found a hill that consisted of the remains and corpses of my countrymen. They were naked. Dogs and ravens were eating them, as if they were criminals and arsonists. This is how the heroes who died for their fatherland are disgraced".[86] It was not this overwhelming experience of mass warfare that buttressed Jahn and his young volunteers but the type of warfare, well-known in the eighteenth-century military theory, that received new attention after 1789—small and guerrilla wars.[87] This was the type of war that seemed to sit well with Prussian reformers.

The principal advocates of Prussian military reform, Gerhard von Scharnhorst and August von Gneisenau, envisioned a citizen militia, *Landwehr* and *Landsturm*, whose patriotic zeal and individual motivation would complement the professionalism of the standing army. The bond between the landownership and military command, typical of the Prussian army, was to be dissolved and rank-and-file soldiers would no longer be the serfs of landowner-officers. There were two ways to achieve this goal: Emancipate the peasants from their bondage, and extend recruitment outside the traditional military classes (aristocrats and peasants). The abolition of serfdom, proclaimed in the Royal Edict of 1807, should have accomplished the first target; but the technicalities of compensation and political disputes over land transfer greatly prolonged the process, and the self-destructive bond between officer and soldier-peasant lingered on.[88] More radical and effective was the Decree of Universal Conscription from March of 1813. Emulating the French model of a citizen-army, it obligated every male between 17 and 40 to military service, without exception and without the opportunity to transfer the obligation to someone else. As a result, middle-class men now were soldiers, and the Prussian army had a large contingent of men whose socialization and education was strikingly different from those of the traditional military classes.[89]

More than any other unit of the Prussian army, Lützow's troops fit the example called for by von Scharnhost and Gneisenau. They were recruited from the most heterogeneous backgrounds, including men and some women—Krimer mentions two, Dürre only one woman, Anna Lühring[90]—from Prussia, Westphalia, Saxony, Frankfurt, Austria, Mecklenburg, Holstein, Bavaria, Switzerland, the Netherlands, and Belgium.[91] Several came from middle-class and academic families. The shift from the nobility and peasantry to the middle class in the recruiting pool, however, did not abolish the social hierarchy within the troops but, rather, produced a new one. Noblemen still occupied the highest officer ranks, for professional as well as social and political reasons. Then came the cavalry of some 400 men "who are well educated, well-bred, intelligent, some of them from distinguished families, rich young men from middle class and gentry, merchants, students, several medical doctors, foresters, and old soldiers, . . . aristocrats, even a couple of counts."[92] Dürre also included the educated contingent of the infantry, *Büchsenjäger*, into this new "aristocracy." The lowest group consisted of those with less or no education, an obscure background, and no money with which to equip themselves with uniform, weapons, and a horse. "There were peasants and seamen. Some of them made their living on whaling. It is self-evident," as Dürre observed, "that in part these people were going downhill."[93]

During the campaign, Lützow's militia adopted an informal code that obligated them to loyalty to the group and personal courage but also allowed for personal hedonism within the boundaries of group solidarity.[94] Wenzel Krimer, a young Austrian volunteer and infantryman, described camp as a place in which soldiers could spend their time painting, reading, reciting poems and plays, dancing, and exercising.[95] Excessive drinking and sexual relationships were tolerated. Atrocities, typically connected with battlefield behavior, were not unknown to Lützow's guerrillas. Krimer describes his fellow soldiers mutilating French prisoners of war to prevent them from rejoining the ranks after repatriation.[96] This military experience—adventurous, brutal, and cheerful—was anticipated by and reproduced in the gymnastics that Jahn conducted in Hasenhaide.[97]

Although Jahn encouraged Eiselen to introduce military exercises after the war broke out, gymnastics in Hasenhaide after the summer of 1811—the first sports field was inaugurated on July 19—were not directly militaristic.[98] Apparatus gymnastics, which Jahn favored, only contributed indirectly to the physical skills of warfare. More important were gymnastic hikes (*Turnfahrt*) and fighting games that Jahn, who was himself an eager participant in them, had introduced.

One of these was the game Robbers and Wanderers (*Räuber und Wanderer*), in which two equal teams tried to capture as many opponents as possible. Jahn wanted the game to take place on varied terrain, with forests, bushes, and fields.[99] Moreover, the game taught young men to recognize friend from foe, and to trust their friends with their welfare. Instilling a sense of community was Jahn's goal in gymnastics, and his exercises created a community that was freewheeling and immersed in team spirit.[100] It was a unique and an exclusively male experience. If for GutsMuths manliness had been a moral ideal, for Jahn it was also a realm of experience, and one from which women were excluded. As he said: "Soft-hearted mothers and other women only do harm on the sports field."[101] Although there were women among Prussian volunteer troops and Lützow's militia, they were exceptions whose presence was tolerated but strongly discouraged. Consider the concern expressed by Lieutenant von Dittmar when he arrived in the city of Zobten, Silesia, on February 21, 1813, one of the first days in the formation of Lützow's detachment. He announced that he had brought with him 97 volunteer men and four volunteer women, whose presence might give rise to commotion and immorality.[102] Although the number of women participating in the war of 1813–15 was, according to Hagemann, 23, there were not enough for Jahn to include them in the common experience of war.[103]

The sense of community and the experience of male camaraderie provide manifest links between the experiences of gymnasts and those of the *Lützow* detachment. Community and male camaraderie were not Jahn's inventions. What he invented was a new way of enlisting individuals into this community, quite different from the ideal of manliness that GutsMuths promoted. Excited by the patriotic prospects opened by the collapse of Napoleon's power in Germany in the winter of 1814–15, GutsMuths published three long essays on "Patriotic Education" in his own journal, seeing in current events the vindication of his original belief that a boy's education should be based on "reasonable hardening and bodily strengthening."[104] According to his recommendations, "a boy should avoid soft and too warm feather beds from his early years on to become his habit; he should change randomly to different places to learn to easily fall asleep in a feather bed, on a straw mattress or hard bench where an underlay (*Unterlage*) or the hat serve as pillow."[105] No word on games and playing from this celebrated authority on children's games; no thoughts about physical education fostering cheerfulness and happiness from this famous critic of oppressive educational practices that plagued German schools in the eighteenth century.[106] The patriotic war allowed GutsMuths to recast himself an advocate of dietetic hardening. In fact, he discovered military training, *kriegerische Waffenübung*, as an important part of physical education.[107] Boys and young men, he said, should be divided into companies and battalions; they should learn "the martial step, wheeling, and the handling of the rifle," and they should incorporate those movements and codes that came closest to traditional warfare with strict discipline and drill.[108] In 1818, he went so far as to advocate the adoption of *Turnen* as a part of military training.[109]

Jahn could not have been more in disagreement. In the warlike games and hiking tours of 1811, he had thought little of moral rules and discipline.[110] In *Deutsche Turnkunst,* he advised boys simply to find an "original image of masculine vitality" to emulate.[111] His followers, who fiercely attacked what they considered GutsMuths's grave misinterpretation, emphasized the natural Germanic freedom of the gymnast. Franz Passow and Wolfgang Harnisch, gymnastics directors from Breslau, believed they should separate military exercises, *exercitia,* from Jahn's gymnastics, *Turnen*, because *exercitia* were mere drills that instilled subordination, whereas Jahn's gymnastics served the higher purposes of education and self-cultivation of *Bildung*. But they both conceded that gymnastics implied preparation for military service.[112] The real difference between GutsMuths and Jahn was not in military use of gymnastics per se but in what kind of military tactics gymnastic exercise was to serve. Whereas GutsMuths devised his exercises for an active but disciplined rank-and-file soldier in a military formation, Jahn envisioned an active, brutal, and tribal male, fit for guerrilla attacks.

GutsMuths might have been wrong in his interpretation of Jahn's gymnastics, but his remarks still indicate a problem that escalated into a controversy in Prussia in 1818. The myth of Lützow unit stressed the individual courage and patriotism of its soldiers. But, in truth, the detachment was riddled with insubordination. The social structure of the detachment had made it arduous to implement military discipline. In particular, the soldiers from the educated middle class had resisted standard military discipline for its own sake because it was associated with the "stiff performance of the masses."[113] Several, mostly conservative, critics made a similar observation of the gymnasts. Wilhelm Scheerer saw the main problem in the gymnnasts' "scorn of all kind of danger" which "makes them particularly barbaric. This in turn makes them inclined to indecency, excess, and quite often also to that arrogant arbitrariness and stubbornness that is so common among the uncultivated class and has often led to revolts and civil wars."[114] As Henrich Steffens, Johann August Kotzebue, and Karl Wadzeck, eminent critics of Jahn and the gymnastics movement, quite correctly argued, gymnasts were involved in and even directly responsible for a series of provocations, especially in the Wartburgfest in 1817.[115] As a result, Scheerer proposed a return to the old dancing, fencing, and riding controlled by state.[116] For him Basedow's, Salzmann's, and GutsMuths' methods and military academies, *Kadettenanstalten*, were more acceptable than Jahn's gymnastics.[117]

Scheerer's criticism was directed against Jahn's belief that gymnasts were part of a semi-historical and semi-mythological Germanic community that embodied the German national character. In the late eighteenth century, when the physiological, moral, dietetic or educational utility of physical exercise was discussed, the point of reference was ancient Greece.[118] GutsMuths meticulously propounded the Greek exercise but he added a new chapter to the history of gymnastics by setting, in short albeit skeptical remarks, the heroic and robust ancient Germans as counter-images to his phlegmatic and overrefined contemporaries.[119] Even so, the ancient Germanic tribesmen, like American Indians, Eskimos, and Lapps, could not equal the Greeks as physical prototypes. Therefore the new model of physical culture, GutsMuths suggested, should be a combination of the ancient Greek and a primitive *Naturmensch*—a cultivated savage.[120] Jahn overturned GutsMuths's standard-bearer, the exemplary Greek man. Like the physician May in his lectures on dietetics of 1793 or Fichte in his *Addresses* of 1807, Jahn, intoxicated by radical German tribalism, set the Germanic tribesmen as archetypes of health and physical vigor: "The highest and most holy duty of a German boy and young man is to become and keep himself a German man. By doing so he, like our ancestors, those saviors of the world, can vigorously contribute to the best of the people and fatherland."[121]

The introduction of the tribal argument changed the nature of physical exercise. In Jahn's writing, we find few remarks on the utility of particular exercises for health or physiological development. Instead, the benefits of exercise were ranked by their relation to the community, and this community was tribal, rather than nationalistic. Although Jahn was anything but consistent in his terminology, using words such as "*Volk*," "*Vaterland*," "*Stamm*" (tribe), "*Staat*," and even "*Nation*" interchangeably, his scattered historical remarks bear evidence of such an interpretation. In his 1814 pamphlet, *Runenblätter*, Jahn derived the unity of a *Walte* (an administrative unit or domain) from the unity of a "language and tribal community constituted by a shared danger and feeling."[122] He rearticulated clearly this premise in the *Werke zum Deutschen Volkstum* (1833) by arguing that the unity of a people was constitutional and linguistic but, above all, of the "tribal community, living territory, administrative domination, education, people's sentiment, public and private life, commerce and change, controversies with other peoples, but above all common history."[123] When it came to the unity of Germans, Jahn argued, it could be detected in the very meaning of the word *Deutsch* (German) which signified

> the people as the whole of related tribes and clans (*Geschlechtsverein*). Because in the primordial time of peoples' formation, only the formation of a people through inbreeding was known, and because the "multipeoples" (*Mangvölker*) as blends of competing peoples belong to a later time period, the notion of one people, as a higher form of a household, clan, and tribe, [is] the oldest meaning [of the word *Deutsch*].[124]

Traces of Jahn's Germanic tribalism can be found in his exercises. The javelin, for instance, was no longer called *Speerwurf* but *Gerwerfen*, evoking the early Germans.[125] It carried the memory of the tribal community; an act of this exercise became a reenactment of the tribal community.

Closely connected with the Germanic justification of gymnastics was a project that Jahn had started in 1806, when he published a dictionary to enrich the German vocabulary. His intention was to increase the number of meaningful German words by capturing the old, extinct meanings and rehabilitating them for modern users.[126] In 1811, after he had launched his gymnastics venture, his work on the

German language gained new momentum. As he told his friend Feuerstein, he was working on a new specialized vocabulary: "My gymnastic association takes a lot of time, because the beginning is always difficult. Moreover, the whole language must be recreated because the Germans cannot use mere artificially invented technical terms."[127]

Jahn was aware of a special feature of the German language that allowed him to build on his tribal project:[128] "The fullness, rigor, and subtlety of particles are the key to an unlimited vocabulary. These particles can be used as *prefix, medial syllable, and suffix*. They can be treated as permanent instructions for word formation."[129] This was a key not only to the history of language but also one to its future. Jahn made effective use of the discovery that the word was an individual image, a microcosm, a homogeneous space that can be governed only if we know its root.[130] By creating compound words, this space could be expanded almost infinitely. The word *Turnen* was such a root.[131] Its usefulness was obvious in comparison with *Gymnastik* or *Leibesübungen*, which allowed either few or no formations. Whereas *Gymnastik* had practically no socially significant connotations (with one important exception, the *Gymnasium*), *Turnen* had an enormous power to conjure up an elastic social texture around the idea of physical training. It signified not only the space (*Turnplatz,* /sports field) but also clothing (*Turnkleidung*), social units (*Turngemeinde*), social relationships (*Turnfeinde,* /enemies of *Turnen*, *Turnfreunde,* /friends of *Turnen*) and metaphysics (*Turngeist,* /spirit of *Turnen*).[132] Special exercises, such as hiking (*Turnfahrt*), the vaulting-horse (*Schwingen*) and balancing (*Schweben*), were marked with specifically German words. Johannes Zeidler has identified in his study on the language of German gymnasts more than 1,200 related words introduced by 1819. Jahn had created most of them, especially those with the root *Turn*, which alone accounted for 112 words.[133]

Jahn's decision to "return" to what he imagined to be the old Germanic vocabulary had significant social consequences because the vocabulary he developed and systematized can be fully understood in the context of what was non-Germanic, i.e., French or—to a lesser degree—Jewish. The established forms of physical exercise (dancing, fencing, and riding) had a centuries-old history of sophisticated usage dominated by French instructors, French instruction manuals, and French terminology. In dancing, especially, French was the language of professional discourse. Vieth used it, and half a century later dancing instructors such as Paul Bruno Bartholomay and Theodor Hentschke, and even Franz Anton Roller were still using it. In riding or in vaulting on the pommel-horse, the terminology was also French at the time Jahn started his project.[134] Fencing likewise belonged to the tradition of French exercise.[135] But unlike social dancing, which Jahn and his disciples despised, fencing soon was redesigned and redefined in German terms. Eiselen, who had been fencing director at Hasenhaide, created a new German terminology of fencing that he modeled on what had been used by Kreußler in the late seventeenth century. German vocabulary not only made fencing more acceptable and accessible to gymnasts but also incorporated it into the continuum of meanings and symbols used by Jahn's gymnastics. The results were published in 1826 in Eiselen's booklet, *Outlines of the German Rapier.*[136] It was obvious that Jahn and his tribalism project benefitted from Francophobic images. German words and physical exercises that had been adopted for Germany now were clearly anti-French.

Jahn's antisemitism, however, had a specific meaning with regard to physical exercise. Jahn's contemporaries associated Jewishness with cosmopolitanism, a euphemism for a landless community. Although this was antithetical to Jahn's image of a community united through a common land, a common language, and quasi-historical memories of a common tribal past, opposition to the imagery of the French language was far more powerful and useful in unifying the gymnastics community than the vaguely and poorly understood experiences of being Jewish. Indeed, some gymnastics clubs allowed sons of Jewish families to attend and even to become members.[137] Nevertheless, antisemitism played its part in the gymnastics movement because Jahn envisioned a Christian community that excluded Jews.[138] The event that most forcefully promoted antisemitism among gymnasts, the meeting at the Wartburg, was unequivocally Christian. Occasioned by the tercentenary commemoration of Luther's ninety-five theses, the leaders of *Burschenschaften*, of whom several were active gymnasts, called a large-scale meeting in 1817. Its focal point was the burning of anti-Germanic books. Maßmann, who was active in the *Burschenschaften*, was in charge of throwing the books onto the fire. Among others, he threw in *Germanomanie* (Obsession with Germanness), a critical work by Saul Ascher, a well-known Jewish writer.[139] Later, in the 1830s, Maßmann's antisemitic instincts received public attention when he engaged Heinrich Heine, a converted Jewish author, in a bitter dispute over Jewishness.[140]

The borders of Jahn's community are now visible: Women and Jews were excluded or unwelcome, whereas the French were the archenemy, foes of the tribal community of Germans. But what made the gymnastics movement the wellspring of social agitation and revolt that its critics and the authorities believed it to be? A deeper reason for the public irritation with the gymnastics movement was in the internal organization of the gymnastics community.

Jahn understood the tribal community of gymnasts as an egalitarian brotherhood. He and his followers repeatedly claimed its camaraderie, cheerfulness, and friendliness. Rules of dress and address also expressed gymnastic egalitarianism, including the use of "thou" (*Duzen*) instead of the more formal "you" (*Sie*). And this was noticed by those who gathered in Hasenhaide to witness gymnasts at their exercises. The gymnasts wore a neutral uniform of loose gray shirts and linen pants.[141] In Berlin, there were sons of aristocratic and even princely families among the gymnasts, and the political message of the uniform did not go unnoticed. One appalled observer was Henrich Steffens, a professor of physics at the University of Breslau and an important figure in Berlin cultural circles. He was disturbed by the democracy of the gymnastics community, which threatened to transgress existing social boundaries. He recognized the challenge the movement posed to the feudal structure of Prussia and Germany and pointed out the cultural damage that "untamed equality" could cause.[142] In the gymnastics community, social differences were ignored and the complicated practices of mutual recognition in the social code of the German upper and middle classes, became irrelevant when uniform dress and the use of "thou" made all appear equal. Just as threatening was the greeting *Gut Heil* whenever gymnasts met.[143] In consequence, the gymnastic community seemed all the more threatening to persons like Steffens, who had developed a completely different code of bodily conduct and who now saw the body reduced to an image of muscular strength and dexterity.

Yet the egalitarianism of Jahn's gymnasts was not unprecedented. At the Dessau *Philanthropinum* in the 1780s, friendly relationships were encouraged between students and teachers.[144] Moreover, in the early gymnastics movement the active gymnasts were often students of local *Gymnasiums*. In Breslau, home of one of the biggest clubs in Prussia before 1819, the gymnasts were between 8 and 20 years old. In most of the chapters listed by Schneider in his statistical reports of gymnastics clubs, the members were from this age group.[145] Among these young enthusiasts, inspired by images of tribal community, a vision of the unity of all Germans, a casual tone was not difficult to implement. As Düding shows, Jahn saw the importance of "thou" in instilling a close and intimate sense of solidarity among the gymnasts. Yet it was used exclusively only among young gymnasts, whereas the uses varied greatly between adults and boys and among adults. Jahn seems to have used "thou" rarely in his correspondence with the loyalists of the movement.[146]

## Gymnastics in Context

The self-conception of the gymnastics movement relied on the forgetfulness of history. According to its own historical understanding, the exercises of German tribesmen or medieval townsmen had been forgotten by the seventeenth and eighteenth centuries.[147] The gymnastics movement believed itself a revival movement memorizing and reenacting the ancient Germanic mastery of the body. However effective this self-conception, it does not explain fully the success of Jahn's gymnastics as a historical phenomenon. Although it continued to affect the ways that Germans, including the educated middle class, cultivated their bodies, the modes of cultivation varied greatly and often were something quite different from what Jahn and his assistants had intended. The ideas and definitions of a Jahn, an Eiselen, a Maßmann started to blur and break down when decisions actually were implemented on how Jahn's gymnastics could be applied to established curriculums or when the gymnasts of Leipzig, Vaihingen, Stuttgart, Tübingen, Hamburg or Dresden, organized in their local clubs and chapters started their own programs of gymnastic exercises—which may or may not have been exactly as Jahn proscribed them. So the perception of gymnastics had a history of its own, with an important impact on how GutsMuths, Jahn, and their followers spread their influence and how the authorities reacted to the gymnastics movement.

Since the 1770s, state authorities had recognized gymnastics as a key element of the educational reforms that *Philanthropismus* had launched in Dessau and Brunswick. When the Prussian and Bavarian governments started to reform their educational systems after 1800, GutsMuths took the initiative and wrote a long memorandum to the Prussian minister of education, von Massow. To his disappointment, he received only a polite, even sympathetic, response, but no commitment to his program.[148] The door, which recently had been half-opened to a broad recognition of physical education, was closed. Then in 1809, in the middle of a reformist fervor, the right man seemed to have taken the office: Wilhelm von Humboldt became the head of the department of the educational and cultural affairs. Humboldt was not a flag-waving advocate of gymnastics, but his personal experience contributed to its revival.[149] Between 1809 and 1810, the Humboldts' son, Theodor, was educated at Plamann's institute, in which Jahn was teaching and von Humboldt recognized its excellence in "physical education and care."[150] Some of his closest colleagues, moreover, had a positive, albeit from a distance, appreciation of physical education. Friedrich August Wolf, who had considerable influence on Humboldt and his close assistant Johann Wilhelm Süvern, understood *Bildung* as the "cultivation of the body and the mind leading to the perfection of humanity."[151] Humboldt also acknowledged the importance of physical education when reform of the military academy of Liegnitz was under discussion.[152] It was obvious that he, the spokesman for educational reforms, approved physical training as part of the standard education.[153] Süvern, who between 1809 and 1819 prepared school legislation, agreed with Humboldt that gymnastics should be retained on all levels of the Prussian school system: elementary schools, council schools (*Stadtschule*), and *Gymnasiums*. Although the proposal of 1816 did not stipulate physical exercise as mandatory, in the final proposal for the Law on Higher Education in 1819 an agreement on the issue was reached and a forum seemed open for a broad institutional recognition of gymnastics.[154] But the proposal of 1819 never became law; and although it served as a guideline for the higher education in Prussia, the situation after the Carlsbad Decrees of 1819 ignored gymnastics, which were banned in Prussia.[155]

Despite the partial, albeit intermittent, recognition of gymnastics by Prussian authorities, leading figures of neohumanism in Prussia and Bavaria paid remarkably little attention to physical exercise—with the exception of Friedrich Thiersch, professor of philology at the University of Munich. No major neohumanistic treatise on physical exercise or gymnastics is known. Nor was gymnastics a topic worthy of comment in private exchanges, apparently. Only after 1816, when Frederick William III took a public stand for Jahn and his project, did leading neohumanist intellectuals and philosophers such as Georg Wilhelm Friedrich Hegel and Friedrich Schleiermacher, visit Hasenhaide and begin to think favorably of Jahn's cause.[156]

If Jahn's recognition by the neohumanistic establishment had limits, what was the status of his work in the public perception? In one of several official reports on Jahn and his movement, August Ferdinand Bernhardi described Jahn's activities and public reaction to the gymnastics movement in Prussia, particularly in Berlin in 1818.[157] Although Bernhardi understood Jahn's political aspirations and his critique of the establishment, he pointed out the limits of Jahn's influence. In cold fact, fewer people were interested in or even aware of *Turnen* than what friends and foes of the movement assumed:

> The lower class practices Jahn's gymnastics hardly at all. It is interested in, if anything, exercise related to tightrope walking and "strongman performances." The higher and especially the highest estates have a particular distaste for the very essence of Jahn's gymnastics, community and camaraderie. In the middle class there are fewer indifferent opinions, more foes and more friends, especially the former.[158]

Bernhardi was a well-informed observer. Several descriptions from the provinces associated gymnastics with tightrope walking and acrobatics, amusements of the lower class. In Leipzig, gymnasts performed their exercises on the Roßplatz next to tightrope walkers and skaters.[159] This association was not accidental. Jahn had established gymnastics as a vehicle for public performance and, as some critics noticed, it required mastery of acrobatics. When the young student Stüve reported from Berlin that he had participated in gymnastic exercise, his mother admonished him. Local critics of the gymnastics movement in Osnabrück had shown, Mrs. Stüve warned her son, how perilous most of these exercises were.[160] Gymnastics also was seen as immoral and obscure, as early critics in Hamburg pointed out.[161] Rather than a respectable field of physical education, they considered *Turnen* next to dubious public entertainments such as gambling and legerdemain, which were allowed only outside the city gates.[162] As late as 1838, Maßmann felt it necessary to remind his readers that Jahn's gymnastics were not a vain imitation of tightrope walking.[163] However far from the truth these views might have been, they persisted and shaped the public image of Jahn's gymnastics.

The Carlsbad Decrees of 1819 and subsequent ban on Jahn's gymnastics did change public perception of the movement by refusing it official recognition. Gymnastics leaders countered by inventing new forms of gymnastics to circumvent the proscription. Tribal unity and the reenactment of tribal community through public performances were now effectively precluded. Support came from scattered student fraternities and groups that secretly continued to cultivate gymnastics in Jahn's spirit, especially in Hanau, Frankfurt am Main, Offenbach, Hamburg, and Tübingen.[164] In the Hapsburg territories, where Jahn never managed to find a noticeable following, gymnastics remained a private, individual activity. It was not recognized as a collective exercise until 1838.[165]

Jahn and his followers dominated gymnastics in Berlin, but in German provinces their vision often was challenged.[166] Local gymnastic activities, although inspired by Jahn, had their own characteristics, determined by local politics and a variety of substitute gymnastics that took root after the ban on Jahn's movement. Small towns such as Tübingen had few if any problems in adopting gymnastic symbols, such as the gray gymnast's uniform and the general use of "thou."[167] The gymnastics leader Karl Völker solved the conflict between town and gown, always present in university towns, through a simple plan: Students and young men of the city practiced on separate days, thus avoiding personal contacts and acts of recognition and rejection across the social divide.[168] In Hamburg, where the gymnastic club grew out of an older institute of physical education directed by a retired officer named Nicolai, old and new traditions were carried on hand in hand—or made compatible through compromise. For example, there was an older teacher of Nicolai's institute, Lampe, who retained his position after 1818 when the new director, Wilhelm Beneke, took over. In principle, as a leading gymnast, Lampe should have used "thou" with his new students. This, however, never happened. Lampe simply was exempted from the rule and students continued to address him with the formal *Sie*.[169] Harnisch, a gymnastics leader from Breslau, also did not accept the use of "thou."[170]

The attire of gymnasts often gave rise to dispute. Unless one deliberately ignored the political connotations of gymnastics emblems, the dress was likely to evoke social and political friction. Friedrich Wilhelm Klumpp, a gymnastics leader and teacher at a *Gymnasium* in Stuttgart, prescribed a paramilitary uniform for his young gymnasts in Swabian Vaihingen and Leonberg.[171] In a city such as Hamburg, which had a well-controlled dress code in the eighteenth century, gymnastics attire was most likely to be confronted with skepticism, even resentment, by the patrician class. Although the men from the stock exchange tolerated the public wearing of the German coat (*Deutscher Rock*), they did not embrace it. Several forbade their apprentices and journeymen, who were under their paternalistic control, to wear it. Dr. Gurlitt, the director of the school system, was an even stronger opponent of the democratic gymnastics attire.[172] But unlike the merchants, his authority could not prevent students from dressing in the German coat, and gymnastic clothing became normal within the academic community.[173]

If the conflicts over gymnastics in the provinces were different from those at the center, so was the observation of doctrinal purity. Klumpp credited Campe's novels and later Salzmann's educational experiments for his early interest in education. These also had introduced him to GutsMuths's *Gymnastik*, which he continued to use as a guide and a source of inspiration for teaching of physical exercise, even after 1816, when Jahn's ideas became public.[174] In far-away Vaihingen discrepancies between gymnastics authorities were indistinguishable; Klumpp did not see much difference between GutsMuths's and Jahn's approaches. For a teacher, GutsMuths's book, clear and graphic in its outlines and more pronouncedly educational than Jahn's ideological booklet, was simple to implement.[175] The influence of *Philanthropismus* was even more significant in private education, and it bolstered the cause of exercise and physical education. Liberal autobiographies from 1780 to 1850 show that *Philanthropismus* important to the

German elite until the middle of the nineteenth century.[176] The early education of August Ludwig Reyscher, later a professor of law at the University of Tübingen, combined readings recommended by the neohumanists and exercises derived from manuals of Pestalozzi and Campe.[177] Regardless of his mother's enthusiasm for Goethe and Schiller, *Philanthropismus* also was the main inspiration for Robert von Mohl, a professor of law, a leading liberal thinker, and a founding father of modern political science whose early education included a considerable amount of physical education, wrestling, and playing.[178] The continuing influence of *Philanthropismus* also explains, apart from the general interest in physical exercise, the popularity of GutsMuths's ideas in complement to Jahn's more flamboyant and politically passionate program.

The linkage of *Philanthropismus* and Jahn's gymnastics became even more striking after Jahn's program was banned in 1819. While Jahn's gymnastics did not vanish altogether—even in Berlin, Eiselen would continue with his gymnastic institute—it was now limited to indoor training.[179] Under such changed circumstances, it was GutsMuths's more educational and politically neutral program that gained momentum. Gymnastics retreated from public fields to educational institutes or other places far enough from public observance to avoid provoking political disturbances. When the gymnastics club of Hamburg obtained its first training ground in 1828, it was on the bastion Groß-Ericus, far away from the city center.[180] Friedrich Buek now could recommend for any tourists visiting Hamburg that they watch the gymnastics exercises of "this harmless association that has not given excuses for any political persecution."[181] And by the 1820s, new conceptions of gymnastics started to align Jahn's and also GutsMuths's programs with dancing and with physical education of girls and young women.

## Manliness or Elegance

The state of war that had existed continuously since the French Revolution had a profound impact on gymnastics. It either provided the experience upon which physical exercise rested, or it was the ultimate goal for which gymnastics should prepare a man. But war was not the only source of experiments that became so common in the 1820s. When GutsMuths and Jahn declared the cultivation of manliness to be the only basis of German gymnastics, classical dancing had been the main target of their criticism. So dancing instructors set out to defend their traditional status as the guardians of aristocratic and academic cultivation of the body by appropriating the techniques of gymnastics as a part of their professional practice. Franz Anton Roller was the most famous of them.

Formerly a professional dancer in a Viennese ballet, Roller had landed in Leipzig in 1799 as a dancing instructor. Like most in his profession, Roller was a man of the minuet. He came close to promoting what GutsMuths and Jahn had identified as the negative and effeminate influence of a French, therefore contemptible, cult of charm and frailty.[182] But his defense of the minuet incorporated a wider concept of physical exercise. In 1805, Roller founded an institute for gymnastics in Reichel's garden in Leipzig.[183] We do not know much about its activities. But we do know that when Roller took a position as instructor of dancing and gymnastics in the elite Saxonian school Schulpforte in the same year, he continued to redefine dancing as physical exercise.[184] Eduard David Helmke, himself a dancing master as well as the biographer of Roller, gives a vivid description of a carnival ball that Roller organized at his school in 1812. Its theme was ancient Greece. The dancers, all boys, were divided into two groups representing Greek soldiers in full armor and weaponry. After a compliment to the audience, the two troops began their performance, which included complicated drills with spears and dance solos. The finale was a fierce but undecided battle between the groups.[185] Not unexpectedly, Jahn gave full approval to Roller's experiment. This was a kind of dancing he could accept in his gymnastics program because it separated the genders and created a model of purely masculine dancing.[186]

In 1816, after two months of personal consultation in Berlin, Jahn entrusted Roller to introduce gymnastics at the Schulpforte.[187] Roller, who almost until his death in 1844 remained involved with the instruction of gymnastics and dancing at his school, was loyal to Jahn's program. Yet he went beyond Jahn's intentions. Roller considered pure gymnastics one-sided, gauche, even ungraceful, and in need of refinement and cultivation. Only a dancing instructor, in his estimation, could provide this higher sense of body image and body culture.[188] With imperceptible but important modifications, Roller shared Jahn's vision of a cultivated male body. But most dancing instructors did not share Roller's moderate enthusiasm for gymnastics and raised critical voices against its headlong spread.[189] Despite this, Roller showed—and his dancing master colleagues agreed, albeit lukewarmly—that dancing and *Turnen* were not mutually exclusive. By separating the genders institutionally and conceptually, he had, in fact, invented a strategy to expand the influence of educational gymnastics.

Gymnasts seem to have been less interested in the new, polished, and socially acceptable type of dancing. Instead we find them engaged in a variety of merry activities that circled around social dancing. Consider what might happen during a hiking tour, for example. Reyscher, a student in Tübingen in the early 1820s, took off with his comrades on a hiking tour (*Turnfahrt*) in the Black Forest. The students came to a small village, Stammheim, where they found a friendly reception. The night was spent engaging the local girls in a ballroom. In the morning more dancing and drinking followed, activities that Jahn had not prescribed for a sound and healthy hiking tour.[190] Gymnastic meetings (*Turnfeste*) themselves often involved much that was outside the immediate control of supervisors. Normally these included public competitions, professional meetings, and socializing, often including a public ball as the finale. At the annual convention of the *Allgemeine Turnverein* of Leipzig, a ball was held every year after 1848.[191]

Whereas Jahn's tribal gymnastics, GutsMuths's educational gymnastics, and Roller's program at the Schulpforte had been designed for the education of boys, some instructors saw possibilities in these regimens for the education of girls. In 1828, Phokion Heinrich Clias, a Swiss native and an advocate of physical exercise, introduced calisthenics for girls that brought together his experiences as a gymnastics teacher in Switzerland, France, and England.[192] His exercises for girls were not derived from dancing and graceful carriage but from the gymnastics program to strengthen the body and increase its dexterity.[193] He did for girls' education what GutsMuths had done for boys' education, turning the separate programs into a gender-neutral physical education. By comparison, L.F. Kümmerle, dancing instructor at the *Catharineninstitut* in Stuttgart, concentrated on female carriage (*Anstand*). According to Kümmerle, the achievment of *Anstand* was the purpose of dancing. He tried to integrate it with more abstract exercises, such as swimming and balancing.[194] He considered this moderate gymnastics, deprived of aggressive features, to be decorous method for forming the female body.

Though GutsMuths' and Jahn's gymnastics have been described correctly as the gymnastics of manliness, the elements that made the greatest inroads into male culture came from dancing, from the realm of elegance and grace.[195] How did these two cultures, male gymnastics and "feminized" dancing, relate to each other? For Jahn, manliness was educational, the vehicle for overcoming one-sided intellectualization and the overrefinement of modern man. One should reinvent "masculinity," claimed Jahn, by engaging the young man and his development in his real life.[196] This was hardly an original idea. In the common wisdom of the early nineteenth century, a stoic and aggressive notion of manliness, *Männlichkeit*, overshadowed the paradigm of tranquil self-knowledge that Johann Heinrich Zedler had provided as the standard interpretation in 1739: "In moral perspective is manliness a position in which one initiates and does nothing but what is proper for someone whose mind is mature."[197] By the turn of the nineteenth century, manliness became associated with the execution of one's will. Johann Christoph Adelung defined it "as a resolute and earnest being, ability to reasonably calm one's fear,"[198] whereas Campe extended its scope to characterize "the manliness of physical shape, [T]he manliness of facial features" and the entire moral habitus of a real man, as distinct from a woman.[199] Jahn transferred these into the Germanic past, back to the old German tribes who now became the true expression of manliness.

It is, however, not the folkloric ideal of manliness that Jahn institutionalized. His version was influenced by the war experiences of 1813–15. Ute Frevert has suggested that Jahn's conception of manliness, increasingly militaristic, was built into the German cultural code during the *Vormärz*.[200] Daniel Alexander McMillan has noticed, however, a shift from the early gymnastics movement, which valorized the man as a brave soldier, to the later movement of the 1840s, which defined manliness as characteristic of a virtuous citizen.[201] The conditions of this change, I suggest, were largely dictated by two fundamental conditions and choices. First, guerrilla life was the primordial experience of the gymnastics movement. Once this experience receded, its memories faded, and its worship restricted by the ban of 1819, the gymnastics ideology became susceptible to new influences. Second, Jahn's response to his war experience was decidedly tribal. It was not based on natural rights. It did not create a political movement, much less a political mass movement. Instead it constructed a historically and linguistically extended community of Germans, a community whose members necessarily shared the essential features of their ancestors.

All these elements, the short climax of Jahn's movement and its increasing receptivity to new influences turned it toward a new kind of gymnastics during the 1820s. Through the integration of dancing, fencing, and girls' gymnastics into the repertoire of *Turnen*, the culture of manliness was infiltrated by the ideas of elegance. Rather than solving the increasingly complicated equation, Maßmann, in his desperate defense of *Turnen*, tried to clarify what gymnasts could not emulate, namely "1) the vanity of a tightrope walker, . . . 2) the sweetness of a dancing master, . . . 3) the stiffness of a corporal and his military exercise."[202] Yet for Roller, Klumpp, and several local followers of Jahn, these borderlines were anything but clear. *Turnen* was only one of several forms of gymnastics that shaped the middle-class body. After the Carlsbad Decrees of 1819 and the subsequent ban on Jahn's gymnastics movement, it was, in fact, GutsMuths's gymnastics that gained a new momentum. It was not narrowly collectivistic; it did not raise aspirations to national unification; and, above all, it was readily applicable to such different purposes as education and military training.

## Notes

1. Karl Friedrich Koch, *Die Gymnastik aus dem Gesichtspuncte der Diätetik und Psychologie, nebst einer Nachricht von der gymnastischen Anstalt zu Magdeburg* (Magdeburg: Creuß'sche Buchhandlung, 1830), V.

2. Ernst Eiselen, a disciple and colleague of Friedrich Ludwig Jahn, was the most active advocate for German gymnastics in the 1820s. In 1831, supported by high officials of the Prussian administration, he applied for a license to teach gymnastics teachers. See Klemens Wildt, *Daten zur Sportgeschichte*, vol. 2, *Europa von 1750 bis 1894* (Schorndorf bei Stuttgart: Hofmann, 1972), 45.

3. Friedrich Ludwig Jahn and Ernst Eiselen, *Die deutsche Turnkunst* (Berlin: Sportverlag, 1960), 161; Christian Friedrich Geisler, *Turnfreund. Eine Sammlung hochachtbarer, aus alter und neuer Zeit, für den Werth und die Nothwendigkeit absichtlicher, wohlgeordneter Leibesübungen der Jugend* (Berlin: G.C. Nauck's Buchhandlung, 1819), IX.

4. "Die Wiederbelebung der alten Tanzkunst," Koch, *Gymnastik*, 281–82.

5. Christa Kleindienst-Cachay, *Die Verschulung des Turnens. Bedingungen und Folgen der Institutionalisierung der Leibesübungen in den öffentlichen Schulen* (Schorndorf: Karl Hoffmann, 1980), 130, 185.

6. Willi Schröder, *Burschenturner im Kampf um Einheit und Freiheit* (Berlin: Sportverlag, 1967); Dieter Düding's excellent *Organisierter gesellschaftlicher Nationalismus in Deutschland (1808–1847). Bedeutung und Funktion der Turner- und Sängervereine für die deutsche Nationalbewegung* (Munich: R. Oldenbourg Verlag, 1984), esp. 57–75,

studies the forms of sociability and social organization in the gymnastics movement, but is mainly informed by the theories of political history and Germanic nationalism (*deutsche Nationalbewegung*) between 1808 and 1847. On the so-called third wave of the German gymnastics movement, after 1860, see Michael Krüger's *Körperkultur und Nationsbildung. Die Geschichte des Turnens in der Reichsgründungsära—eine Detailstudie über die Deutschen* (Schorndorf: Verlag Karl Hofmann, 1996), esp. 416–22, which, again, sees *Turnen* in the light of German political history. At the same time, Krüger understands gymnastics shaping a distinctive German habitus. See especially McMillan, "Germany Incarnate," Abstract and 20–22. On the influence of gymnastics on the formation of German nationalism in the second half of the nineteenth century, see Svenja Golterman's *Körper der Nation. Habitusformierung und die Politik des Turnens 1860–1890* (Göttingen: Vandenhoeck & Ruprecht, 1998).

7. Still the best analysis of physical education in *Philanthropismus* is Hajo Bernett's concise *Die pädagogische Neugestaltung der bürgerlichen Leibesübungen durch die Philanthropen* (Stuttgart: Karl Hofman, 1960). Of the large number of studies on German sport, Wolfgang Eichel, ed., *Geschichte der Körperkultur in Deutschland,* vol. 2, *Die Körperkultur in Deutschland von 1789 bis 1917* (Berlin: Sportverlag, 1969) and its contender from West Germany, Horst Überhorst, ed., *Geschichte der Leibesübungen,* vol. 3, 1, *Leibesübungen und Sport in Deutschland von der Anfängen bis zum ersten Weltkrieg* (Berlin: Bartels & Wernitz, 1980) are theoretically stimulating but empirically hardly more compelling than Edmund Neuendorff's massive *Geschichte der neueren deutschen Leibesübung vom Beginn des 18. Jahrhunderts bis zur Gegenwart* (Dresden: Wilhelm Limpert, 1930), of which volumes 1–3 deal with the history of physical exercise in Germany before 1860. More systematic is Hans Groll's *Die Systematiker der Leibesübungen. Vergleichende Systemkunde der pädagogischen Leibesübungen* (Vienna: Österreichischer Bundesverlag für Unterricht, Wissenschaft und Kunst, 1959).

8. Henning Eichberg, *Leistung, Spannung,* passim.

9. Christiane Eisenberg, *"English Sports" und deutsche Bürger. Eine Gesellschaftsgeschichte 1800–1939* (Paderborn: Ferdinand Schöningh, 1999), 111, 116. On the formation of German masculinity and gymnastics, see Daniel Alexander McMillan, "'. . . die höchste und heiligste Pflicht . . .' Das Männlichkeitsideal der deutschen Turnbewegung 1811–1871," in *Männergeschichte—Geschlechtergeschichte. Männlichkeit im Wandel der Moderne,* ed. Thomas Kühne (Frankfurt: Campus Verlag, 1996), 90, and Ute Frevert, "Das Militär als 'Schule der Männlichkeit.' Erwartungen, Angebote, Erfahrungen im 19. Jahrhundert" in *Militär und Gesellschaft im 19. und 20. Jahrhundert,* ed. Ute Frevert (Stuttgart: Klett-Cotta, 1997), 145–73.

10. For instance, Neuendorff sees in the rise of genteel gymnastics the demise of physical exercise proper. This negative history readily supports Jahn as the founding father of "real" gymnastics, who reformed the discipline and restored its lost value. See Edmund Neuendorff, *Geschichte der Deutschen Leibesübung,* vol. 1, *Vom Beginn des 18. Jahrhunderts bis zu Jahn* (Dresden: Wilhelm Limpert-Verlag, 1932), 84.

11. Eichberg, *Leistung, Spannung,* 28. Cf. Volker Saftien, *Ars Saltandi. Der europäische Gesellschaftstanz im Zeitalter der Renaissance und des Barock* (Hildesheim: Olms, 1994), 376–77, who sees a tendency toward increasing use of geometric order in the Baroque dance. Instead of being suppressed, Saftien argues, one's natural mobility gained new opportunities to express itself through new configurations.

12. Bruno Mahler, "Die Leibesübungen in den Ritterakademien" (PhD diss., University of Erlangen, 1921), 8–10. Although Bleeck tries to argue that there was virtually no difference between curricula in military academies and *Gymnasiums*, his evidence is not conclusive beyond the academies of Lüneburg, see, Klaus Bleeck, *Adelserziehung auf deutschen Ritterakademien. Die Lüneburger Adelsschulen 1655–1850*, vol. 1 (Frankfurt am Main: Peter Lang, 1977), 121–30. On gymnastics at military academies, see also Neuendorff, *Geschichte der Deutschen Leibesübung*, vol. 1, 127–33. An exhaustive, though mechanically organized, account of German military academies and aristocratic educational institutes in the nineteenth century can be found in Bernhard von Poten's *Geschichte des Militär-Erziehungs- und Bildungswesens in den Landen deutscher Zunge*, vols. 1–5 (Berlin: Hofmann & Co., 1889–97).

13. Ludwig Mester, *Die Körpererziehung an den Universitäten. Eine historisch-systematische Untersuchung über die Bedeutung der körperlichen Übungen für das Universitätsleben der Reformation, der Aufklärung und das Neuhumanismus* (Langensalza: Julius Beltz, 1931), 21.

14. Wilhelm Henze, "Leibesübungen und Körpererziehung in der Gründungszeit der Universität Göttingen," in *Von den ritterlichen Exercitien zur modernen Bewegungskultur. 250 Jahre Leibesübungen und Sport an der Universität Göttingen*, ed. Wolfgang Buss (Duderstadt: Mecke Druck und Verlag, 1989), 24–26. The position of an *Exercitienmeister* was normally lower than that of an ordinary professor but higher than a *Privadozent* (an untenured professor without permanent income). Cf. Mester, *Die Körpererziehung*, 37–41.

15. Mester, *Die Körpererziehung*, 33.

16. For a classical formulation see, for instance, Johann Adolf Karl Roux, *Gründliche und vollständige Anweisung in der deutschen Fecht-Kunst auf Stoss und Hieb* (Jena: Wolfgang Stahls Buchhandlung, 1798), 3.

17. On fencing, see Mester, *Die Körpererziehung*, 54–57. An adequate study of fencing is yet to be written. On social aspects of fencing, especially on dueling and student dueling, *Mensur*, see Frevert, *Ehrenmänner*, esp. the chapter "Studentischer Comment und Verbindungswesen bis zur Mitte des 19. Jahrhunderts." Kevin McAleer's *Dueling. The Cult of Honor in Fin-de-Siècle Germany* (Princeton: Princeton University Press, 1994), esp. 120–27, provides a short but stimulating account of *Mensur* from the eighteenth century to the 1930s.

18. Hannes Strohmeyer has described the rise of gymnastics as a shift from the six non-naturals to physical education (*Leibeserziehung*) in his "Von den 'sex res non naturales' zur 'Leibeserziehung.' (Ein Beitrag zur Begriffsgeschichte von 'Leibeserziehung')" in *Sportwirklichkeit. Beiträge zur Didaktik, Geschichte und Soziologie des Sports*, eds. Reinhard Bachleitner and Sepp Redl (Vienna: Österreichischer Bundesverlag, 1981), 134–37.

19. Krüger, *Diät oder Lebensordnung*, 413; Tissot, *Gesundheit der Gelehrten*, 106, 150–54. Cf. also Jahn, *Norma Diaetetica*, 163–64.

20. Christa Kersting has shown most convincingly how the rise of pedagogy is closely related to the lasting influence of dietetical discourse, see Kersting, *Die Genese der Pädagogik*, 9–10, 123–26, 216–21.

21. Peter Villaume, *Von der Bildung des Körpers in Rücksicht auf die Vollkommenheit und Glückseligkeit der Menschen oder über die physische Erziehung insonderheit* (1787) (Dresden: Wilhelm Limpert Verlag, 1929), 43, 77–78.

22. Villaume, *Bildung des Körpers*, 57–59, 134.

23. "Wo ist der Punkt, von welchem man sagen könnte: Weiter kann der Mensch nicht kommen," Villaume, *Bildung des Körpers*, 6.

24. Villaume mentions several Greek exercises and games in his "Von der Bildung des Körpers in Rücksicht auf die Vollkommenheit und Glückseligkeit der Menschen, oder über die physische Erziehung insonderheit," in *Allgemeine Revision des gesammten Schul- und Erziehungswesens von einer Gesellschaft praktischer Erzieher*, vol. 8, ed. Joachim Heinrich Campe (Wolfenbüttel: Gräffer, 1787), esp. 377–85, 407–22.

25. Villaume, *Bildung des Körpers*, 7, 134–35.

26. Villaume, *Bildung des Körpers*, 219–34.

27. Villaume, *Bildung des Körpers*, 241–45.

28. Johann Christoph Friedrich GutsMuths, *Gymnastik für die Jugend. Enthaltend eine praktische Anweisung zu Leibesübungen. Ein Beytrag zur nöthigsten Verbesserung der körperlichen Erziehung* (Schnepfenthal: Buchhandlung der Erziehungsanstalt, 1793), 97. This critique of the dietetic-moral regime of physical exercise was GutsMuths's point of departure.

29. I rely on two biographies of Vieth, Karl Peters, *Gerhard Ulrich Anton Vieth. Der Werdegang eines Jeverländers zum bedeutenden Schulmann und Turnpädagogen* (Jever: Mettcker & Söhne, 1962), esp. 67–107, 183–212, and Gerhard Lukas, *Gerhard Ulrich Anton Vieth. Sein Leben und Werk* (Berlin: Sportverlag, 1964), passim.

30. Peters, *Gerhard Ulrich Anton Vieth*, 114–15.

31. Peters, *Gerhard Ulrich Anton Vieth*, 162

32. He was aware of Johann Christoph Friedrich GutsMuths's work, *Gymnastik für die Jugend*, which had been published a year earlier.

33. Vieth, *Versuch einer Encyklopädie*, vol. 2, 14–15.

34. Vieth, *Versuch einer Encyklopädie*. Vol. 2, 251 and Table III in the addendum. Vieth emphasized the social benefits of skating. "The movement is not so shaking that it would prevent conversation. Side by side, arm in arm friends can enjoy together all that only a promenade can provide," Vieth, *Versuch einer Encyklopädie*. Vol. 2, 255.

35. See Eichberg, *Leistung*, 40. If we treat the history of physical exercise as a succession of different systems, then Vieth was indeed an outdated enthusiast, as Eichberg maintains. Clearly, this approach is problematic. It constructs a teleology from genteel exercises to "bourgeois" gymnastics, games, and sport, one that assumes gymnastics, games, and (by the end of the nineteenth century) sports would have become dominant. But during the first decades of the nineteenth century, aristocratic exercises, which Vieth promoted, were even more popular than "bourgeois" exercises and gymnastics.

36. Vieth, *Versuch einer Encyklopädie*, vol. 2., 7.

37. *Nachrichten aus Schnepfenthal für Eltern und Erzieher*, vol. 2 (Leipzig: Siegfried Lebrecht Crusius, 1788), 43–44. See also Schröder, *GutsMuths*, 58.

38. *Nachrichten aus Schnepfenthal für Eltern und Erzieher*, vol. 1 (Leipzig: Siegfried Lebrecht Crusius, 1788), 66; *Nachrichten aus Schnepfenthal*, vol. 2, 41.

39. As the title of the book *Mechanische Nebenbeschäftigungen für Jünglinge und Männer. Enthält eine praktische auf Selbstbelehrung berechnete Anweisung zur Kunst des Drehens, Metallarbeitens und des Schleifens optischer Gläser. Als Anhang zur Gymnastik* (Leipzig, 1801), indicates, there was a close relationship to gymnastics.

40. There has been an increased interest in GutsMuths. Hajo Bernett's concise presentation is stimulating in its emphasis on GutsMuths's cultural innovations, such as measurement, see Bernett, *Die pädagogische Neugestaltung*, 70–90. But its focus is on the late eighteenth century, though GutsMuths' influence on education increased during the nineteenth century. Concerning the biography of GutsMuths, Ulrich Popplow's "Johann Christoph Friedrich GutsMuths. Erzieher—Forscher—Mensch," *Leibesübungen* 8 (1959) is still one of the best, together with Clemens Menze's "Die pädagogische Bedeutung von GutsMuths," *Leibeserziehung* 7 (1959). Willi Schröder's *Johann Christoph Friedrich GutsMuths. Leben und Wirken des Schnepfenthaler Pädagogen* (Sankt Augustin: Academia-Verlag, 1996) is a useful historical essay. Yet a fuller understanding of the theoretical, pedagogical, and societal ramifications of GutsMuths' work is needed.

41. GutsMuths, *Gymnastik 1804*, 5. Eisenberg's, "*Sports*," 100, argues that the educators of Schnepfenthal invented a bourgeois style of physical exercise, displaying economic efficiency and moral integrity. GutsMuths's intention, however, was to create pure education.

42. Schröder, *GutsMuths*, 81–84, shows interesting connections between Hufeland's macrobiotics and GutsMuths's theory of gymnastics: both of them had medical foundation and rejected what they considered the culture of sensitivity and over-refinement They remained, however, separate projects. GutsMuths's gymnastics was useful for moral education but not identical with it or with any moral regimen.

43. Although he avoided public reflection on the formal quality of his works and left no private notes on the classification, his extensive oeuvre allows an insight into these reductions.

44. There were twenty-one of them.

45. Schröder, *GutsMuths*, 53–56, mentions the ancient Greek and the popular tradition as GutsMuths' main sources and sees GutsMuths as the reinventor of the Olympic games, ibid, 59.

46. Villaume, *Bildung des Körpers*, 232.

47. See Bernett, *Die pädagogische Neugestaltung*, 70–72, who argues that GutsMuths' invention of measurability is an expression of a capitalistic logic of accomplishment.

48. GutsMuths, *Gymnastik 1793*, 222–25.

49. Cf. Eisenberg, "*Sports*," 100.

50. GutsMuths, *Gymnastik 1793*, 233.

51. Roux, *Gründliche*, 3–4. The book contains only a short passage on the educational benefits of fencing.

52. Roux, *Gründliche*, 3.

53. According to Anton Friedrich Kahn, *Anfangsgründe der Fechtkunst* (Göttingen: L. Schultze, 1739), 31, the geometrical approach was in decline by the middle of the eighteenth century. Cf. Eichberg, *Leistung*, 67.

54. GutsMuths, *Gymnastik 1804*, 147–55.

55. GutsMuths, *Gymnastik 1793*, 370.

56. GutsMuths, *Gymnastik 1793*, 372–74.

57. GutsMuths, *Gymnastik 1804*, 183.

58. GutsMuths, *Gymnastik 1804*, 273–74.

59. Games that GutsMuths had compiled in his *Spiele zur Uebung und Erholung des Körpers und Geistes für die Jugend, ihre Erzieher und alle Freunde unschuldiger Jugendfreuden* (Schepfenthal: Verlag der Buchhandlung der Erziehungsanstalt, 1796), followed pedagogical and anatomical principles. The first category, games of motion (*Bewegungsspiele*), were divided by mental and bodily faculties. The second category, sedentary games (*Ruhespiele*), were also divided according to observation, judgment, attention, memory, fantasy, taste, and reason, see GutsMuths, *Spiele*, esp. 42–46.

60. Ursula Weidig, "GutsMuths-Bibliographie," in *Festschrift zum 200. Geburtstage von Johann Christoph Friedrich GutsMuths* (s.l.: Ministerrat der Deutschen Demokratischen Republik, 1959), 97–98. On the reception and influence of GutsMuths' thought, see Schröder, *GutsMuths*, 135–47.

61. Johann Heinrich Pestalozzi, "Über Körperbildung als Einleitung auf den Versuch einer Elementargymnastik, in einer Reihenfolge körperlicher Übungen," in *Sämtliche Werke*, vol. 20 (Zürich: Orell Füssli Verlag, 1963), 47–68. As editor Emanuel Dejung shows, Pestalozzi wrote only parts of the text. Central passages on specific exercises came from Johann Niederer. On the exercises, see Pestalozzi, "Über Körperbildung," esp. 58–60, 65–68.

62. Philipp H. Geiss, *Das Leben des Turnpädagogen Adolf Spieß (1810–1858). Ein Beitag zur Geschichte des deutschen und des schweizer Schulturnens* (Idstein: Schulz-Kirchner, 1991), 69.

63. See Christiane Eisenberg, "Charismatic National Leader. Turnvater Jahn" *The International Journal of the History of Sport* 13, no. 1 (1996): 14, 23. Applying Max Weber's theory of the routinization of charisma, she sees in the gymnastics movement after Jahn a shift toward bureaucratization.

64. During the third revival of German gymnastics, in the 1860s, this became a critical issue dividing the gymnastics community into hostile camps.

65. "Zierlichkeit ist in einem verweichlichten Zeitalter am ersten zu entraten," Jahn, *Die deutsche Turnkunst (1960)*, LIV.

66. There was substantial interest in fencing among Jahn's followers, causing him to write to Eiselen from Paris on October 3, 1815, that he would bring a fencing manual to Eiselen, Jahn, *Briefe (1930)*, 83.

67. Jahn had discovered this term in 1814, in a manual published in 1698: *Voltigieren* was here translated as *Schwingen*. See Jahn to Eiselen, Frankfurt am Main, June 30, 1814, in *Die Briefe F.L. Jahns*, ed., Wolfgang Meyer (Dresden: Wilhelm Limpert-Verlag, 1930), 77.

68. Friedrich Ludwig Jahn and Ernst Eiselen, *Die deutsche Turnkunst* (Dresden: Wilhelm Limpert-Verlag, 1928), 204–5, 228–29, 249–50.

69. Düding, *Organisierter*, 67. In his statistics of 1818, Schneider, a clerk working for the Prussian government, reports 4,462 gymnasts in Prussia, Schneider, "Statistische Übersicht von Gymnasten und Turnplätzen in Preußen," in *Unbekannte Briefe von Friedrich Ludwig Jahn und Hugo Rothenstein als Quellen zur Frühgeschichte des Turnens*, ed. Hans Langenfeld and Josef Ulfkotte (Oberwerries: WTB, 1990), 76–78. Düding's figures for Prussia come from Neuendorff; for all of Germany, he uses Jahn's own estimation, made in 1818. See Jahn to Vieth, Berlin, April 11, 1818, in Jahn, *Briefe (1930)*, 124.

70. On the situation in Munich, see Alois Huber, *München im Jahre 1819*, vol. 1 (Munich: Zängl, 1819), 330, and on the lands of Hapsburg, Hermann Wagner, "Zur Geschichte des Turnwesens in Oesterreich," *Deutsche Turn-Zeitung* 10 (1884): 88.

According to Emil Kneschke, *Leipzig seit 100 Jahren. Säcularchronik einer werdenden Großstadt. Ein Beitrag zur Sozialgeschichte seiner Heimath* (Leipzig: Hartknoch, 1870), 427, "Leutzsch and Gohlis were the areas in which practicing gymnastics continued." I could not find support for this statement. Düding and McMillan exclude Saxony from the first wave of the gymnastics movement, see Düding, *Organisierter*, 67, and McMillan, "Germany Incarnate," 94.

71. Düding, *Organisierter*, 137–38; McMillan, "Germany Incarnate," 92–94.

72. Otto Beneke, *Hamburgische Turnanstalt von 1816. Erinnerungen aus der Zeit ihres Entstehens und Aufblühens* (Hamburg: Johann August Meißner's Verlags-Buchhandlung, 1866) , 8.

73. Beneke, *Hamburgische Turnanstalt*, 19.

74. Carl Schneider, *Die Hamburger Turnerschaft von 1816, von ihrer Begründung bis zur Gegenwart*. Anläßlich des 75jährigen Bestehens der Turnerschaft im Auftrage des Turnrathes (Hamburg: Hamburger Turnerschaft, 1891), 161. Schneider has compiled this figure from the economic records of the club. While it may not be completely accurate, it provides a good estimate.

75. Joachim Burkhard Richter, *Hans Ferdinand Maßmann. Altdeutscher Patriotismus im 19. Jahrhundert* (Berlin; New York: Walter de Gruyter, 1992), 88.

76. Schneider's statistical report of 1818 mentions only 136 gymnasts regularly attending the exercise in Berlin, Schneider, "Statistische Übersicht," 76.

77. Düding, *Organisierter*, 233.

78. For Jahn, the King of Prussia and the emperor of Austria were both acceptable leaders. Peter Brandt, "Einstellungen, Motive und Ziele von Kriegsfreiwilligen 1813/14: Das Freikorps Lützow" in Jost Düffler, ed., *Kriegsbereitschaft und Friedensordnung in Deutschland 1800–1814*. Jahrbuch für historische Friedensforschung. 3. Jahrgang 1994, 228.

79. Karen Hagemann, "Of 'Manly Valor' and 'German Honor': Nation, War, and Masculinity in the Age of the Prussian Uprising Against Napoleon" in *Central European History* 30 (1997), 187–220 and the literature there.

80. Cf. McMillan, "Germany Incarnate," 112, who sees the Pietistic features of Jahn's enterprise. See also Düding's excellent analysis of the gymnastic lyrics and songs during the years 1815–18, which reveal a striking combination of divine mission and emotional agitation, Düding, *Organisierter*, 107. On North German Pietism see the synoptic chapters of Martin Brecht, "Philipp Jakob Spener, sein Programm und dessen Auswirkungen," and his "August Hermann Francke und der Hallische Pietismus," in *Geschichte des Pietismus. Vol. 1. Der Pietismus vom siebzenhten bis zum frühen achtzehnten Jahrhundert* (Göttingen: Vandenhoeck & Ruprecht, 1993), 281–398, 440–539. On the separate Pietist movement in Wurttemberg, see Hartmut Lehmann's *Pietismus und weltliche Ordnung in Württemberg vom 17. Bis zum 20. Jahrhundert* (Stuttgart: W. Kohlhammer Verlag, 1969), esp. 22–65 and 117–34. Lehmann argues, following Koppel S. Pinson's dictum, that Pietism, especially its Wurttemberg variation, contributed significantly to the rise of German "nationalism," anchoring the idea of a spiritual fatherland as it was transformed into a secular one.

81. McMillan, "Germany Incarnate," 118–26. Cf. Düding, *Organisierter*, 57, who sees Jahn's movement as an archaic form of community, without democratic perspectives. Düding has noted Jahn and his followers' aspirations to promote the unification of Germany, culturally and linguistically as well as politically. More problematic is the conclusion that McMillan has drawn that the social forms and theories developed by Jahn amounted to a

liberal or protoliberal position with an ostensibly constitutional and democratic message and mission. On the development of German language in the eighteenth century, see Wolfgang Ruppert, *Bürgerlicher Wandel. Die Geburt der modernen deutschen Gesellschaft im 18. Jahrhundert* (Frankfurt am Main: Fischer, 1984), 45–47.

82. Rudolf Ibbeken, *Preußen 1807–1813. Staat und Volk als Idee un Wirklichkeit* (Berlin: Grote, 1970), 443. Obviously the figures fluctuated during the war. The official chronicle of the conflict, *Das Preußische Heer der Befreiungskriege*. Vol. 2. *Das Preußische Heer im Jahre 1813. Der Große Generalstab. Kriegsgeschichtliche Abteilung II* (Berlin: Ernst Siegfried Mittler und Sohn, 1914), estimated the number of Lützow's troops at 3,600 men on August 9, 1814.

83. In his autobiography, the Viennese physician Wenzel Krimer gives a detailed account of his experiences in the *Lützowsches Freikorps*, especially in the chapter "In Sachsen." The book was edited by Adolf Saager in 1913. It gives a fairly balanced and detailed picture of events, emphasizing heroism without ignoring the atrocities. See Wenzel Krimer, *Erinnerungen eines alten Lützower Jägers 1795–1819.* Vol. 1. (Stuttgart: Lutz, 1913), 284–307. See also Christian Eduard Leopold Dürre, *Aufzeichnungen, Tagebücher und Briefe aus einem deutschen Turner- und Lehrerleben*, ed. Ernst Friedrich Dürre (Leipzig: Strauch, 1881), 112–56, in which the same events are described in more reserved terms. Dürre, a close associate of Jahn and an active gymnast in Berlin, described from the perspective of 65 years—he died in 1879—the events of the war, commenting mainly on their political implications.

84. "Was glänzt dort vom Walde im Sonnenschein?/Hör's näher und näher brausen./Es zieht sich herunter in düsteren Reih'n,/und gellende Hörner schallen darein/und erfüllen die Seele mit Grausen./Und wenn ihr die schwarzen Gesellen fragt:/Das ist Lützows wilde, verwegene Jagd!/Was zieht dort rasch durch den finsteren Wald/und streift von Bergen zu Bergen?/Es legt sich in nächtlichen Hinterhalt;/das Hurra jauchzt und die Büchse knallt,/es fallen die fränkischen Schergen./Und wenn ihr die schwarzen Jäger fragt:/Das ist Lützows wilde, verwegene Jagd!/" Theodor Körner, "Lützow's wilde Jagd," in *Sämmtliche Werke*, vol. 1. (Berlin: Grote, 1892), 26–27.

85. Part of Lützow's detachment fought in the battle of Leipzig.

86. "Auf dem offenen Hofe der Bürgerschule fand ich einen Berg, der aus Kehrigt und Leichen meiner Landsleute bestand, die nackend lagen und von Hunden und Raben angefressen wurden, als wenn sie Missethäter und Mordbrenner gewesen wären. So entheiliget man die Ueberreste der Helden, die dem Vaterlande gefallen sind!" Georg Heinrich Pertz, *Das Leben des Ministers Freiherrn vom Stein. Vol. 3: 1812 bis 1814* (Berlin: Reimer, 1851), 442.

87. On small wars, their use and theory during the Napoleonic Wars, see Werner Hahlweg, *Guerrilla. Krieg ohne Fronten* (Stuttgart: W. Kohlhammer Verlag, 1968), 50–60.

88. After 1816, especially the transfer of land and compensation for it became increasingly complicated and burdensome for peasants, Reinhart Koselleck, *Preußen zwischen Reform und Revolution. Allgemeines Landrecht, Verwaltung und soziale Bewegung von 1791 bis 1848* (Stuttgart: DTV, 1989), 490–92.

89. Gordon Craig, *The Politics of the Prussian Army 1640–1945* (London: Oxford University Press, 1964), 53–81, is still a stimulating analysis of the intertwining of politics, social history, and military organization in Prussian army reforms. On the political and cultural consequences of this reform, see Ute Frevert, "Das jakobinische Modell: Allgemeine Wehrpflicht und Nationsbildung in Preußen-Deutschland" in *Militär und Gesellschaft im*

*19. und 20. Jahrhundert* (Stuttgart: Klett-Cotta, 1997), esp. 17–27, and Hagemann, "Of "Manly Valor," 187–220.

90. Krimer, *Erinnerungen eines alten*, 272; Dürre, *Aufzeichnungen*, 118–19. Dirk-Alexander Reder's instructive study of female patriotism during the war of 1813–14 shows the several ways women could contribute to nationalism, and also the obvious limits of what was considered acceptable. One of these was the battlefield, ibid., "'Natur und Sitte verbieten uns, die Waffen der Zerstörung zu führen . . .' Patriotische Frauen zwischen Frieden und Krieg" in Jost Düffler, ed., *Kriegsbereitschaft und Friedensordnung in Deutschland 1800–1814*. Jahrbuch für historische Friedensforschung. 3. Jahrgang 1994, 174–75. He gives the number of known female soldiers as 17, whereas Karen Hagemann says it was 23, Hagemann, "Heldenmütter, Kriegerbräute und Amazonen. Entwürfe 'patriotischer' Weiblichkeit zur Zeit der Freiheitskriege" in Ute Frevert, ed., *Militär und Gesellschaft im 19. und 20. Jahrhundert* (Stuttgart: Klett-Cotta, 1997), 196.

91. Dürre, *Aufzeichnungen*, 134; Krimer, *Erinnerungen eines alten*, 284–88.

92. "Von Bildung, Erziehung, Einsicht, selbst aus den höheren Ständen, reiche Bürgersöhne, Gutsbesitzer, Kaufleute, Studenten, namentlich viele Mediziner, Förster, altgediente Soldaten, . . . Adelige, darunter zwei Grafen," Krimer, *Erinnerungen eines alten*, 272.

93. "Es waren unter ihnen Bauern und Schiffsknechte, unter letzteren einige, die wiederholt bei dem Wallfischfang gedient hatten. Es versteht sich von selbst, daß ein Theil dieser Leute ziemlich verkommen waren," Dürre, *Aufzeichnungen*, 133–34.

94. Krimer, *Erinnerungen eines alten*, 273, 278.

95. Krimer, *Erinnerungen eines alten*, 274.

96. Krimer, *Erinnerungen eines alten*, 284.

97. Hagemann, "Manly Valor," 214, finds in Körner's poetry several traces of this playful approach to the imagery of war.

98. "Tell him [Dürre] already that I would very much appreciate his efforts to let the gymnasts do real military training, first without weapons but then with a spear. He is very well in command of the Prussian school of military training and has worked as a trainer." Jahn to Eiselen, Frankfurt am Main, June 30, 1814, in Jahn, *Briefe (1930)*, 77. On the sports field, see Dürre, *Aufzeichnungen*, 81.

99. Dürre, *Aufzeichnungen*, 80.

100. Dürre, *Aufzeichnungen*, 85. See also Karen Hagemann, "Heran, heran, zu Sieg oder Tod! Entwürfe patriotisch-wehrhafter Männlichkeit in der Zeit der Befreiungskriege," in *Männergeschichte—Geschlechtergeschichte. Männlichkeit im Wandel der Moderne*, ed. Thomas Kühne (Frankfurt: Campus Verlag, 1996), 59.

101. "Zärtliche Mütter und andere Verwandtinnen sind auf dem Turnplatze nur im Wege," Friedrich Ludwig Jahn and Eiselen, Ernst, *Die deutsche Turnkunst zur Einrichtung der Turnplätze* (Berlin: Auf Kosten der Herausgeber, 1816), 232.

102. *Preussische Heer*, 209.

103. Hagemann, "Heldenmütter, Kriegerbräute," 196.

104. Johann Christoph Friedrich GutsMuths, "Was müssen Aeltern, erzieher und Lehrer als Freunde des deutschen Vaterlandes bey der Erziehung der Ihrigen von jetzt an thun, und das Schicksal unseres Vaterlandes und die freie Selbständigkeit unseres Volks auch für unsere Nachkommen zu sichern?" in *Neue Bibliothek für Pädagogik, Schulwesen und die gesammte pädagogische Literatur* January 1814 and 1815, 17.

105. "Vermeide der Knabe das weiche, zu stark erwärmende Federbette von früh an aus Gewohnheit; er wechsele vielmehr bald so bald so, und finde überall den erquickenden Schlaf, bald im Federbette, bald auf dem Strohsacke, bald auf der härtern Bank, wo die erste Unterlage, selbst der Hutkopf statt des Kopfkissens dient," GutsMuths, "Was müssen Aeltern," 18.

106. Johann Christoph Friedrich GutsMuths, "An den Herrn geheimen Kanzley-Sekretär Brandes in Hannover. Gegen dessen Behauptung die Revolution in der Erziehung sey am verminderten Sinne des Vergnügens Schuld" in *Braunschweigischer Journal* June 1791, 317–18

107. GutsMuths, "Was müssen Aeltern" January 1814 and 1815, 25.

108. GutsMuths, "Was müssen Aeltern" January 1814 and 1815, 26.

109. Johann Christoph Friedrich GutsMuths, *Turnbuch für die Söhne des Vaterlandes. Beigebunden: Katechismus der Turnkunst* (Wiesbaden: Sändig, 1973), Vorbericht. On the dispute between Jahn and GutsMuths, see Manfred Lämmer, "Vorwort," in GutsMuths, *Turnbuch.*

110. In the *Turnkunst,* Jahn argued against military exercise (*Drillerei*) as part of *Turnen.* See Jahn, *Die deutsche Turnkunst (1816)*, 219.

111. Jahn, *Die deutsche Turnkunst (1816)*, 234.

112. Wilhelm Harnisch, *Das Turnen in seinen allseitigen Verhältnissen* (Breslau: Lenz, 1819), 76; Lämmer, "Vorwort."

113. "Stramme Auftreten der Massen," Dürre, *Aufzeichnungen*, 129.

114. "Schafft bei ihnen zugleich eine große Rohheit, und mit dieser den Hang zur Unsittlichkeit, zur Ausschweifung, ja nicht selten jene freche Willkür, jenen *Insubordinationsgeist*; der bei der ungebildeten Menschenklasse überall vorherrschend ist, und oftmals schon in Aufruhr und Bürgerkrieg geendet hat," Wilhelm Scheerer, *Turn-Fehde, oder: Wer hat Recht?* (Berlin: Krause, 1818), XIII.

115. Scheerer, *Turn-Fehde*, XV.

116. Scheerer, *Turn-Fehde*, XIV.

117. Scheerer, *Turn-Fehde*, 20.

118. In Villaume, the turn to the ancient Greeks was combined with a watered-down interpretation of Rousseau's naturalistic argument; in modern times, he argued, nature was still the best teacher, but it was to be harnessed by "the necessary vices" of civilization, such as clothing and manners, which were used as guides to improvement while the work of nature was perfected, see Villaume, "Bildung des Körpers," 246, 299–341.

119. GutsMuths, *Gymnastik 1793*, 33, 48–50.

120. GutsMuths, *Gymnastik 1793*, 155.

121. Jahn, *Die deutsche Turnkunst (1928)*, 252. See also Jahn, *Deutsches Volksthum*, 250–52. May, *Fastenpredigten*, vol. 1, Vorbericht. On Fichte, see his *Reden an die deutsche Nation* (Hamburg: Felix Meiner, 1955), esp. Chapter IV, in which he defines the "seed" of Germans: "The *Deutsche* (German) is, first of all, a Germanic tribe (*Stamm der Germanier*)," Fichte, *Reden*, 58. He elaborates in Chapter VII, and in Chapter IX that the tribe becomes the basis of public education and physical education, Fichte, *Reden,* 157.

122. Friedrich Ludwig Jahn, "Runenblätter (s.l.,1814)," in *Werke*, vol. 1, ed. Carl Euler. (Hof: Verlag von Rud. Lion, 1884), 408–10.

123. Friedrich Ludwig Jahn, "Werke zum deutschen Volkstum (1833)," in *Werke*, vol. 2,2, ed. Carl Euler. (Hof: Verlag von Rud. Lion, 1887), 487.

124. Jahn, *Werke zum deutschen Volkstum*, 503.

125. See Jahn, *Die deutsche Turnkunst (1928)*, Chapter IX on throwing (*Werfen*).

126. Jahn's short compilation included lists of "missing synonyms" (*Fehlende Sinnverwandtschaften*) in Adelung's dictionary. None of them related to physical exercise, Johann Friedrich Ludwig Jahn, *Bereicherung des hochdeutschen Sprachschatzes versucht im Gebiethe des Sinnverwandtschaft, ein Nachtrag zu Adelung's und eine Nachlese zu Eberhard's Wörterbuch* (Leipzig: Adam Friedrich Böhme, 1806). After this first publication he started to use Friedrich Ludwig Jahn as his professional name.

127. Jahn to Feuerstein, July 25, 1811, in *Die Briefe Friedrich Ludwig Jahns gesammelt und im Auftrage des Ausschusses der Deutschen Gymnastschaft*, ed. Wolfgang Meyer (Leipzig: Paul Eberhardt, 1913), 34.

128. Düding, *Organisierter*, 89–90. The politics of language, so crucial to Jahn's project, has been analyzed only sporadically. Düding, for instance, points out Jahn's strong interest in the German language. An essential power of gymnastics, or *Turnen*, was in its distinctive vocabulary, the so-called *Turnsprache* (turn-language).

129. "Die Fülle, Schärfe und Feinheit der *Worthilfen*, [die] als *Vorlinge, Inlinge* und *Endlinge* gebraucht werden und wie stehende Schriften der Wortbildung anzusehen sind, geben den Schlüssel zu dem unendlichen Sprachschatz," Jahn, *Die deutsche Turnkunst (1960)*, LVIII.

130. The same idea can be found in Wilhelm von Humboldt's early text, "Die Sprache als Ausdruck eigentümlicher Geistesform," in *Schriften zur Anthropologie und Bildungslehre*, ed. Andreas Flitner (Frankfurt am Main: Ullstein, 1984), 117.

131. Ironically, Jahn misinformed about the etymological root of *Turnen*. It was derived from the medieval tournaments (*Turniere*), which orginally came from French. Jahn had thought the term originated in German and passed from it into French. See Johannes Zeidler, *Die deutsche Turnsprache bis 1819. Untersuchungen zur Geschichte der deutschen Sprache*.(Halle: Niemeyer, 1942), 44.

132. Zeidler, *Die deutsche Turnsprache*, 112–13.

133. Zeidler, *Die deutsche Turnsprache*, 111–15. Cf. Eisenberg, "*Sports*," 113.

134. According to Vieth, the terminology of vaulting was predominantly French by the end of the eighteenth century. He used its language extensively, Vieth, *Versuch einer Encyklopädie*, vol. 2, esp. 202–25, on riding, see, Vieth, *Versuch einer Encyklopädie*, vol. 2, 430–37.

135. Although avoiding French sentences, Roux, *Gründliche*, 138, still used expressions such as "Legirt der Feind auf die Quart-Koupee-Finte," meaning a feint from right to left, used to deprive the adversary of his sword.

136. Ernst Eiselen, *Abriß des Deutschen Stoßfechtens, nach Kreuslers Grundsätzen dargestellt* (Berlin: Dümmler, 1826). This short manual followed the system of Heinrich Wilhelm Kreußler, as did the *Anfangsgründe der Fechtkunst* by Kreußler's disciple Anton Friedrich Kahn. Kreußler, fencing master at the University of Jena, was the last great advocate of the old German art of fencing with a saber (*Hieb*). On Kreußler's reception and influence, see Johann Adolph Karl Roux, *Die Deutsche Fechtkunst, enthaltend eine theoretisch-praktische Anweisung zum Stoßfechten*. Zweyte verbesserte und vermehrte Ausgabe (Leipzig: Johann Ambrosius Barth, 1817), V–VI.

137. Even Jahn's group had a Jewish member. See McMillan, "Germany Incarnate," 100. During the hiking tour to Silesia, Jahn's antisemitism was plain when a Jewish boy could not bear the heat and fell behind from the main group.

138. As McMillan has argued, "Germany Incarnate," 99, it is difficult to find systematic antisemitism in Jahn's writings. But the signs are clear in the *Deutschen Volksthum*, where Jahn describes the Christian origins of German spirit and culture. To enforce his case Jahn quotes from Schlötzer's 1791 article, which started with the assertion: "Originally Christianity was a transcendental public religion of the people. The founding fathers of this religion were thus in opposition to . . . the Jewish priests and their religious enthusiasm." See, Jahn, *Deutsches Volksthum*, 153.

139. Richter analyzes Maßmann's antisemitism in *Hans Ferdinand Maßmann*, 7. He points out that Maßmann's antisemitism was evident only in occasional outbursts. This is partly true but leaves open the question of what role the Jews and images of Jewish culture played in the early gymnastics movement. Obviously the Jews were useful but not as important as images of France and the French.

140. Richter, *Hans Ferdinand Maßmann*, 8.

141. Jahn, *Die deutsche Turnkunst (1816)*, 226–28.

142. Henrich Steffens, *Caricaturen des Heiligsten*, vol. 1 (Leipzig: Brockhaus, 1819), 411–51. Steffens defended a limited, constitutional aristocracy in *Caricaturen des Heiligsten*, vol. 2 (Leipzig: Brockhaus, 1821), 187–93. His rejection of the gymnastics movement was critical because of the high esteem in which he was held among the intellectuals of Berlin. Schleiermacher, who considered Jahn's ideas promising, was especially saddened by Steffens' views, see Carl Euler, *Friedrich Ludwig Jahn. Sein Leben und Wirken* (Stuttgart: Verlag von Karl Krabbe, 1881), 571. Cf. Mester, *Die Körpererziehung*, 89. Helge Hultberg, *Den ældre Henrich Steffens 1811–1845* (Kopenhagen: Retzels Boghandel, 1981), esp. 30–33, points out that Steffens, a romantic individualist, was frightened by Jahn's collectivism and his desire to destroy the individuality of his students. This interpretation is shared by Jeismann, *Das preußische Gymnasium*, vol. 2, 62–63.

143. On customs among gymnasts, see Edmund Neuendorff, *Geschichte der neueren deutschen Leibesübung vom Beginn des 18. Jahrhunderts bis zur Gegenwart*, vol. 2, *Jahn und seine Zeit* (Dresden: Limpert, 1932), 413–15.

144. The rules of the gymnastics organizations stipulated that "the heartiest and most faithful love seals together all the inequal members of a good family [. . .]. Our relationship can and will also be this way, regardless of the class differences determined by social circumstances. The director is a director only in respect to the institute, a professor is professor only *ex cathedra*, but at social events we are all friends." See *Landeshauptarchiv Sachsen-Anhalt (Außenstelle Oranienbaum)* "Acta, enth. einzelne Sachen über das Philanthropin zu Dessau, dessen Lehrer, dessen Einrichtungen und sonst Anhängendes. 1771–80." C 18b, 34I: Gesetzmäßige Constitution des philanthropischen Erziehungs-Instituts zu Dessau, Fol. 120.

145. Schneider, "Statistische Übersicht," 76–78. Schneider's statistical reports were based on information submitted by the clubs themselves and compiled by a government office. In 1818, when Jahn's gymnastics movement already was under scrutiny, the clubs had no self-interest in reporting attendance of older members who as mature members would be implicated and whose activities would make the clubs appear more political than what they wanted. The percentage of older members remained low because the majority of chapters were centered on a school or attracted the student body of a local institution of higher

education. This was the case in Berlin, Hamburg, Tübingen, Stuttgart, Leipzig, and Breslau.

146. Düding, *Organisierter*, 82. According to McMillan, "Germany Incarnate," 245–47, "thou" was used by young gymnasts in the early gymnastics movement. In the second wave, in the 1840s, this form of address spread to all members.

147. Edmund Neuendorff, *Geschichte der neueren deutschen Leibesübung vom Beginn des 18. Jahrhunderts bis zur Gegenwart*, vol. 1, *Geschichte der deutschen Leibesübung vom Beginn des 18. Jahrhunderts bis zu Jahn: mit einem Grundriss der Geschichte der deutschen Leibesübung von den Urzeiten bis zum Beginn des 18. Jahrhunderts* (Dresden: Limpert, 1930), esp. 81–102. Neuendorff, a long-time director of the Preußischen Hochschule für Leibesübungen in Berlin, was an authority within the gymnastics movement in the 1920s and 1930s. As a member of the NSDAP since 1932, he was the leader of the Deutschen Turnerschaft and responsible for the exclusion of Jews from the organization in 1933. The leading historians of the German gymnastics movement almost exclusively come from the movement itself, so Carl Euler, Karl Wassmannsdorff, and, more recently, Horst Ueberhorst. Cf. Eisenberg, *"Sports,"* 84.

148. Eichel, ed., *Geschichte der Körperkultur*, 46.

149. McMillan, "Germany Incarnate," 70, see von Humboldt as an advocate of gymnastics in educational reform.

150. Wilhelm von Humboldt to Caroline von Humboldt, Berlin, January 14, 1809, in Wilhelm von Humboldt, *Wilhelm und Caroline von Humboldt in ihren Briefen*, vol. 3. *Weltbürgertum und preußischer Staatsdienst . . . 1808–1810* (Berlin, Ernst Siegfried Mittler und Sohn, 1909), 69–73. Humboldt, who was skeptical at first, said nothing negative about Plamann's institute. In 1810, however, he moved Theodor to the Friedrisch-Werdersche *Gymnasium* in Berlin because "it is very good and appropriate for his current level of knowledge and for his age." Wilhelm von Humboldt to Caroline von Humboldt, Berlin, April 7, 1810, in von Humboldt, *Briefen*, 373. Euler, *Friedrich Ludwig Jahn*, 148. For Jahn's employment at Plamann's institute, the years vary from 1809, Carl Euler, *Geschichte des Turnunterrichts* (Gotha: Thienemann, 1891), 85, to 1810, Neuendorff, *Neuere deutsche Leibesübung*, vol. 2, 33.

151. "Cultura et corporis et animi ducens ad perfectionem humanitatis," Paulsen, *Geschichte des Gelehrten Unterrichts* 218–28.

152. Although Humboldt saw intellectual education, as it was taught in the *Gymnasium*, as the most appropriate form of education, he still approved physical education, when appropriate to local and economic circumstances. He even approved some ideas of *Philanthropismus* because "the instruction in these exercises [i.e., dancing and fencing] does not have the positive impact on health that gymnastic exercises can have, almost free, under the guidance of a teacher like the ones we have in Schnepfenthal," see Humboldt, Wilhelm von, "Über die Liegnitzer Ritterakademie. 7. September 1809," in *Gesammelte Schriften*, vol. 10 (Berlin: B. Behr's Verlag, 1903), 169.

153. Wilhelm von Humboldt, "Bericht der Sektion des Kultus und Unterrichts an den König—Dezember 1809," in *Schulreform in Preußen 1809–1819. Entwürfe und Gutachten*, ed. Lothar Schwiem (Weinheim: Beltz, 1966), 47.

154. According to Johann Wilhelm Süvern, "Unterrichts-Verfassung der Gymnasien und Stadtschulen. Vom 12. Jan. 1816," in *Schulreform in Preußen 1809–1819. Entwürfe und Gutachten*, ed. Lothar Schwiem (Weinheim: Beltz, 1966), 60, 97, "instruction in singing and gymnastics takes place after normal school day."

155. Johann Wilhelm Süvern, "Entwurf eines allgemeinen Gesetzes über die Verfassung des Schulwesens im preußischen Staate," in *Schulreform in Preußen 1809–1819. Entwürfe und Gutachten*, ed. Lothar Schwiem (Weinheim: Beltz, 1966), 133–34, 136, 138. See also Euler, *Geschichte des Turnunterrichts*, 141.

156. Schleiermacher took physical exercise seriously. In his lectures on education, which he started after the ban of *Turnen*, gymnastics had its own locus in the system of Bildung. See also Mester, *Die Körpererziehung*, 83–86. Schleiermacher had a close personal connection to Eiselen and Ernst Moritz Arndt, Professor of History at the University of Greifswald and an avid supporter of Jahn's gymnastics movement.

157. I follow Euler's summary of this report, Euler, *Friedrich Ludwig Jahn*, 544–53. Bernhardi was supportive of *Turnen* but critical of what he saw as Jahn's extremism.

158. Euler, *Friedrich Ludwig Jahn*, 552.

159. Adolf Lippold, *Erinnerungen eines alten Leipzigers. Humoristische Chronika aus Leipzigs jüngerer Vergangenheit*, vol. 1 (Leipzig: Lenz, 1893–95), 8. Compare to Schnepfenthal experiences in tightrope walking in August 1794, *Nachrichten aus Schnepfenthal. Für die Eltern und Freunde der dasigen Zöglinge* 1794, 71.

160. Johann Stüve to his mother, Berlin, May 5, 1818, in *Unbekannte Briefe von Friedrich Ludwig Jahn* , 69–70.

161. Beneke, *Hamburgische Turnanstalt* , 22.

162. Friedrich Georg Buek, *Wegweiser durch Hamburg und die umliegende Gegend* (Hamburg: Pethes & Besser, 1836), 221.

163. Hans Ferdinand Maßmann, *Die öffentliche Turnanstalt zu München. Nebst Anlagen über Einrichtung von Turnanstalten und Beyträgen zur Geschichte älterer deutscher Leibesübungen* (München: Lindauer'sche Buchhandlung, 1838), VII. Although there is no direct evidence, Maßmann's defense of Jahn might have been occasioned by the comments of Johann Christian Jahn (not related to Friedrich Ludwig Jahn), who in remarks on physical education in German *Gymnasiums* in 1836 compared Jahn's gymnastics to tightrope walking and acrobatics (which he regarded as dangerous) and supported moderate gymnastics. See his "Die in dem voranstehenden Aufsatze besprochene Anklageschrift des Herrn Med.-Raths Lorinser," *Neue Jahrbücher für Philologie und Paedagogik oder kritische Bibliothek für das Unterrichtswesen*. 16 (1836), 456–83.

164. Düding, *Organisierter*, 145, 211. On Hamburg see Schneider, *Hamburger Turnerschaft*, 39.

165. Hermann Wagner, "Zur Geschichte des Turnwesens in Oesterreich," *Deutsche Turn-Zeitung* 12 (1884): 105–6.

166. McMillan, "Germany Incarnate," concentrates on Saxony. See also Kleindienst-Cachay's study on Württemberg, *Die Verschulung des Turnens*. On the local organization of gymnastics, there are recent studies of Bavaria by Stefan Illig, *Zwischen Körperertüchtigung und nationaler Bewegung: Turnvereine in Bayern 1848-1890* (Köln: SH-Verlag, 1998), of Pomerania by Wolfgang Müller, *Turnen und Sport in Vorpommern* (Erfurt: Sutton, 1999), and of Hesse by Harald Braun, *Geschichte des Turnens in Rheinhessen. Ein Beitrag zur wechselseitigen Beeinflussung von Turnen und Politik* (Alzey: Verlag der Rheinhessischen Druckwerkstätte, 1986).

167. *Gesetze für die Turnergemeinde zu Tübingen* (Tübingen: Richter und Eberhardt, 1819), 9–10.

168. Max Eifert, *Geschichte und Beschreibung der Stadt Tübingen* (Tübingen: Ludwig Friedrich Fues, 1849), 219.

169. Beneke, *Hamburgische Turnanstalt*, 28.

170. Euler, *Friedrich Ludwig Jahn*, 567.

171. Friedrich Wilhelm Klumpp, *Eine Selbstbiographie* (Essen: Bädeker, 1838), 45.

172. Beneke, Hamburgische Turnanstalt, 16, 20.

173. Beneke, *Hamburgische Turnanstalt*, 16.

174. Klumpp, *Eine Selbstbiographie*, 5, 16, 32, 44.

175. *Philanthropismus* also played a part in Köhnke's effort in 1805 to found an institute for physical exercise in Hamburg, Markus Christian Köhnke, *Erinnerungen aus meinem Leben nebst Bemerkungen über mancherlei Gegenstände* (Ottensen: Perthes-Besser & Mauke, 1839), 150.

176. Uwe Zimmermann, in his extensive research on liberal autobiographies, has found the influence of the *Philanthropismus* to be significant. My reference is based on Zimmermann's personal account on July 18, 1995.

177. A[ugust] L[udwig]. Reyscher, *Erinnerungen aus alter und neuer Zeit (1802 bis 1880)* (Freiburg in Breisgau und Tübingen: Mohr, 1884), 14.

178. Robert von Mohl, *Lebenserinnerungen (1799–1875)*, vol. 1 (Stuttgart; Leipzig: Deutsche Verlags-Anstalt, 1902), 68.

179. On Eiselen's institute, see Neuendorff, *Geschichte der neueren deutschen Leibesübung*, Vol. 3, 8–19.

180. Schneider, *Hamburger Turnerschaft*, 39.

181. Buek, *Wegweiser durch Hamburg*, 96.

182. Jahn, *Die deutsche Turnkunst (1960)*, LIV–LV; GutsMuths, *Gymnastik 1793*, 206.

183. Eduard David Helmke, *Almanach der neuesten Modetänze auf das Jahr 1833. Für Freunde und Freundinnen der höheren Tanzkunst* (Merseburg: Fr. Weidemann, 1835), 100. On Roller's life, see the careful depiction of Marion Kant, "Nachwort," in Franz Anton Roller, *Systematisches Lehrbuch der bildenden Tanzkunst und körperlichen Ausbildung* (1843) (Leipzig: Zentralantiquariat der DDR, 1989), IV–IX.

184. A curriculum from 1838–39 shows that whereas gymnastics was practiced during the summer term, dancing took place every week throughout the year. Dance instruction did not follow customary grade divisions; instead students were divided into 14 groups according to their level of proficiency; see Carl Kirchner, *Kurze Nachricht von der Königlichen Landesschulen Pforta* (Leipzig: Vogel, 1839), 27, 41–42.

185. Helmke, *Almanach*, 106–108. See also Kant, "Nachwort," IX.

186. "Both sexes have to learn dancing separately. The example of Schulpforte shows that it works and can produce great dancers," Jahn, *Deutsches Volksthum*, 264. As Kant shows, "Nachwort," XI–XII, Roller shared, at least in 1817, Jahn's ideas of a purely masculine gymnastics, purified of all effeminate features.

187. Helmke, *Almanach*, 101, gives 1817 as the year, whereas Euler maintains the introduction happened in 1816, Euler, *Friedrich Ludwig Jahn*, 459. See also Jahn to Zernial, s.l., June 6, 1816, in Jahn, *Briefe (1930)*, 89.

188. Roller, *Systematisches Lehrbuch*, IX–X. See also Kant, "Nachwort," XIII–XIV, who sees too many similarities between Jahn's and Roller's programs.

189. See J.H. Gourdoux-Daux, *Die Tanzkunst als Bildungsmittel der Jugend oder Methodik, Grundsätze und Elementar-Kenntnisse dieser Kunst, mit Hinsicht auf die Art sich in guter Gesellschaft zu zeigen un zu benehmen.* 3rd ed. (Wien: Verlage der C. Haas'schen Buchhandlung, 1830), esp. IV–V. It is most likely that the critical tone comes from the Viennese translator, Paul Bruno Bartholomay, who in his *Die Tanzkunst in Beziehung auf die Lehre und Bildung des wahren Anstandes und des gefälligen Aeußern* (Giessen: Selbstverlag, 1838), 14, repeats many of these remarks.

190. Reyscher, *Erinnerungen*, 56.

191. Gasch, *Festschrift*, 7–11.

192. On Clias, see Johann Adolf Ludwig Werner, *Das Ganze der Gymnastik oder ausführliches Lehrbuch der Leibesübungen nach den Grundsätzen der bessern Erziehung zum öffentlichen und besondern Unterricht* (Meissen: Friedrich Wilhelm Goedsche, 1834), 18–20.

193. Phokion Heinrich Clias, *Kalisthenie. Oder Uebungen zur Schönheit und Kraft für Mädchen* (Bern: Jenni, 1829), 7.

194. L.F. Kümmerle, *Praktische Anleitung zu Leibesübungen für Mädchen. Nebst einem Anhang über die Haltung des Körpers und über die Anfangsgründe der Tanzkunst* (Stuttgart: Metzler, 1832), 26–48; Franz Anton Roller, "Leibchen für Damen, zu Beförderung einer schöneren Haltung des Körpers," in *Erstes Toilettengeschenk. Ein Jahrbuch für Damen* (Leipzig: Georg Voss, 1805), 78.

195. See McMillan, "Germany Incarnate," passim. See also Teresa Sanislo, "Models of Manliness and Femininity. The Physical Culture of the Enlightenment and Early National Movement in Germany 1770–1819" (PhD diss., University of Michigan, 2001), 179–82.

196. Jahn, *Die deutsche Turnkunst (1816)*, 209. Cf. Jahn, *Deutsches Volksthum*, 184, in which he also saw bodily *Bildung* in aesthetic terms.

197. Johann Heinrich Zedler, *Grosses vollständiges Universal-Lexikon aller Wissenschafften und Künste*, vol. 19. (Halle & Leipzig: Johann Heinrich Zedler, 1732–54), 173.

198. Adelung, *Grammatisch-kritisches Wörterbuch*, vol. 3, 64.

199. Campe, *Wörterbuch*, vol. 3, 205.

200. Ute Frevert, "Soldaten, Staatsbürger. Überlegungen zur historischen Konstruktion von Männlichkeit," in *Männergeschichte—Geschlechtergeschichte. Männlichkeit im Wandel der Moderne*, ed. Thomas Kühne (Frankfurt: Campus Verlag, 1996), 76. See also Hagemann's close reading of war lyrics written during 1813–15. They disseminated patterns and images of manliness, Hagemann, "Heran, heran," 64.

201. McMillan, ". . . die höchste," 90. On antisemitism in the gymnastics movement, especially in Ernst Moritz Arndt, see Léon Poliakov, *Geschichte des Antisemitismus. VI. Emanzipation und Rassenwahn* (Worms: Verlag Georg Heintz, 1987), 184–88. Poliakov argues that Jahn indirectly contributed to the spread of antisemitism by constructing an image of aggressive male habitus. It is, however, debatable whether this habitus had the continuity and social and geographic extent that Poliakov implies. Cf. also George Mosse, *Die Nationalisierung der Massen. Politische Symbolik und Massenbewegungen in Deutschland von den Napoleonischen Kriegen bis zum Dritten Reich* (Frankfurt/M: Ullstein, 1976), 157, who distinguishes between the relative tolerance of the early gymnastics

movement and the openly antisemitic movement of 1848.

202. Maßmann, *Die öffentliche Turnanstalt*, VII.

# Chapter Five

# Dance

In the years between the French Revolution and the Congress of Vienna, political modernism was born. For Germans, those years meant the end of the Holy Roman Empire and the promise of a more enlightened, egalitarian society and political system. *Turnvater* Jahn and his gymnasts had been vocal advocates of modernism's promises by defiantly opposing the hierarchical structures and practices of the *ancien regime*. For Jahn's opponents, the ban on *Turnen* meant a return to normality. But was it simply a return to *ancien regime*? From the numbers, the answer might be yes. The years between 1820 and 1850 saw the publication of an unprecedented number of instructional manuals for fencing, riding, and, particularly, dancing.[1] This suggests the tremendous tenacity of the old practices of the body. More people than ever attended balls, *thés dansants*, and dancing clubs. Dancing and walking were arguably the most common bodily practices during the three decades before the Revolution of 1848. Why and how did dancing achieve and retain this position? And who were the dancers?

Current research on social dance in the early nineteenth century has defined a juncture of configurational shifts and social transformations. In its most polished form, this juncture associates the evolution from the minuet to the waltz with the transition from court culture to bourgeois culture. The waltz, according to Reingard Witzmann, was a dance of the urban bourgeoisie, and its appearance by 1800 signified a social revolution comparable to the political one ten years earlier.[2] But the influence of the waltz did not stop with the urban bourgeoisie. The first decades of the nineteenth century established the waltz as the standard dance among all urban classes. The Congress of Vienna made it acceptable as a court dance.[3] The obvious contradiction in terms, that a bourgeois dance was appropriated by other classes, calls for a closer look at the social setting in which the waltz evolved. Rudolf Braun and David Gugerli treat the waltz as a metaphor of bourgeois virtues of work, dynamic mobility, and striving. The complexity of the waltz and its social reception, they argue, was the result of a symbolic class struggle between the declining but defiant aristocracy and the rising bourgeoisie with its atavistic urge to cultivate itself.[4] But what qualities of the waltz made possible this contest of appropriation? How did the waltz facilitate the enforcement of a typically bourgeois code of conduct? Henning Eichberg's studies on the development of motional configurations in the occidental world since the sixteenth century attempt to answer this question. Eichberg shows that, in the beginning of the nineteenth century, dancing configuration became egalitarian after the waltz was introduced as a couples dance, replacing the complex and regulated figures of the minuet, cotillion, and contredanse. The waltz, argues Eichberg, was a democratic dance allowing an unlimited number of couples who could move freely about the floor.[5]

Eichberg's and Braun and Gugerli's explanations leave us with an additional question whether the political contest over the social appropriation of the waltz overlaps with its democratic and universalistic configuration. Rather than describing the social options for a class to use the symbolic capital of the waltz, we should look at the processes in which this capital was used and activated in the entrances to ballrooms and invitations to dance. These processes were not class struggles but acts of mutual recognition.[6] In an interesting way, the history of ballroom dance shows that, in the first half of the nineteenth century, the educated middle class adopted the conditions of mutual recognition typical of court society.

What is mutual recognition? In traditional Western societies, recognition depended on pride and honor. Whether an aristocrat or a member of a guild, a man's value was measured against his carefully defined and nurtured social status, recognizable in his deeds and habitus. A woman, unless a widow, normally was excluded from this male code; her honor was defined in terms of chastity and marital fidelity.[7] This system was legally protected through codes of dress, codes of honor and dueling, and regulations of guilds and universities. Although the mutual recognition of one's social status that these customs and regulations provided was constantly contested, the stability and predictability of one's social trajectory was still considerable.[8] After the first third of the eighteenth century, philanthropic and social associations challenged and changed this traditional pattern of mutual recognition. Unlike military contingents, guilds, and academic faculties, associations placed their members in situations in which they felt the unpredictability of social relationships and the vulnerability of their social status, i.e., their honor and pride. Although a member's social status was constantly at stake in an association, some activities seem to have been more meaning-laden than others. Dancing was among the most important. It exposed members to a potentially unpredictable situation that related to his or her body but ultimately had significant emotional and social consequences. A surprising fact of early nineteenth century social history is that an increasing number of people of aristocratic and bourgeois origin were willing to pay the price of lost predictability and expose themselves to a potential loss of face. Why? How did they organize their social relationships? These are the two questions that I try to answer in this chapter. It begins with a short exploration of the development of dance as a discipline before the early nineteenth century in order to show how this "science" of mutual recognition underwent a productive crisis of legitimacy. Then I turn to the social environment of dancing, the urban clubs in which it flourished. Finally, I analyze how dancing became a practical configuration of mutual recognition in ballrooms and dance clubs.

## The Discipline of Dancing

In Baroque society, dancing expressed respect. The display and acceptance of respect was the particular art of court society that reached its maturity in Versailles under Louis XIV. German princes eagerly imitated the Sun King and imitation Versailles soon arose in major and minor principalities, making French court culture the German standard. One of the most vocal advocates of this aristocratic culture of respect was Christian Thomasius, a professor of law at the University of Halle.

Thomasius's importance to a history of the body is embedded in his particular idea of ethics and political philosophy. Unlike most postscholastic philosophers of the Aristotelian or Cartesian school, Thomasius was interested in the pragmatic aspects of his philosophy. During the formative years between 1688 and 1700, he was preoccupied by questions of the politics of the court.[9] Instead of postulating an ethical utopia, void of evil and corruption, Thomasius embraced a realistic ethical theory based on the inevitable corruption of human nature. He was deeply involved in the Pietist movement, and the Pietist leadership vigorously rejected the very idea of secular ethics, which it regarded as "worldliness," a sin for any Christian. To circumvent the critique of his allies, Thomasius started to emphasize the importance of the *adiaphora*, indifferent things that were neither virtues nor vices, yet, indispensable:

> Our abstinence from things that do not go against common sense but are treated as harmful is, on one hand, a decoration for a tranquil person because these things contribute very little to the good order of social life. On the other hand, these things also provide tools—because one obtains common characteristics—to persuade people to associate with us. And we also realize that we would make a mistake if we not allow these things to influence us. This would violate our intentions and the real virtue.[10]

*Adiaphora* were the cement of social bonds. Among them were the practices that Thomasius called decorum, i.e., "ease of manner, courtesy, good manners, sense of propriety."[11] These played an important role: They were the tools of sustaining the system of honor. To be sure, Thomasius distinguished between internal and external honor. Internal honor was identical with virtuousness; it was, strictly speaking, the realm of wisdom and ethics. But his attention was directed toward external honor, the "visible gestures" (*äusserliche Zeichen*) by which others show respect toward us.[12] Decorum was thus an ensemble of visible gestures that were potentially harmful for moral conduct, principally indifferent, but socially fundamental.

The discussion of decorum was closely associated with the body, the instrument of the visible gestures. How critical Thomasius's position was, became apparent in 1698, when he found himself in a heated debate over school reform. Starting in 1696, August Hermann Francke, a leading Pietist and a close friend of Thomasius, had run a secondary school for the sons of nobility and upper bourgeoisie, *Paedagogium Regium*, in Glaucha near Halle. In order to obtain the permit for his school, Francke had compiled its regulations, which he circulated among his allies for comments in 1698. A year later, Thomasius, as one of Francke's trusted commentators, published his thoughts in the *Bericht von Einrichtung des Paedagogii zu Glaucha an Halle*.[13] In a paradigmatic format, this text embraced the ingredients that made up the cultivation of the body during the long eighteenth century. When Francke defined the school's purpose as the inculcation of genuine piety, instruction in sciences and humanities, and cultivation of decorum, Thomasius asked whether moral education and especially the cultivation of decorum were properly placed in this plan. In the traditional education of nobles, decorum was thought to occur in dancing, about which Francke mentioned nothing. Thomasius asked whether Francke accepted the so-called "dance of honor" with the bride or whether he completely banned dancing.[14] Thomasius knew quite well what he was asking, for in 1697, Francke had published a pamphlet that condemned dancing because too many theological problems arose when religious scholars confronted instances of dancing in the Bible. It was not dancing as such but its side-effects that were the target of Francke's critique. Dancing was suspect for its erotic possibilities, but this was not Francke's primary concern; he recoiled from it as the epitome of vanity, the valorization of worldly honor, and the rejection of the honor of God.[15] It was a distraction from the substantial occupation of a Christian, a waste and abuse of Christian time. In this sense, dancing, as an historically defined practice, negated the honor of God, and the body, especially the dancing body, was the locus of sin and immorality.

Religious writing against dancing was not unknown but the force and breadth of this outburst was unprecedented. Between 1693 and 1720, fifteen major works were published against dancing in Germany. Most of them came from the Pietist circles of Francke and Spener.[16] This debate set the tone and provided the arena for dancing masters who, influenced by French dancing, started to formulate dancing as a discipline by 1700. It was the tension between the practices of the court and this Pietist critique that gave rise to a systematic theory of dancing.[17]

In defending dancing against its critics, Johann Pasch, a disciple of the French dancing master Charles Louis Pierre Beauchamp and a leading dancing instructor in Leipzig, situated dancing between ethics and acting. For a professional like Pasch, this balance could be maintained only through a set of rigorously constructed rules. Dancing was to be a discipline (*Wissenschaft*) that formulated and applied mathematical and philosophical principles to regulating the natural instincts of human bodies.[18] For this purpose, the classical French school of dancing had defined three main areas of the human body and its movements: *port-de-bras* (the movements of arms), the movements of legs and feet (*passepied*), and the dynamic combinations of these two (figures). Regardless of whether dancing was for performance or participation, dancers were to concentrate on applying universal principles in all three areas. Through the movements of arms, steps, and figures, and consequent control of the passions, the dancer could find the most accurate expression of his body and social status. A good dancer could convey the moral quality of mind and nature by creating and embodying what Pasch called a harmonious air (*wolanständiges Air*).[19]

Classical dancing, as the masters Pasch, Samuel Rudolph Behr, Gottfried Taubert, and Johann Leonhard Rost (Meletaon) envisioned in their dancing manuals, had three different functions.[20] Dancing was an effective means of controlling bodies.[21] It also was an instrument of expression: As Volker Saftien argues, dance was a means of intensifying life.[22] Finally, as a combination of social control and artistic expression, dance was an effective tool of education. Dancing instructors, employed by universities and noble and patrician families, were the true educators, functionaries of moral cultivation.

During the golden age of the French dancing school, from the late seventeenth century to the French Revolution, European courts and the aristocracy emulated the example of Louis XIV and his dancing instructors, Beauchamp and Raoul Auger Feuillet. The minuet was the archetype. Appearing before 1660 in the court of Louis, the minuet soon became one of the two standard dances of the court repertoire—the courant was the other.[23] By the middle of the eighteenth century, it was the most popular ballroom dance in Europe. In Germany, the minuet was adopted as the signature dance of formal balls and remained so until the second decade of the nineteenth century.[24] From its beginning, the minuet had the reputation as a complicated and difficult dance. The combinations of steps and figures in this dance were almost inexhaustible and each of them required the meticulous following of complex rules. Why, then, did it remain dominant and for so long resistant to changes of style and fashion? One explanation, supported by current scholarship, sees the minuet as a paradigmatic dance of court society. As the dance of the nobility, the minuet demonstrated the cultural hegemony of this class over the upper segments of the bourgeoisie. But during the second half of the eighteenth century, it was commonly taught to children of burgher families. The young Goethe had minuet lessons in Frankfurt:

> From my early childhood, my father taught me and my sister to dance. For such a serious man, that was in itself something extraordinary. My father did not let this bother him but taught us in most exact way how to take right positions and steps. Once he had introduced us to the secrets of minuet, he took his *flûte-douce* and played us something in three/four time, and we tried to follow as well as we could.[25]

Moreover, the minuet was an educational dance. It dominated the moral education of noble and patrician youth to the extent that some of its configurations were identical with standards of social conduct. For instance, the initial pose of the minuet, was a standard gesture of aristocratic and patrician greeting.[26] For dancing instructors, the increasing complexity and applicability of social dances raised the importance of their profession. They were the arbiters of what Pasch called the first impression of the body, "the first thing that we see in a person."[27] These dancing instructors, especially those who upheld their professional standards, became gatekeepers to social recognition.

Around 1800, when the waltz replaced the minuet as the dominant ballroom dance, dancing instructors and the educated laity realized how strong and effective had been the minuet as an educational template. Opposition of the dancing profession to the new dance was fierce. In countless writings on dancing after 1780, we find hardly any positive account of the waltz.[28] Goethe's early impression of the waltz and Schiller's poetic remarks on dancing were rare exceptions to this wave of professional and public outrage. The critics labeled the waltz as unhealthy, immoral, indecent, and too physical. Salomo Jakob Wolf believed that "the waltz was one of the main sources of bodily and mental weakness" of his time. Without rejecting dancing as such, he recommended that "all the balls should be opened and finished by a minuet. Therefore the minuets, allemandes, polonaises, and petites anglaises with few couples and without waltzes should take preference over all other dances."[29] Much of the criticism that had been launched against dancing a century earlier was now just as convenient a tool for rejecting the waltz.

This rupture in the dancing culture seems to parallel the political and social upheavals of the time. Several scholars have connected the change from the minuet to the waltz to the transformation from an aristocratic regime to a bourgeois one.[30] Yet, in important ways, the subsequent decades point toward continuity rather than rupture. Several commentators and writers persisted in their loyalty to the minuet long after it had disappeared from common ball repertoires. Theodor Hentschke, a young dancing instructor from Stralsund, complained in 1836 that minuet's decline had recast dancing as "careless whirling."[31] As late as 1843, Franz Anton Roller showed nostalgia for the lost greatness of the minuet: "The bodily *Bildung* and the sense of propriety that was produced [by the minuet], furnished the balls of high society with a special excitement, because of the then dominant dance. Everyone attempted to distinguish himself, and dancing instruction then lasted longer in years than nowadays in months."[32] Hentschke and Roller suggested an explanation for the remarkable tenacity of the minuet. As a social configuration, it combined functions that were separated or excluded from the waltz and other ballroom dances of the nineteenth century. It was the educational value of the minuet that created this tenacity. Through the waltz and other quick dances, such as the écossaise, dancing lost most of its methodical features. Being relatively simple and requiring few or no figures, these dances did not require strenuous formal instruction. Helmke dismissed the waltz as a dance that could be learned in no time by oneself.[33] Dancing was becoming pure entertainment, threatening moral education as well as the standards and incomes of dancing masters.

The disappearance of the minuet from ballrooms gave rise to a curious tension. Whereas the real attraction of dancing was increasingly bound to entertainment, the dancing masters refused to accept the inevitable and continued to promote the minuet throughout the first half of the nineteenth century. This tension is graphically expressed in the development of dancing as a discipline. Since the end of eighteenth century, two major forces shaped the discipline of dancing: first, the simplification and purification of its object, the body in movement; second, the reduction of the discipline of dancing.

In court dance, the functions of the moving body allowed for maximal use of the limbs. In the minuet and in its compliments, a swift and graceful swing of the arms was an essential element expressing, in combination with steps, one's passions.[34] Toward the end of the eighteenth century, the use of arms went into decline. According to Vieth, a great advocate of the minuet, the arms were to be passive. They should rest naturally and with ease on the sides to avoid any impression of affectation.[35] The waltz brought little change because in it, and other modern dances, the arms contributed to motion; in a dance such as a schottische, it added to the momentum of the dancing body. Only in the ballet did *port-de-bras* retain its function as the instrument of human passions. Consequently, the ballet became the primary vehicle for the display of passions, whereas ballroom dancing, the "lower dances," emphasized speed and indifference to exhaustion, resulting in entertainment.[36] This de-emotionalization of social dancing was complemented by a strict control of facial expressions, or, rather, its exclusion from the representational techniques. For instance, Franz Xaver Nadler, the Bavarian court dancer, recommended a friendly but unmoved and calm face for a cultivated dancer. Hentschke took the same standpoint.[37]

While *port-de-bras* declined and facial expressions were neutralized, the attention shifted to the steps and positions of the feet. By the end of the eighteenth century, the ten basic positions for the feet had been established. Of these, five were good (*gut*) (See Figure 5.1.) and usable in social dancing, whereas the other five false (*falsche*) positions were relegated to ballet. In the minuet, due to its multiple complicated figures, generally only four of the five "good" positions were employed. Numbers two and three dominated, because the minuet step was a combination of these positions.[38] In the waltz, due to its whirling configuration, two kinds of steps were used: the promenade step (*Pas zum Promenieren*) and the whirling step (*Pas zum Drehen*). The first consisted of a sequence of position number four, while the whirling step could be analyzed as a combination of positions four, two, and three.[39] The "problem" with the waltz, however, was its obscure and "inaccurate" way of combining these positions. Vieth did not even bother providing a detailed choreographic description of the waltz. It was simply endless whirling until dizziness.[40] Instead of reducing or simplifying the choreography of classical dancing, the new dynamic dance made the customary conceptualizations and normative codes more obsolete.

The minuet retreated from ballrooms. Yet the waltz, which during the first decade of the nineteenth century replaced it as the standard dance, was not the same *Ländler*, as it was called, that we find among Bavarian and Austrian peasants in the 1760s. After cultivated circles in Vienna had started to dance it, the waltz began to lose its original suggestive characteristics. Witzmann has documented in detail how the Viennese dancers replaced such typical features of the *Ländler* as lifting and hopping steps by dragging steps and whirling movement. During the following fifty years the waltz turned from a group dance of paired dancers to a dance of individual couples.[41] In the so-called *Deutscher*, the couples danced in a row or circle. In the 1780s, the tempo began to increase to such an extent that in the *Langaus-Walzer* the individual couples detached themselves from the group. After bringing almost unanimous criticism from dancing masters and dietetic writers, this waltz then was replaced by the more tranquil and solemn Viennese waltz, the dance of the Congress of Vienna.

The transformation of the waltz into a respectable ballroom dance shows why straightforward equations of the waltz with the bourgeoisie and embourgeoisement has to be interpreted with caution.[42] The reaction against inserting more complex elements into this simple peasant dance is evidence of the waltz's growth over time. Three different but closely related techniques were used. Audience and dancers were separated by limiting the number of dancing couples, which reduced everyone else in the ballroom to the status of observers. The equality of couples, inherent in the proto-waltz, was subverted by the introduction of a leading couple (*Vortänzer*) who guided the course of the dance and controlled the order in which the couples used the floor. Finally, the simple structure of the waltz was changed by adding special figures such as those commonly employed in the contredanse. Several authors, often adherents of the classic minuet, actively promoted these complex elements.[43] They helped to elevate the waltz as a more complex, sophisti-

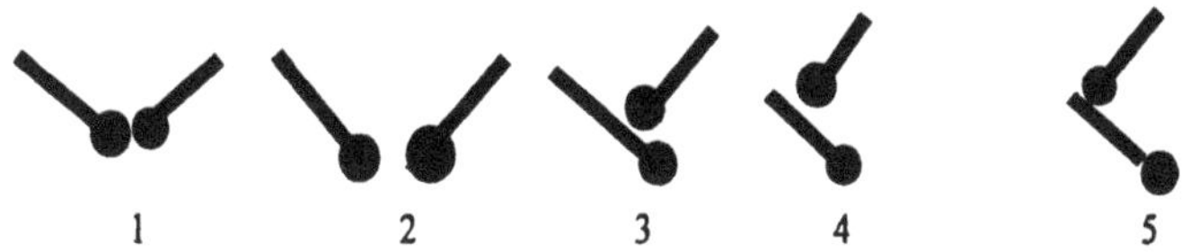


Figure 5.1. The Five Elementary Good Positions of Dancing, Nadler, *Kallischematik*, 59; Eichberg, *Leistung*, 171. In this illustration the dots signify the heels of a dancer who is facing away from the audience.

cated, and respectable dance but they could not compensate for the cultural and educational losses inherent in the decline of the minuet. The minuet had been a form of recreation but also a device of moral education; it had mediated between ballet and public entertainment. The waltz was considered neither a genuine ballet dance nor an acceptable and effective instrument of moral education. As the waltz took hold of the public fancy, there occurred an increasing institutional divide between the professional ballet and ballroom dancing, which, again, enhanced this configurational separation. In 1807, Roller tried to explain this development by pointing out how the number of small theaters with a ballet had dramatically declined since the late eighteenth century. The high aesthetic standards of professional dancing championed by the famous French choreographer at the Württemberg court, Jean Georges Noverre, and his followers, overwhelmed the financial and artistic resources of smaller ballet companies. With these small troupes gone, were also the rank and file of professional dancers who often had found additional income as dancing instructors.[44] Although smaller theater groups did not completely vanish and continued to include dancing in their performances—for instance, Hentschke and his wife, both dancing instructors, began their careers as actors, in the 1830s—Roller correctly reminds us that the higher professional standards for ballet had inserted new divisions into dancing.[45]

There was no shortage of ideas for restoring the unity of dancing. For instance, a proposal in the *Journal des Luxus und der Moden* from 1802 looked back to the pantomimic dances of the ancient Greeks to find an alternative to the waltz, which, according to the author, was harmful to morality and health, though it was German and therefore better than a French dance, i.e., the minuet.[46] Roller, similarly, choreographed some of his dances for students at the Schulpforte according to Greek and Roman themes and figures.[47] Yet this neohumanistic homage to the classical world underlined the irrevocable fragmentation and specialization of dancing. By 1820, we can see four separate and essentially independent discourses taking shape: discipline of appearance (*Anstandslehre*), dancing choreography, gymnastic dancing, and walking.

After the minuet disappeared from the ballroom, the dancing instructors did not abandon it. They continued to employ the minuet in the discipline of appearance.[48] The minuet, explained in detail in most dancing handbooks, was not expected to be danced but it provided the prerequisites for the correct behavior of a dancer and a cultivated person.[49] The minuet exemplified personal bearing (*Anstand*) and established the standards for a polished carriage.[50] However, the conservation of the minuet within the new discipline of appearance presented obvious problems. The public's perception of personal bearing had changed after the first decade of the nineteenth century. As early as 1819, August Hermann Niemeyer insisted that real personal bearing must come from the innate nature of man and should not be "artificially implemented."[51] A few years later, the *Rheinisches Conversations-Lexicon* declared war on the superficial and artificial personal bearing that promoted beautiful images but not real morality.[52] This criticism, directed against the eighteenth-century codes of court society and patrician culture, was potentially devastating for the discipline of appearance. It questioned whether dancing was at all necessary for truly moral (*anständig*) conduct. In 1828, Helmke, as one of the authorities of dancing, responded to this challenge by publishing a manual titled *Neue Tanz- und Bildungsschule*. Beginning with bold neohumanistic rhetoric, Helmke claimed that "the genuinely noble personal bearing must not be empty public representation but an expression of an inwardly and thoroughly intellectually cultivated human being."[53] Furthermore, this inwardness was universal, based upon one's pride in being human, which "rejects the caste feeling."[54] However, this promise of universal recognition of all decent human beings was soon recalled when Helmke had to concede that the complexity of social situations determined how pride in being human was expressed and recognized.[55] Dancing masters largely agreed that, according to the concrete etiquette of greeting, it was still social status that prescribed the modes of bodily conduct and expression. Cultivated friends should be greeted, an anonymous writer suggested, by taking off one's hat and nodding without a verbal greeting; cultivated acquaintances, a greeting with simply taking off one's hat; the uncultivated lower class, a verbal greeting only; the dishonorable, no greeting at all.[56] This social division differed from the traditional greetings and air of the minuet only in one sense: *Bildung* had now ranked as a deciding characteristic of social distinction. Consequently, those who possessed *Bildung* were to be greeted through a nonverbal compliment. Social bonds had again found their gestural correlatives. Whereas the appearance of the body indicated one's genuine *Bildung*, it could enforce the appearance of nonexisting *Bildung* as well.

Closely related to the new discipline of appearance were efforts to develop gymnastic dancing. With the decline of the minuet, dancing instructors had lost an effective argument in support of their role as moral educators. Challenged by the gymnastic movement, dancing instructors also saw their position as physical educators threatened. Between 1805 and 1843, dancing instructors at manèges (*Hohe Schulen*) and progressive *Gymnasiums* published a series of texts that defended dancing as the primary discipline of physical education. Roller's advocacy of *Turnen* at the Schulpforte was perhaps the most enthusiastic reception of the new gymnastic dancing. Andreas Schönwald, a dancing master in the manège of Freiburg, developed a more moderate and traditional program that emphasized the minuet, personal bearing, and the requirements of good balance.[57] From this combination came Bartholomay's program, which was highly critical of Jahn's gymnastics.[58] It was also an important source for the development of girls' gymnastics by Kümmerle and the Saxonian educator Johann Adolph Ludwig Werner.

After all these aspects were peeled away from traditional dancing, something was left over that could be called the discourse of pure social dancing. Deprived of most of its educational, moral, and gymnastic functions, it confined itself increasingly to the simple pleasure of dancing. New dances of greater or lesser staying power were introduced, such as the écossaise-waltz, *chaîne*, and galop.[59] Nevertheless, the entertainment and novelty aspects of dancing were of little moment when dancing instructors laid claim to what they understood as their contribution to *Bildung*—the vision of personal bearing.

The disciplinary specialization of dancing leads us to the surprising conclusion that the minuet would have been the most appropriate dance for the habitus of *Bildung*. As Roller remarked, "the minuet was for a long time the instrument to cultivate the body. In fact, it is an excellent tool for this purpose."[60] We can detect all the essential components of *Bildung* in its complicated configurations: personal development, the labor of spirit through the complicated steps and figures, a highly sublimated erotic undertone, and, finally, a sophisticated code of mutual recognition. Nevertheless, by the time the educated middle class had adopted the code of *Bildung*, the minuet was on the wane, vanishing from ballrooms. The waltz, whose steps found hardly any response in the ideology of *Bildung*, replaced it. It was too simple, too easy to learn, too obviously erotic, and it had a tinge of egalitarianism. Despite strenuous efforts to elevate it, the waltz quickly became an entertainment, in which physical bearing mattered little. It was lacking in the social components of mutual recognition so essential for the classical minuet.

## Cities and Clubs

We have observed the rise of the science of dancing and witnessed its transformation between 1770 and 1820. And we have seen the increasing fragmentation of dancing into separate fields of knowledge with rules and codes of their own. One is now tempted to ask how the science of dancing was applied. The historical significance of dancing for middle-class conduct can be discovered in the ways it shaped certain environments and, more important, how changes in the discipline of dancing became possible through changes in those environments. A clue to this peculiar relationship can be found in the simultaneous demise of the minuet and the rise of social clubs in German cities and towns. There is evidence that by 1800 dancing had become a central activity of these social clubs. In this and the subsequent two sections, I want to show how the loss of configurational power in dancing, to which the disappearance of the minuet was the chief contributor, was replaced by control over the space in which dancing took place.

Dancing was not a uniquely urban activity. Peasants as well as their lords certainly took pleasure in reproducing or transgressing their social worlds through dancing. Yet by the end of the eighteenth century, cities had become home to dancing, which took place in taverns, public or private masquerades, and ballrooms. And the cities saw a new type of society founded in the 1760s. Owning or renting houses in central locations, they sheltered small libraries with good collections of journals and newspapers, reading rooms, and facilities for social life. By the 1780s, the number of these reading societies (*Lesegesellschaften*) had reached 200, comprising a variety of associations first in Northern German cities and hometowns and, somewhat later, in Southern Germany and the Austrian territories.[61] By 1800, more than 430 reading societies had been founded.[62] The sheer number and geographical span of reading societies made them an important medium of civic communication. Recent studies have demonstrated how these reading societies disseminated literature and offered public lectures.[63] Less attention has been paid to activities that were a self-evident part of these societies: conversation and recreation. A great number of reading and other societies, and from the beginning of the nineteenth century a majority, were formed for socializing. In their weekly and annual calendars even the most serious societies, such as the *Patriotische Gesellschaft* in Hamburg, always included conversation and pastimes.[64] Marlies Prüsener has discovered that, by the turn of the century, most of the reading societies shifted their interest from reading and transmission of information toward convivial activities: Concerts, games, billiard, and balls started to dominate their programs.[65] At the same time, a host of social clubs were founded all over Germany, with names such as "Harmony," "Casino" or "Museum." These clubs and the rapidly transformed reading societies became the basis for men's networks that Lothar Gall has seen as the carriers of the classless bourgeois society.[66] But, as we will see, they were neither classless nor exclusively male. Much of their organizing energy was consumed in defining the social and financial limits of membership, and women were involved in most of their activities. And the activity that was especially attractive to women was dancing.

In analyzing the social clubs as dancing environments, I cannot claim to exhaust the endless variety of local experiences in the fragmented German lands, so I have concentrated on six cities: Tübingen, Mannheim, Hamburg, Leipzig, Munich, and Vienna. Together they provide significant insight into how the educated middle class socialized in Germany.[67] These cities had important common features as well as major differences in how they shaped the everyday workings of social clubs. Location and size are crucial, as are the presence or absence of court, university, and an active commercial life.[68] Finally, some of the most profound differences in the social structure of these cities can be understood in terms of political, juridical, and religious regulations.

The founding of social clubs can be seen as a wave that advanced from North to South.[69] Whereas Hamburg saw its first social club, Klub Einigkeit, in 1761, Munich had to wait until 1802 and Vienna until 1840 before social clubs and reading societies found a permanent seat inside their walls. The great divide, however, did not follow the traditional distinction between the Protestant North and the Catholic South. It followed the political borderline of the Austrian lands. Though Josephinian Vienna could easily have competed with Berlin and Hamburg in the variety of societies and clubs it fostered—the first "Casino" in Vienna was founded in 1784—the increasingly anxious administration of Francis II brought that to an abrupt end in 1798. All the associations were abolished and the Austrian aberration started.[70] Social and cultural life in post-Josephinian Austria wilted under uncompromising political control and censorship. There was almost no possibility for voluntary associations, including the dancing clubs, after the regime dissolved an explicitly apolitical society, Ludlamshöhle, in 1826, after nine years of harmless activities.[71] This obvious difference between the Austrian lands and the rest of Germany did not cause a substantive cultural rift. Rather, because of the peculiar restrictions of their political life, the Austrians, and especially the Viennese, created a unique everyday culture that had a significant impact on how the rest of Germany shaped its body culture. To compensate for the lack of clubs the Viennese developed, or rather preserved, an array of spectacles and public entertainments.[72] The greatest cultural invention of this environment—the waltz, a particularly spectacular dance—would have been unlikely to emerge from the small ballrooms and clubs of Hamburg and Leipzig.

The case of Vienna already suggests that religion plays a less significant part in the cultural divide between North and South than has been previously assumed.[73] This observation is further confirmed by the Munich experience. The first social clubs, "Museum" (1803) and "Harmonie" (1804), were founded relatively late if we compare Munich with the Northern metropolises of Hamburg (1761) and Leipzig (1772). The notorious abolition of the secret societies of the Illuminates in 1787 included reading societies.[74] Yet during the first two decades of the nineteenth century, Munich developed one of the densest and most elaborate networks of societies and social clubs in Germany.

As much as Vienna was the embodiment of political control, it also epitomized the immense cultural and financial power of the court. It shared this feature with Munich and partly with Mannheim, which during the early years of the nineteenth century still lived on its memories of the lost court. Whereas aristocratic aspirations could be found in all three cities, the differences were obvious. Unlike Vienna, Munich and Mannheim developed, somewhat delayed, lively club life; both saw their first social clubs founded during the first decade of the nineteenth century. In Vienna, the first families of the aristocracy offered private and exclusive balls.[75] But in Munich the relatively poor aristocrats compensated for their lack of income through the active social life in their sophisticated clubs, Harmonie and Museum.[76]

Commerce or academia characterized Tübingen, Hamburg, and Leipzig. Tübingen was a small university town in which the senate of the university equaled the city council in political power. It was a town in which professors and students set the social tone, often against the wishes and interests of the "lower town" of artisans and workers. Although the city had some commercial significance—as the seat of families such as Cotta and Osiander, it was a center of book printing, publishing, and retailing—the absence of traditional burghers, let alone a modern bourgeoisie, was apparent. The cultural weight of Württemberg's leading university, however, could compensate for what the cosmopolitan and wealthy bourgeoisie created in a city like Hamburg that, as the center of the old Hanseatic League, lacked significant academic tradition. In 1822, the Museum of Tübingen, a united reading society of professors and students, opened in a new building located right next to the gate of Lustnau, outside the city wall. The Museum was notably similar to the Harmonie of Hamburg, combining erudition with socializing and conversation.[77] Finally, with the early foundation of social clubs and reading societies—Harmonie was founded in 1772—Leipzig combined commercial activism with an academic tradition in a way unique among German cities. It had the most active social clubs of all these cities, matched only by Munich after the 1830s.

The social clubs served as nodes in the complicated network of middle- and upper-class bonding. Along with family and friendship circles, the social clubs were the basis of the social infrastructure of urban life.[78] In addition to the daily and weekly opportunities to socialize, they offered annual and monthly concerts, festivities, and balls. The carnival period, from late January through early April, summer holidays, royal festivities, New Year's celebrations, and annual meetings were the high points of the year. Yet the arenas for these feasts were often not the social clubs themselves but ballrooms, restaurants, spas, squares, and parks. Vienna was the city most noted for this kind of spectacle. Two royal ballrooms, Redoutensäle, a host of exclusive private ballrooms, and the popular park of Brigittenau served as sites for weekly or seasonal festivities and recreations. Most of the other cities had nothing comparable to the Viennese Redoutensäle. In Munich, the royal family attended the carnival masquerades in the Royal Theater and occasionally in the Museum and the Harmonie, providing them with a sheen of public recognition and control.[79] Cities that lacked a court and its aesthetic and moral guidance, especially the bigger cities, found compensation in private ballrooms. In Hamburg, the Apollo-Saal and the Elb-Pavillon were as celebrated as the Hotel de Saxe or the Hotel de Pologne in Leipzig. Unlike the lavish private Apollo-Saal in Vienna, these ballrooms could not have survived without a supporting club to organize its balls and provide a loyal and stable clientele. The connection was often close, as Buek writes about the Apollo-Saal in Hamburg:

> the late protonotary, Dr. Anderson, established in 1804 . . . the "Salon d'Apollon" next to the French Theater. He connected these two institutions. . . . Especially on holidays from October until March, the Apollo-Union meets there. It is a club founded by local respectable families and unmarried young men to promote socializing and dancing.[80]

In Leipzig, the connection between the Erholung club and the Hotel de Pologne was looser but still important. The club organized its annual masquerades in this famous hotel and restaurant for nearly twenty years, between 1829 and 1855.[81] The balls of another prominent club, the Tunnel, were divided among the Central-Halle, Hotel de Pologne, Hotel de Prusse, and the New Rifle-Club House or *Schützenhaus*.[82] The *Tanzkränchen* (Dancing Circle) of Tübingen, also without a permanent ballroom, took a decidedly entrepreneurial approach by looking for the cheapest and most decent restaurant.[83]

During the summertime, spas provided opportunities for socializing and recreation. Besides the permanent guests, some spas regularly had visitors who would come over a weekend to look for interesting conversations, the sight of royal families and celebrities, and opportunities for dancing. Several cities had their home spas. Leipzig favored Lauchstädt; Radeberg, Tharand, and Meißen encircled Dresden;[84] the residents of Hamburg visited Travemünde and other spas on the coast; the notables of Vienna frequented Baden; and even Tübingen had a network of minor local spas, such as Blasibad and Niedernau, which provided opportunities for conversation, promenading and dancing.[85] On Sundays, the so-called *Conventionstagen*, the cultured class of Mainz and Frankfurt frequented Wiesbaden, a summer resort with a wide reputation.[86]

In the middle-class world of the early nineteenth century, the number of dancing occasions and environments seemed inexhaustible. There were traditional settings of peasant or bourgeois origin, weddings and harvest festivals. Distinguished court balls, public masquerades, court masquerades, private balls, English assemblies, dancing master balls, and student balls gave, as Fink has discovered, other important opportunities for dancing.[87] When we consider that the number of spas, with their balls, *thés dansants*, and assemblies, had been rapidly increasing since the late eighteenth century, the diversity of dancing opportunities appears even wider. Yet the social clubs occupied a central role in this picture. None of the other dancing environments could display such specific aspiration for social inclusiveness and a simultaneous, instinctive tendency to exclusiveness. Social clubs were, above all, the arena of explicitly formulated norms of social recognition and constant challenges to these norms, and dancing was at the center of this tension. I will now take a closer look at how dancing served this purpose and how it formed the practice of social recognition.

## Inside the Ballroom Doors

The Tanz-Gesellschaft at the Gewandhaus had one of its regular balls on November 30, 1817. The directorate of the society had every reason to expect a successful evening. With the most prominent ballroom in Leipzig, the club had quickly recovered from the hardships of the Napoleonic wars. Gone were the miseries of the year 1810, when Napoleon's continental system forced the cancellation of the balls.[88] The memories of the frightening battles and plundering of 1813 had faded. The only lasting effect of those devastating years seemed to be the dizzying new dance introduced to respectability at the Congress of Vienna—the waltz. Encouraged by this excitement, the directorate had promised to organize seven balls during the winter season of 1817–18.[89] The ball of November 30 was supposed to be the last one before the New Year's Eve Ball, the high point of the year.

Sometime during the evening—our sources do not tell whether it was before or after the first dance—a group entered the ballroom. The leader of the group, Karl Theodor Küstner, the scion of an established local family, was a doctor of law and the director of the newly opened city theater. He had very good reason to expect a joyous evening and merry encounters with the rest of the society of which he had become a member a little more than a month earlier.[90] For the first time, the commercial and intellectual capital of Saxony had received a permanent theater, and Küstner had had a triumphant beginning since performances had started on August 26, 1817.[91] After a performance of Ferdinando Paër's oper *Il Sargino*, he had decided to take some of his most eminent actors, Christine Böhler and Eduard Stein, to the Sunday ball of the Tanz-Gesellschaft.[92] But the evening came to a sorry end. Soon after the group entered the ballroom, the rest of the society—sixty members, their families and guests—made their unhappiness about the newcomers known. At the request of some members, the directors of the ball (*Vorsteher*) intervened and made it clear to Küstner that his friends were not welcome. They were asked to leave without delay, and they obviously did.[93]

A tense correspondence followed between the dancing club, Küstner, and members of the Theaterverein. Baron von Haugk, a prominent member of the club, informed Küstner that the presence of the actors upset several members of the Gewandhausball. Küstner was outraged. In a letter of December 18, 1817, he mentioned that two of the actors, Böhler and Stein, had been angry enough over the incident to resign from his theater. Küstner himself was about to follow suit, because it was impossible to "live without social respect (*allgemeine Achtung*)."[94] The disagreement escalated to a confrontation between the Tanz-Gesellschaft des Gewandhauses and the Theaterverein. The actors claimed that their recognition as artists "by virtue of their profession and the necessary intellectual *Bildung*" was at stake. As artists, Küstner said, they were entitled to "respectable demonstrations of recognition."[95] This obviously had not happened. From the perspective of the ball directors, the situation appeared quite different. Küstner had chosen companions whose respectability was not impeccable, i.e., they did not conform to the "particular spirit of propriety" cultivated in the club.[96] Who, then, were respectable and, therefore, eligible to attend? The correspondence does not provide a direct answer. All we know is that neither Theodor Küstner nor any of the actors left Leipzig until 1828.[97] Yet the incident provides an insight into the process of social recognition: who could attend the balls of the Tanz-Gesellschaft im Gewandhaus? For a social club such as this one there were four critical aspects that determined membership and eligibility for attendance: residency, gender, religion (especially whether one was Jewish), and social class.

We can assume that the presence of nonmembers and outsiders had annoyed the regular members. Yet the culture of social clubs in Germany and the statutes of the Tanz-Gesellschaft itself do not support this. Even reading societies that primarily concentrated on reading, borrowing, and circulating books, journals, and newspapers encouraged visitors. In no open club were they rejected, so the question is simply about the means of integration. In Vienna, which lacked a network of societies and clubs, the first and necessary step of social contact was a letter of recommendation. According to Karl Johann Braun, such as a letter to a good family was enough to introduce the bearer into the network of families, who then readily invited the newcomer to *thés dansants* or dinners.[98] In other cities, a recommendation may not have so readily opened the doors of the leading households but was still an asset in establishing a first contact in the city. Through such a connection, the visitor was taken into a local club or a reading society.[99] Besides his exotic and informational value to a local society, a foreign guest had a special status.[100] As the bylaws of the Museums-Gesellschaft in Tübingen defined it: "especially for concerts, casinos, balls, and other social events at the Museum, no non-member of the club may enter. Women and visitors are excluded from this restriction."[101] The special treatment of visitors from outside of the city became more obvious as reading societies geared their programs toward sociability after the 1810s. In Munich and Leipzig, guest status was normally granted to foreign, nonresident visitors, whereas local people had to apply for regular membership and pay considerable monthly or annual fees. Frohsinn, a middle class and family-oriented social club, allowed guest status only for those who had resided in Munich less than a month. Some clubs, such as the Kleine Erheiterung, whose members were mainly artisans and established tradesmen, limited visitor attendance to three times.[102] These restrictions implied, however, a problem imminent to a society whose activities consisted of regular, almost weekly, balls and social "evenings." Friedrich Johann Lorenz Meyer, a critical and astute observer of Hamburg, mentioned in 1801 that

> the generous hospitality that the foreigners ascribe to Hamburg would greatly benefit if cultivated men and women of scholarly or merchant class would establish permanent clubs. They could meet regularly once a week in a mixed setting to games, music, dance, lectures, and free conversation.[103]

But this vision did not always meet the needs of reality. In Frohsinn, a prominent club in Munich, sociability was definitely limited when social life was essentially shouldered and enjoyed only by member families and their occasional guests. If outsiders could go there, according to Lewald, he would hardly find an "unreserved" lady for dancing.[104]

The Tanz-Gesellschaft was all this. It was a social club for those interested in dancing. It was a family club. Yet it also encouraged its permanent members to bring their guests. And unlike the clubs in Munich, the Tanz-Gesellschaft did not set limits on whether visitors should be residents or foreigners.[105] So, obviously, the fact that recent residents of Leipzig accompanied Küstner was not the reason for members' outrage.

Related to the question of visitors, but sometimes more controversial, was the status of women. One of Küstner's was an actress from his company, Böhler. At the time she was still unmarried, though three years later she married a famous actor at the Stadttheater, Eduard Genast.[106] But a young unmarried actress at a ball had some peculiar obstacles to overcome. To be sure, the bylaws of the Tanz-Gesellschaft did not forbid the attendance of women. For a dancing club, that would have been untenable. Yet among the permanent members there were very few women. Women visitors were expected to belong to the families of the permanent members.[107] This tells us something significant about the workings of social clubs, dancing, and the social recognition of women.

Women held a stronger position in rising bourgeois society than that commonly assumed by scholars of the period. The peculiar structure of families and family circles, as Trepp and Habermas have discovered, provided them with social opportunities denied them by the wider society.[108] In looking beyond the boundaries of the informal and intimate spheres in which they resided, we should expect to find a culture in which women had a decorative role, if any. Yet a closer analysis of the papers of reading societies and social clubs reveals surprising rifts in this male-dominant social world. In 1801, Meyer had criticized the societies in Hamburg as "male clubs that purposely excluded women."[109] In Leipzig, Harmonie defined itself as "a male club dedicated to sociability."[110] Most of the clubs allowed women only as indirect members through their husbands or fathers. In Munich, however, practically all societies and clubs had special rules of admission for widows. The Frohsinn club allowed widows to attend at no cost for a half year after the death of a spouse who had been one of its permanent or honorary members. "If they still wish to visit the club after this time period," say its rules, "they are, however, obliged to follow the regulations for widows."[111] These included a reduced annual membership fee at two fl. 42 kr., as compared with five fl. 24 kr. for regular male members.[112] These do not specify, however, whether a dues-paying widow enjoyed the rights of full membership, as, for instance, whether they could be candidates for office or vote in the club's elections. Although the bylaws did not explicitly exclude them from such activities, it is probably safe to assume that full membership was highly unlikely for women. The family was the basic unit of the club, and most of its regulations were designed accordingly.

Nonetheless, the condition of female participation in the social clubs was changing. Meyer's criticism, not the first but one of the most vocal, tried to view traditional social bonding in the new perspective of gender awareness. Yet it would be a misconception to see in Meyer an early advocate of women's emancipation, for at issue was not political equality but the social workings of the civil society in general and reading societies in particular. This question had been raised two years earlier in an anonymous article in the *Berlinisches Archiv der Zeit und ihres Geschmacks*, whose author, identified as Schleiermacher, strongly argued for women's participation and even leadership in social clubs. Unlike men, who possessed expert knowledge of general interest and would be tempted to engage in semi-professional discussions, women were creatures of their own domain, the domestic sphere, which had the least general, that is political, importance. So, women, Schleiermacher argued, had a natural inclination for promoting disinterested social interaction. Meyer agreed that only women could elevate the tone of male clubs in Hamburg, which were plagued by shop-talk and mediocre conversation.[113]

Schleiermacher was convinced that his theory would be best served through conversation, which would become the genuine carrier of sociability. This view reflected not only the philosophically informed public opinion but also the reality of social life among the educated middle class around 1800. The reading societies were becoming more recreational, whereas new clubs such as Museum and

Harmonie in Munich lived on conversation and socializing. And then dancing started to find its way into the clubs. This development made it easier for women to attend club activities and to define their tone and social life. After all, you cannot have a dancing club without a female presence.

The increasing presence and intellectual engagement of women in social clubs became an issue. Yet how difficult it was to find a reasonable solution can be seen in a controversy around women participants in Mannheim.[114] In August 1803, when a respected book dealer, Mathias Fontaine, sent a circular to 270 notables of his city, he envisioned a reading society, Casino, in which "several people regularly meet, in order to get to know each other better, entertain and educate themselves."[115] The society, which the authorities swiftly approved, included practically anyone who had a name in Mannheim. Rather than a social club, Casino was a reading society that could boast of 95 subscribed journals and newspapers and a rich library. It was an arena of debate on world and local politics. This was not considered an appropriate setting for women and their participation was rejected on grounds of the high renovation costs that such participation would have required. But in a city that nourished strong, albeit fading, memories of a splendid aristocratic culture and that, moreover, had a salon led by Duchess Stephanie, the exclusion of women from the club would have been untenable in the long run. Yet their participation in Casino became an issue in 1808, and a dissenting group, unable to agree with the proscription on women founded Museum, a society for "the purpose and the pleasure of cultivated sociability," in the following year. Unlike Casino, which stressed political discourse and erudition, Museum focused on literature, music, conversation, and games. With Duke Carl and Duchess Stephanie as protectors, Museum offered an aesthetic and conversational program in which women played a prominent role.[116] But within four years, the era of freedom and equality was over. Casino and Museum united into Harmonie, which again put women in a dependent position. Widows and unmarried adult women could apply for membership only through a male member's sponsorship. The new club left some venues open for female participation by organizing biweekly *thés dansants* and formal balls.[117] Not until 1848, however, did women achieve equal status with male members.

A similar kind of development took place in other cities. We have already seen what happened at the Tanz-Gesellschaft in Leipzig. With the Ballgesellschaft Concordia (1800), Leipzig had two clubs for dancing by the turn of the century. In other cities, it took another twenty years, until after the Napoleonic Wars ended, to establish such clubs. In Hamburg, which had a host of male-centered social clubs by the turn of the century, organizations with more convivial programs of dancing and games, and women participants emerged with Erholung (1813) and Apollo-Casino (1828). And suddenly they were all over. In Munich, the Frohsinn club was founded in 1813; the Altengland started its extravagant meetings six years later; in Tübingen, the Tanz-Sängerkränzchen der Sängerkranz-Mitglieder began to organize its balls in 1829; even Vienna had a social club for its intellectuals for a short time, Ludlamshöhle (1817–26).[118] Finally, Mannheim also welcomed a recreational club when the new Casino-Gesellschaft was founded in 1835. According to its bylaws, it had two goals: to serve as a gathering place for men after work and to organize balls.[119]

After the late 1820s, the number of dancing clubs increased rapidly. In particular, Leipzig, Munich, and Hamburg had an abundance of them. Only a few would live long enough to celebrate their centenaries, like the Ballgesellschaft Concordia in Leipzig, but their sheer number testified to a unique social network. They provided opportunities for women to expand their horizons beyond the family network to semi-public associations. Terpsichore in Munich is a good example. It was founded in 1840 to create opportunities to dance and socialize, rather than to engage in political discourse.[120] Women were needed to participate because of the chronic lack of dancing partners, despite the female relatives that accompanied their husbands and fathers. The club felt it necessary to announce that "widows and unmarried women who belong to the cultured class and have an untarnished reputation" were permitted access. This was far more of a concession than the standard invitation to widows. It was also more inclusive than the elitist caveat of the Museum-Gesellschaft to accept "distinguished female artists" on their own without a patron.[121] Yet the limits also were clear. Regardless of their contribution, even Terpischore granted women the status only of associate members with limited rights to vote and participate in decision-making.[122]

We return to the case of the actress Böhler. At Museum-Gesellschaft or Terpsichore in Munich, she obviously could have attended in her own right. Yet Böhler had been brought to a dancing club in which women had a necessary but far from independent role—there was one exception, Pauline Dufour-Ferouce, a longtime regular member of the Tanz-Gesellschaft.[123] But as a young actress who was not a relative of Küstner, she was immediately open to the suspicion that she might be a person who did not have a "good reputation." That his guest was an actress was significant and, obviously, critical, to recognition at the *Gewandhausball*, for the disapproval of the directors and the membership were directed against the whole entourage, not only against Böhler.

The third possible explanation could be that Böhler, or one of the other guests of Küstner, were Jewish. In Leipzig, Jews quite commonly were excluded from the reading societies and most of the social clubs. The bylaws of Erholung explicitly excluded Jews.[124] The Erheiterung rejected "confessors of the Mosaic Religion."[125] In Munich, Frohsinn did not allow Jews.[126] In Hamburg the situation was no different. Garlieb Merkel witnessed an incident in 1798:

> The most striking expression of aversion against the Jews happened in the last months of that year [1798], at the Harmonie, a club of the enlightened men of Hamburg. A local Jewish merchant, a fine man with excellent education, let himself be offered membership. His friend, who saw the difficulties that a Jew might experience, avoided mentioning this circumstance in the application. He called him simply Martin M_r and the application was accepted easily. Some days after the acceptance, his Jewishness became known and suddenly every-

> thing was in an uproar. Most members demanded that he be expelled without delay, whereas some would have had him be advised quietly that it was wise to stay away. A couple of members thought him to be a decent man with a good reputation whose membership could not be annulled because of his religion. To this suggestion, one received an answer that the club did not want to have anything to do with the "damned Jews."[127] This public farce would have very likely embarrassed the club and the city if a cunning politician had not found a solution. He suggested that a necessary condition for membership be that every candidate gives his baptism name. Since there were rumors that the gentleman's name was not Martin but Mendel, the candidate would have to submit his baptism records before he could be considered as a member. This shows, if anything, that even in crudeness there can be some cleverness. Though I do not know how the issue was finally solved.[128]

One's name could open venues for social, or even public, recognition. But here it became an effective tool for the denial of recognition. This rejection took place in a setting in which two parameters of the modern world met: the bourgeoisie and the public sphere. What the associations shared was a distinguished bourgeois spirit. In Leipzig and Hamburg, which scarcely had any aristocratic residents, this was obvious. In Munich, Frohsinn, the commoners' equivalent of Harmonie and Museum, followed suit. Whether this bourgeoisie was feudal, premodern, or even enlightened, it often perceived Jews as an economic and social threat.[129]

Yet German Jewry, especially the wealthiest families, played an increasingly important role in the organization of sociability—both within and outside the dominant culture. By 1800, several Jewish families, often allied with strong royal and imperial houses, had developed an eminent social profile. The salons of Rahel Varnhagen von Ense and Henriette Hertz in Berlin and Fanny von Arnstein in Vienna had established themselves as the most distinguished social arenas, frequented by the von Humboldts, the Schlegels, Schleiermacher, Tieck, and Schelling.[130] To a lesser degree, some wealthy Jewish families in Hamburg, such as Heine, Assing, and Steinheim, had opened their homes to literary and intellectual circles by the 1820s.[131] But salons were private, and Jews were not so much recognized by others as they recognized the others, desperately looking for signs of gentile acceptance.[132] It is, however, this aristocratic or patrician pattern of Jewish-Christian socializing that we can detect somewhat later, working toward the integration of the Jewish bourgeoisie into cultured Christian society. In 1835, Lewald reports that in Munich, which had a small but wealthy Jewish community, Museum accepted Jewish members, and Jewish families also provided the "most popular soirees" in town.[133] At the same time, we can find another, although troubled, indication of increasing integration. In Tunnel, a carnival club in Leipzig, a debate arose about whether it should accept Jews as members, although the masquerade of January 20, 1837, still featured the emancipation of women and Jews as a source of humor. Heinrich Laube, a prominent member of the club and an advocate of the emancipation of Jews, vigorously defended their membership.

Because of opposition, however, this did not take place before the Revolution of 1848.[134]

When rejected by gentiles, Jews often organized separate social clubs. Scattered evidence suggests that in the beginning of the century there were, besides Jewish philanthropic societies, a number of social clubs for Jewish men. In Munich, an exclusively Jewish club, Concordia, existed in the 1820s.[135] The Jewish community in Mannheim founded a social club, Ressource, by the same time.[136] In Bamberg, the Jews founded their own Casino-Gesellschaft in 1850.[137] In Hamburg, the biggest Jewish community in Germany, a vibrant network of associations existed since the late seventeenth century. They were, however, predominantly utilitarian and philanthropic in their goals. We do not know, for instance, whether the Jewish club Freundschaftszirkel had a social function in addition to its philanthropic activities.[138] However, its sister clubs, Gesellschaft der Freunde (Association of Friends), in Berlin and Breslau, were famous for their social life.[139]

Returning to the ball of the Tanz-Gesellschaft im Gewandhaus, it is unlikely that religion did play a crucial role in their eviction. Nowhere in the accounts is Jewishness raised as an issue; None of the members of the entourage was of Jewish origin or, what is more important, was recognized as Jewish. Nor can we find anything in the bylaws of the club that would show explicit discrimination against Jews. The Tanz-Gesellschaft carefully cultivated its sophisticated spirit and had established its reputation as the most distinguished ballroom of the city. It was closer to the cosmopolitan and aristocratic air of Museum in Munich—which allowed Jewish attendance—than to the bourgeois parochialism of Erholung in Leipzig—which explicitly rejected Jews.

The last hurdle that the entourage confronted was the social fabric of the Tanz-Gesellschaft. The bylaws of the Tanz-Gesellschaft defined the membership in a rather curious way: "Because this club provides only bourgeois private entertainment (*bürgerliches Privat-Vergnügen*), persons of aristocratic origin, military officers, and all young gentlemen who are students and their private tutors cannot become members. Yet they are very welcome as guests of a permanent member."[140] When we consider that the bylaws also excluded servants—unless they accompanied a member—a peculiar social picture begins to take shape. Since nobility, students, and the laboring class were excluded, the groups eligible for membership can be found among wealthy merchants, high officials of the city and state administration, and professors. The association carefully nurtured this patrician membership until 1817, when it dropped and replaced §13 with a vague statement of "members of bourgeois origin who have a local residence."[141] But the door was still open to exclusive interpretations. We know, for instance, that the club accepted noblemen, such as von Haugk, who was a longtime member, whereas the stipulation of *wohnhaften* (local residency) effectively excluded foreign students, for resident students would come with their families.[142] In 1844, Bechstein and Kleinknecht still advertised the balls in the ballroom of Gewandhaus as the most lavish and exquisite ones in Leipzig. But they were *vornehm*, exclusive, to the extent that a popular tourist guide saw the members of the Tanz-Gesellschaft as the "most distinguished families" of the city.[143]

The social fabric of the Tanz-Gesellschaft was not uncommon for societies in Leipzig. The Harmonie accepted aristocrats only as associate members. Their full membership was first proposed in 1829, except to Saxonian army officers, who were to retain associate status. After long deliberations, the bylaws of 1845 finally included all those who belonged to the cultured classes (*gebildeten Ständen*).[144] In most German cities—with the exception of Vienna, which did not have any—membership in reading societies had long been tailored accordingly. Rather than separating the bourgeoisie and the nobility, these clubs increasingly (though tacitly) encouraged to the assimilation of the nobility with the upper segments of the bourgeoisie. In Hamburg, the Harmonie embraced men from all social classes, though for eligibility one had to submit one's full name and social status or profession.[145] The Museum in Munich accepted all men who passed the requirements of *Bildung*, residency, and the strong endorsement of a permanent member.[146] But in a city like Munich, which from the 1830s on had a rapidly expanding network of social clubs, exclusion did not cause much social damage. Recognition by a less prestigious club whose standards of *Bildung* were, if not lower, then at least different, always could compensate for rejection by a Museum or a Harmonie. One could, for instance, become a member of Frohsinn, which provided "pleasant and useful entertainment whose cornerstones are morality, personal bearing, and dignity." Only those who were interested in pure socializing and recreation frequented clubs like Kaufmanns-Casino.[147]

In smaller towns, the possibilities for a diverse network of clubs were limited. In Tübingen, the three reading societies that emerged by the end of the 1810s soon merged their resources into Museums-Gesellschaft. While the aristocracy was essentially absent, social tensions concerning membership emerged between the academics and the tiny community of tradesmen. In a proposal for a reading society in 1817, a professor of medicine, Wilhelm August Georgii, defined its membership inclusively. It should comprise tradesmen (*Geschäftsmänner*), as well as scholars with a position and scholars without a position, i.e., students. "A genuine association," argued Georgii, "does not recognize any other reason for exclusion than the one which is based on the rude ignorance of cultivated etiquette, obvious lack of education and, in a derived sense, lack of *Bildung*. All these deficiencies indicate notorious impropriety."[148]

Yet the inclusiveness was carefully limited. Instead of a unified and democratic membership, Georgii suggested a class system of four socially and culturally separate groups: professors and dignitaries, students of the university, students of the Evangelical seminary, and students of the Catholic seminary.[149] These groups should have separate meetings, governments, and selection of members. Georgii's proposal, which was essentially adopted in the organization of the Museum-Gesellschaft in 1822, simply omitted lower-ranking city-dwellers. Artisans, not to mention day-laborers, were effectively outside the social network.

So, to return to the Leipzig Tanz-Gesellschaft incident, the situation at the ball by mid-December 1817 seems rather peculiar. Küstner had accused the society of a lack of *Bildung*, or rather, the failure of the guards to consider that artists might have a place in its *Bildung*. Küstner believed that the directors of the ball did not show appropriate respect toward the actors. What Küstner himself, and his companions, too, failed to realize was that there might be another basis for respect—that *Bildung* might be such a new mode of recognition that all those who satisfied their social needs of mutual recognition through dancing did not share it, or did not realize that residency, gender, religion, and social class could be condensed in the nebulous term of *Bildung*. And if they did, they suddenly were confronted with another problem: How was one to know if someone else possessed *Bildung*?

## An Invitation to Dance

After overcoming various social and physical barriers and gaining entrance to the ballroom, participants were subjected to additional social observation. They were neither excluded nor rejected but tolerated. Here is a picture of an evening at the ball. After leaving his overcoat in the cloakroom and perhaps changing to dancing-shoes, the newcomer took a first glance into the ballroom. The music had hardly started, but the first women who had fainted already had been guided outdoors to recuperate. Waiters hurried between tables to serve those who had pre-ordered dinner.[150] This bustling surface was anchored by the solid appearance of those charter members who, after an exchange of approving nods and greetings with their peers, had seated their friends and families at their customary tables.[151] Yet the appearance of harmony and social distance was challenged once the dance started and partners had to be engaged.

We have already identified some of the elements of this challenge. After the last decades of the eighteenth century, the decline of the minuet and rise of the waltz had imported a new sense of intimacy into the ballroom. As Küstner's troubles indicate, the educated middle class had its reservations about the extent to which this new intimacy was offered. Without rejecting it, the cultivated dancers created a set of behaviors to preserve a genteel antagonism between physical intimacy and social distance. In this section, I will first take a look at the ball programs to identify to what extent the new intimacy was present at the balls. Then I will turn to three different and, I argue, most important strategies to handle the undermining conflict: avoidance, non-engagement, and invitation.

Table 5.1. German Ball Programs in the 1820s, Länger, *Terpsichore*, 176–78

| *Program 1* | *Program 2* | *Program 3* |
|---|---|---|
| 1. Waltz | Waltz | Waltz |
| 2. Écossaise | Écossaise | Écossaise |
| 3. Waltz | Waltz en Russe | Waltz |
| 4. Quadrille | Douze | Triolet |
| 5. Waltz | Waltz | Waltz |
| 6. Conversation | "Kreuz-Écossaise" | Écossaise |
| 7. Waltz | Waltz | Waltz |
| 8. Seize | Seize | Tempête |
| 9. "Wechsel-Walzer" | Waltz | Waltz |
| 10. Contre Écossaise | Écossaise with six figures | Quadrille |
| 11. Waltz | Waltz | Ladies' Choice |
| 12. Écossaise Waltz | Écossaise Waltz | "Wechsel Walzer" |

In analyzing the debates over the incursion of the waltz, we saw that the intimacy of its couples and the change in dancing configurations threatened the composure of the ballroom. This is confirmed by the balls and assemblies of the early nineteenth century. The waltz dominated ordinary balls, as Christian Länger's ball programs from 1824 (see Table 5.1.) illustrate. So do the few programs that survived from dancing clubs.[152] Some other dances were just as important, interesting, and popular as the waltz, however. The écossaise was a couples dance that, as Roller mentions, could include the waltz in one of its four figures.[153] The quadrille, the *douze*, and the *seize* were contredanses with four, twelve, or six couples, respectively, dancing different figures and occasionally changing partners. These dances were no less intimate than the waltz but offered more variation and even a certain sensual excitement. In the *douze*, for instance, one figure involved a circle of six men and six women. After each dancer's individual figure, the men approached the ladies to their right, rather than their original partners. Throughout the dance, all the dancers went through the set of changing couples. In another variant of the *douze*, the circle comprised four men and eight women.[154] In the triolet, the dancers formed a row in which each man was flanked by two ladies. The trio, not the couple, was the unit.

The number of intimate dances challenged the traditional function of dancing as a form of social recognition. In fact, a fundamental question to the existing social order was how one could find social satisfaction in this confusing mixture of intimacy and social distance. Quite frequently, one could not and one did not want to find it. The story of the Mehlgrube, the oldest and most famous ballroom in Vienna until 1808, shows this vividly.[155] From 1726 until the middle of the century, it was an exclusive venue for the high aristocracy. Official genealogical documents were required for eligibility.[156] In this highly controlled and restricted space, the confusing codes of simultaneous intimacy and social distance could cause only little, if any, nuisance or, for that matter, excitement. However, the lower aristocracy (in the 1750s) and then the bourgeoisie (in 1765) gained access to the Mehlgrube, thanks to the policies of social leveling implemented by Joseph II.[157] Nevertheless, by 1790 the high aristocracy had withdrawn from active dancing to become observers in the passages and hallways of the Mehlgrube and other respectable public ballrooms.[158] Not until the late nineteenth century did they return to public balls and masquerades. The Mehlgrube, once the most desirable arena of social and physical engagement, rapidly lost its status. A city guide of 1827 described it as a dancing hall for "apprentices."[159]

Though particular to the environment of Vienna, examples of aristocratic withdrawal from and avoidance of public balls also can be found in other German territories. The reports from German spas reveal a morass of social conflicts at balls. An account from the Pyrmont spa complained in 1798 that

> those lovers of dance who belong to the bourgeoisie do not gain any satisfaction there. Only the aristocrats dance. They give *Dejeneurs, Goutes Dansants* etc. The bourgeoisie is allowed only to watch. No further comments are needed on how this conforms to the natural laws of good tone and what is the reaction of the bourgeoisie. The contemporary history delivers the best testimony to this state of affairs.[160]

In 1803, there were still separate ballrooms for the nobility and the bourgeoisie in Pyrmont.[161] One summer night at the Liebenstein spa, only the intervention of the Duke and Duchess of Meiningen prevented the division of the ball: By dancing with bourgeois visitors they set the example for their aristocratic entourage.[162] The spirit of exclusion was not universal. Reports from Doberan, a small spa on the coast of the Baltic Sea, depict social bonding in a pastoral idyll.[163] Yet in major spas, dancing remained a form of social distinction for the aristocracy rather than a mode of assimilation and bonding. Rather than improving the situation, the continuing complaints from the bourgeois clientele underscored the contest of differences and recognition as a common feature of major spas until the 1850s. Even in a small spa, such as Ems, one could find "a strange spirit of distinction" and class separation in the late 1820s.[164] In Carlsbad, the tendency was toward increasing differences not only between classes but also toward fostering political fractions within the status groups. As an anonymous commentator noticed, "not only the bourgeoisie and aristocracy are separated but both are themselves divided into a number of factions."[165] But if the intention was to make the bourgeoisie so uncomfortable that they fled the spas, it failed. By the middle of the 1830s, according to Kühne, all the leading spas, including Carlsbad, Gastein, Teplitz, and Spaa, boasted constantly growing numbers of visitors. And these visitors were mainly aristocrats who occupied their urban life with salons and social clubs.[166] Where the tone of distinction was missing, as in Teplitz in the summer of 1842, the result was boredom: "How graphic is the lack of cavaliers who would set the tone, how much we are lacking in rich aristocrats, in buoyant people who have taste and resources enough to create a center for social life."[167]

Beyond the mere quantity of such conflicts is the way they suggest how controversies were absorbed into dancing. When, for instance, the aristocratic families of Munich decided to hold a masquerade of their own in 1816, closed to those who were not "socially qualified for aristocracy" (*turnierfähig*), it was in reaction to the anonymity and randomness of contacts of Mardi Gras celebrations.[168] The culture of avoidance was not a uniquely aristocratic privilege. In fact, we can see increasing pressure not to attend public balls spreading among the educated middle class during the first half of the nineteenth century. According to Bartholomay, the public ball was, in fact, not a ball at all and thus a cultivated person should not attend because it did not conform to the order of personal bearing.[169] Helmke was only slightly more liberal when he maintained that "a public ball is, in fact, not a ball at all but a public dancing event in which everybody can participate. Personal bearing is not recognized at these events, and therefore no cultivated gentleman and no lady who guards her reputation can approach each other."[170] The only option Helmke left for the visitor was a voyeuristic withdrawal to the sides of the dancing floor. All those who subscribed to the codes of personal bearing and *Bildung* could and should follow this mode of negative social recognition.

Once social pressure against the sanctioned intimacy had called for widespread social disengagement, the central institution of dancing, the invitation, became even more complicated. How could one approach another person whom one probably did not know but whose body one was bound to touch? In the exclusive world of the Mehlgrube before the 1750s, the approach to a lady was through a careful investigation of one's family tree.[171] Intruders and dishonorable touches were prevented. And once the doors were opened to the lower echelons, a serious problem became evident: When the ballroom became a public sphere with virtually unlimited access, it no longer provided a safe venue for the expression of social and bodily distance. To this embarrassment, no permanent solution was found. Rather, the more or less tacit subtext to a proper invitation was that the arena was, as Helmke described, a "dancing club," in which "the dancers are not combined randomly (*gemischt*) but only through their own choice. In these clubs, the dancers also feel obliged to show equal and reciprocal respect."[172] Although this interpretation is not directly documented in the papers of the dancing clubs, we still can understand that the socially exclusive conditions of membership confirmed this requirement.[173] Not accidentally, the number of dancing clubs started to rise rapidly from the 1820s on in non-Austrian Germany, fulfilling the desire for appropriate social homogeneity.

After the social enclosure of the lower class—and sometimes the upper class, as in Leipzig—was solved, the next problem was the intimacy and distance between the sexes. Could a woman decline an invitation? On July 24, 1826, Ms. Weber attended one of those midsummer balls organized by the newly founded Museums-Gesellschaft of Tübingen. She was just about to leave after a long and exhausting cotillion when Mr. Leupp, a local student, approached and invited her to dance. Weber, not at all pleased with this unexpected invitation, tried to find a respectable way out by promising to accept only if the dance were a waltz. Leupp, who had calculated that a ball would perhaps not end with a cotillion and, moreover, had heard the conductor promise a final waltz, expected that Weber would honor his invitation.[174] The waltz started. Leupp rushed to his prospective partner only to find that she was not at all willing to join him.

> Her rejection did not immediately discourage me from extending my invitation. By doing so, I asked her to take off her shawl and touched her large shawl with one finger, in order to assure my intention . . . If this happened in obtrusive manner, to which only the witnesses can testify, it was naturally against the rules of propriety. Realizing that all my efforts were in vain, I still attempted to proceed further. At that moment, Mr. Schädtler intruded between the young lady . . . and me. He said to me: "Do not be obtrusive." As anyone can imagine, *these words*, from *this person*, *on this place*, *in front of ladies* were not a matter of indifference to me.[175]

Leupp, deeply humiliated, pushed the intruder so forcefully that he fell on the nearby chairs. The outraged Schädtler complained to the presidium of the Museums-Gesellschaft.

We do not know whether Schädtler received satisfaction or if Leupp was reprimanded. The incident itself is a standard one: A woman declined an invitation to dance. Yet the account is not as standard as the incident itself. It was Ms. Weber herself whom Leupp approached and who refused to honor his request, not her father, brother, or another male relative, as for instance Helmke still prescribed.[176] Ms. Weber seems to have made her own decision, but in a way that might not have been completely appropriate. To some romantic writers, not only a marked aversion but any kind of hesitation on the woman's part was a reason enough to recall one's invitation.[177] The ball of the Museums-Gesellschaft was, however, a closed event; in itself, this should have made any invitation acceptable. A woman who accepted the general invitation to attend a closed ball had promised to dance with virtually any man in attendance, and, as Mädel and Helmke maintained, she could not but accept any invitation to dance.[178] Despite these compelling circumstances, she rejected Leupp's invitation: an obvious discourtesy. What could Leupp do? His next move, physical coercion, was wrong, as Leupp himself admitted. An informal consensus agreed that a woman's body could not be touched without her consent; not because the female body was untouchable—a husband could always use physical punishment against his wife[179]—but because the logic of dancing required mutual willingness. Thus Mr. Schädtler's intervention served, in addition to whatever his private interest may have been, the public interests of the ballroom.

The act of invitation was complex enough to call for effective methods of coping with frequent conflicts and possible humiliation of male pride. Bartholomay describes a procedure that was common, albeit complicated.

> At some balls the ladies are pre-invited (*Vorherengagiren*). In order to avoided confusion, this arrangement is combined at all times with a custom that both gentlemen and ladies carry a special card that mentions all the dances of the evening. Once a lady has accepted an invitation to a dance, one asks her to present her card and signs, if it is not the next dance, one's name next to the invited dance and also her name on one's own card. In this way there will not be any mistakes and one can immediately recognize for which dances the lady is still available.[180]

This prearranged invitation, which in England and the United States became known as the dance card, was a safe way to prevent conflicts and nuisances. But another system was easier and became commonly used by social and dancing clubs. The couples were randomly matched through a lottery. This was especially useful in dances in which the position in a row or circle, rather than the partner, was important. When the Museum of Munich organized a ball on January 7, 1809, the ladies were asked to draw lots to determine their position in the écossaise row.[181] For contredanses and the quadrille, a lottery also was recommended.[182] None of these dances required an intimate and dedicated relationship to a partner. In contredanses and the quadrille, the exchange of partners was customary in the dance. Moreover, in a dance with complicated figures, one's position in the row or circle reflected his or her status. For instance, in the écossaise, the closer one was to the lead dancer, the more important was the role one took in the respective dance. In the Museum of Munich, which had several members from the high nobility, this produced an obvious problem, in view of the increasing attendance of bourgeois members. In the waltz, neither one's position in the social hierarchy nor the changeability of the partner was easy to arrange. And the waltz was the dominant dance after the Napoleonic Wars.

## Social Recognition

The clash between the intimacy of ballroom dances and the persistent need for social distance brought a variety of social strategies, whose characteristics I have described in the preceding sections. In order to understand the nature of these practices and their social importance, I would like to revisit my observations in terms of social recognition. In his recent work, Axel Honneth has reformulated Hegel's ideas of social recognition by describing its three different stages: the private and familial recognition of love, the political and legal struggle for rights, and the ethical longing for solidarity.[183] By introducing the concept of social recognition, Honneth overcomes the narrow meanings of such political and legal categories as liberalism and equality. Recognition, although it is made possible by political and legal struggle, is a social process of identity formation. Although it has been used to describe collective actions and relationships, it is essentially the concept of intersubjective relationships. Dancing is a good example of how intersubjective relationships contributed to the recognition of one's social status and individuality and therefore connected a person to his group, gender, and social class.[184]

In his depiction of the Pyrmont spa and its social system in the eighteenth century, Reinhold Kuhnert has made an important observation. In discussing conflicts between bourgeois and aristocratic guests of Pyrmont, he notices that criticism by the bourgeoisie was never directed against the "legal and political privileges of the aristocracy" but instead targeted the personal (*menschliche*) conduct of the aristocrats."[185] This seems to be true of the intersubjective relationships of dancing during the early nineteenth century as well. The practices of exclusion, avoidance, and engagement used by dancers did not challenge the political order; we cannot find any radical quest for equality in these practices. The status of women and Jews, rather than continuously improving, was subject to fluctuation contingent on the local and national balance of power. Yet we can detect a feature that strikingly characterizes dancing as a form of social recognition: Dancing practices were reciprocal without being equal. In an important way, this characteristic was dependent on the body as the vehicle of recognition.

The social importance of the body was its capacity to convey first impressions. Pasch had written that dancing masters should teach their students "how they shall be courteous and elegant in their manners toward distinguished persons."[186] So the body had two dimensions: It was a vehicle of good behavior, greeting, and compliments and an instrument of expression, a substitute for and extension of language. At the same time, it was an object of veneration or irreverence, an object that made—or failed to make—an impression by virtue of its own shape. It was always quicker and more effective than words. As Ivensen and Roller argued, it was the messenger of the first impressions that, ultimately, gave significant hints of one's moral qualities.[187] From a dancer's point of view both functions were vital: how one was socially recognized and how one recognized the bodies of others.

Schleiermacher challenged this body-centered view of sociability and social recognition by suggesting social interaction that did not lend itself to utilitarian use and provided outlines of a social form that "cultivated people claim as their first and most refined need."[188] He applied Kant's theory of aesthetic perception to a social interaction that should be pursued for its own sake. This interaction had two properties: Everything should contribute to interaction, and everyone could maximize the associations related to one's own ideas.[189] Neither was applicable to a ball.

> A ball is not a form of sociability because each dancer communicates only with the partner with whom he is dancing at the moment. They both treat the rest of the society as only a medium or tool for them. Therefore the English style of dancing with only one partner the whole evening is much more consequent than our style [of changing partners after one or two dances].[190]

Only conversation appeared to fulfill the requirements of sociability, because other means necessarily limited the realization of human potential. Thus Schleiermacher agreed that one could make inferences from the physical appearance, and in fact one often did, but from this recognition one could not proceed to recognition of the human being as a whole. That is to say, the recognition of bodies could not convey a recognition that would be equal to all.

If one argues that the recognition of physical appearance was so repressive, and if dancing were so detrimental to sociability, why should anyone pay attention to the physical appearance of another? Schleiermacher's position, an apology for the salons in which intellectual conversation flourished, clearly implied that one should not pay attention to appearance.[191] But he failed to recognize the other part of the dancing discourse: Bodies were not only tools for compliments, as he seemed to think, but also objects of moral inference and veneration. In so being, they did not have to establish equality but only acknowledge a reciprocal relationship. As we have seen in descriptions of guests rejected and excluded, of how they engaged a partner or avoided dancing altogether, the underlying premise was not equality and security but social asymmetry and insecurity. The process of reciprocal recognition needed social asymmetry. The lower-ranking person was expected to recognize his or her superior, whereas the higher-ranking person could and should recognize his or her inferior only under certain carefully considered conditions, such as that person's visible merits, respectful demeanor, and sincere intentions. This was Schleiermacher's problem. He wanted to create a social environment in which everyone was included who could promote the common goal of mutual understanding and excitement. Exclusion, he said, should be situational and not permanent. It was the equality of mutual tolerance that was to suggest the air of a genuine salon and its conversation.[192] In dancing and social clubs, exclusion (when executed) was permanent, and mutual recognition took place on an agreed-upon level of social asymmetry. This asymmetry, once again, was needed to provide the basis of a process that formed one's self—the process of *Bildung*.

## Notes

1. According to Kurt Petermann's *Tanzbibliographie. Verzeichnis der in deutscher Sprache veröffentlichten Schriften und Aufsätze zum Bühnen-, Gesellschafts-, Kinder-, Volks- und Turniertanz sowie zur Tanzwissenschaft, Tanzmusik und zum Jazz*, vols. 1–5 (München: Verl. Dokumentation Saur, 1978-1987) just fifteen dancing manuals were published between 1800 and 1820, whereas during the following thirty years forty-six manuals came out. Cf. Braun and Gugerli, *Macht des Tanzes*, 229.

2. Reingard Witzmann, *Der Ländler in Wien. Ein Beitrag zur Entwicklungsgeschichte des Wiener Walzers bis in die Zeit des Wiener Kongresses* (Wien: Arbeitsstelle für den Volkskundeatlas in Österreich, 1976), 80, 175–83, does not analyze the social nexus of ballroom dancing but she still supports the interpretation that the new waltz—not the early waltz of the peasant class—was particularly a dance of the urban bourgeoisie.

3. Witzmann, *Ländler*, 80–81. See also, for instance, Braun and Gugerli, *Macht des Tanzes*, 210, and Eichberg, *Leistung*, 158.

4. Braun and Gugerli, *Macht des Tanzes*, 227–36.

5. Eichberg, *Leistung*, 189. Eichberg does not equate "democratic" with the "bourgeoisie" but sees the aristocracy as a participant in this "revolution" of intensification and innovation, Eichberg, *Leistung*, 245–47, 254–56, 278–80. Eichberg's insights are informed by August Nitschke's studies of the historical anthropology of Europe from the late Middle Ages until the twentieth century. See, for instance, August Nitschke, *Körper in Bewegung. Gesten, Tänze und Räume in Wandel der Geschichte* (Stuttgart: Kreuz-Verlag, 1989) and more concisely in his *Bewegungen in Mittelalter und Renaissance. Kämpfe, Spiele, Tänze, Zeremoniell und Umgangsformen* (Düsseldorf: Schwann, 1987), esp. chapters on physical exercise and dancing. Volker Saftien, a disciple of Nitschke, adheres to the same interpretation, although he focuses on the Renaissance and the Baroque, Saftien, *Ars Saltandi*, 372–85. Nitschke and his disciples' configurational studies of the transformation from the minuet to the waltz would profit from an empirical investigation on dancing events, balls, and assemblies. In Monika Fink's *Der Ball. Eine Kulturgeschichte des Gesellschaftstanzes im 18. und 19. Jahrhundert* (Innsbruck: Studien Verlag, 1996), we have that study. It provides a wealth of material and a systematic account of balls between 1700 and 1900 in Switzerland, Austria, and South Germany. Unfortunately, Fink does not analyze systematically how the crucial change from the minuet to the waltz influenced balls and their social setting.

6. Among the German literati, Fichte was the first to systematically use the concept of mutual recognition (*Anerkennung*). In his *Grundlage des Naturrechts* (1796), Fichte defined mutual recognition as the foundation of the theory of right (*Recht*) keeping in mind bourgeois society and carefully excluding feudal connotations of honor, prestige, and reputation, Wolfgang Janke's "Anerkennung. Fichtes Grundlegung des Rechstgrundes," in *Selbstbehauptung und Anerkennung. Spinoza—Kant—Fichte—Hegel*, ed. Helmut Girndt (Sankt Augustin: Academia Verlag, 1990), 96–98. Fichte's interpretation of mutual recognition was symmetric: genuine recognition was possible on the basis of mutual acceptance of the other's right to self-determination. Hegel started to develop the theory of mutual recognition during his tenure in Jena. Unlike Fichte he affirmed its feudal characteristics. Although the young Hegel realized the social equality of mutual recognition, its most paradigmatic elaborations, such as the relationship of lordship and bondsmen and the self-estrangement of the spirit (*Phänomenologie des Geistes*) were strikingly asymmetri-

cal. In his later philosophy, especially in the *Grundlinien der Philosophie des Rechts*, Hegel moved to Fichte's direction and situated mutual recognition in bourgeois society (*bürgerliche Gesellschaft*) within contracts and commercial exchange. Mutual recognition was, again, deprived its asymmetrical characteristics. On Hegel's juridical notion of recognition, see chapters in Helmut Girndt, ed., *Selbstbehauptung und Anerkennung* by Dieter Suhr, "Dialektik der Anerkennung in Hegels bürgerlicher Gesellschaft," esp. chapter "Anerkennung des konkreten Menschen." An excellent introduction to the current discussion on mutual recognition is in Klaus Roth, "Selbstbehauptung und Anerkennung bei G.W.F. Hegel," in *Selbstbehauptung und Anerkennung. Spinoza—Kant—Fichte—Hegel*, ed. Helmut Girndt (Sankt Augustin: Academia Verlag, 1990) esp. 177–80. Roth's approach is informed by legal theory and omits the rhetoric and self-presentational aspects that constituted the feudal practices of mutual recognition and indirectly influenced Hegel's definition of *Anerkennung*. See also Axel Honneth in his *The Struggle for Recognition. The Moral Grammar of Social Conflicts* (Cambridge/Mass.: Polity Press, 1995), which has opened a fresh look into the processes of mutual recognition, pays little attention to the problems of self-presentation and the culture of bodily conduct. See esp. the chapter "Patterns of Intersubjective Recognition: Love, Rights, and Solidarity." Yet the asymmetrical elements, I suggest, are crucial in analyzing the processes of social recognition, and especially those in which the body and its appearance were involved.

7. On the discussion of the notion of honor in women's history see, for instance, Ute Frevert, *"Mann und Weib, und Weib und Mann." Geschlechter-Differenzen in der Moderne* (München: Beck, 1995), 187–201 and the literature given there. Frevert argues that in Germany the code of female honor in the nineteenth century remained subordinated to the husband's, father's, or brother's honor. This observation is correct in view of such legal matters as infidelity, whereas the associational life and the semi-public sphere provided a different social environment in which female honor could display positive and independent characteristics. Invitations to dance and conversation were good examples of this. On women's honor and its relationship to sexuality, see Hull, *Sexuality, State*, 82–84.

8. Friedrich Zunkel, "Ehre," in *Geschichtliche Grundbegriffe*, vol. 2, ed. Otto Brunner, Werner Conze, and Reinhart Koselleck (Stuttgart: Kett-Cotta, 1975), 17–30. Cf. Richard van Dülmen, *Die Kultur und Alltag in der Frühen Neuzeit*, vol. 2, *Dorf und Staat 16.–18. Jahrhundert* (München: Beck, 1992), 194ff. and Wolfgang Martens, *Die Botschaft der Tugend. Die Aufklärung im Spiegel der deutschen moralischen Wochenschriften* (Stuttgart: Metzler, 1971), 300–2, 373–78. See the abundant literature on the history of honor in Early Modern Europe in Sibylle Backmann, ed., *Ehrkonzepte in der frühen Neuzeit. Identitäten und Abgrenzunge* (Berlin: Akademie Verlag, 1998) and esp. Martin Dinges's seminal article on the "Die Ehre als Thema der Stadtgeschichte" in *Zeitschrift für historische Forschung* 16 (1989): 409–40.

9. This was the theme in works, such as *Introductio ad philosophiam aulicam* (1688), *Weitere Erleuterung durch unterschiedene Exempel des ohnlängst gethanen Vorschlags wegen der neuen Wissenschaft anderer Menschen Gemüther erkennen zu lernen* (1692), and *Von der Kunst, vernünfftig und tugendhaft zu lieben. Als dem eintzigen Mittel zu einen glückseligen, galanten und vergnügten Leben zu gelangen. Oder Einleitung zur Sitten-Lehre* (1692). Twenty years later, after a period of Pietist desperation and debate on matters of a juridical nature, Thomasius crowned his works in 1713 with *Kurtzer Entwurff der politischen Klugheit, sich selbst und andern in allen menschlichen Gesellschaften wohl zu rathen und zu einer gescheiden Conduite zu gelangen* (Franckfurth; Leipzig: Gross, 1713).

10. Christian Thomasius, *Von der Kunst, vernünfftig und tugendhaft zu lieben. Als dem eintzigen Mittel zu einen glückseligen, galanten und vergnügten Leben zu gelangen. Oder Einleitung zur Sitten-Lehre* (Halle: Christoph Salfeld, 1692), 102.

11. Christian Thomasius, *Von der Kunst, vernünfftig und tugendhaft zu lieben. Als dem eintzigen Mittel zu einen glückseligen, galanten und vergnügten Leben zu gelangen. Oder Einleitung zur Sitten-Lehre* (Halle: Christoph Salfeld, 1692), 101. See also his *Kurtzer Entwurff der politischen Klugheit*, esp. 97–102. Meticulously crafting a complex table in which each social passion—lust (*Wollust*), greed (*Geld-Geiz*), and ambition (*Ehr-Geiz*)—and its combination with another passion denoted a set of social and bodily characteristics, Thomasius set forth a guide to detecting the secret nature of the soul. The most important application of this technique was the art of cleverness (*Klugheitslehre*). On Thomasius politics of *conduite*, see the outstanding analyses of Manfred Beetz, "Ein neuentdeckter Lehrer der Conduite. Thomasius in der Geschichte der Gesellschaftscthik," in *Christian Thomasius 1655–1728. Interpretationen zu Werk und Wirkung. Mit einer Bibliographie der neueren Thomasius-Literatur*, ed. Werner Schneiders (Hamburg: Meiner, 1989), esp. 201–4 and Frederick M. Barnard, "Rightful Decorum and Rational Accountability. A Forgotten Theory of Civil Life," in *Christian Thomasius 1655–1728. Interpretationen zu Werk und Wirkung. Mit einer Bibliographie der neueren Thomasius-Literatur*, ed. Werner Schneiders (Hamburg: Meiner, 1989), esp. 187–89.

12. Thomasius, *Einleitung zur Sitten-Lehre*, 98.

13. Christian Thomasius [probable author], *Bericht von Einrichtung des Paedagogii zu Glaucha an Halle. Nebst der von einem gelehrten Manne verlangten Erinnerung über solche Einrichtung* (Franckfurt; Leipzig, 1699), 3. Thomasius' anonymously published comments are from January 1699. The printed text was only a part of a more elaborate commentary that Fleischmann has located in the University Library of Bonn. These "Additamenta" contain remarks and questions on the method of moral education (*elegantium morum*), Christian Thomasius, "Additamenta ad notas praecedentes," in *Christian Thomasius. Leben und Lebenswerk*, ed. Max Fleischmann (Halle: Max Niemeyer Verlag, 1931), 419–20. Thomasius was not sure whether Francke's method would be effective in teaching manners if he required equality of all Christians and simple forms of greeting: a handshake instead of a bow in the French style.

14. Thomasius, *Bericht von Einrichtung*, 4–5, 10. In Thomasius's rendering of Francke's proposal the term was the "äusserlichen wolanständigen Sitten."

15. August Hermann Francke, "Was von dem weltüblichen Tanzen zu halten sei, Vorrede, 1697," in *Werke in Auswahl*, ed. Erhard Peschke (Berlin: Luther-Verlag, 1969), 386.

16. On this debate see the bibliographic note in Kurt Petermann, "Nachwort," in Johann Pasch, *Beschreibung wahrer Tanz-Kunst, Nebst einigen Anmerckungen über Herrn J.C.L.P.P. zu G. Bedencken gegen das Tanzen (1707)* (Munich: Reimer Verlag, 1978), III–IV. Friedrich Eberhard Collin's *Der grosse Ernst des thätigen Christenthums aller vergnüglichen Welt- Spiel- und Tanz-Lust entgegen* (Halle: Waisenhaus, 1719) could be added to Petermann's list.

17. Petermann, "Nachwort," II–III. It would be worth a detailed study to follow this debate throughout the eighteenth century. Although Saftien sees the efforts to legitimize dancing as a scientific enterprise as a special German feature there is a broader question of how the Pietism and related religious regimens influenced body culture in German principalities, Saftien, *Ars Saltandi*, 283.

18. Pasch, *Beschreibung wahrer Tanz-Kunst*, 16.

19. Pasch, *Beschreibung wahrer Tanz-Kunst*, 43.

20. Samuel Rudolph Behr, *Anleitung zu einer wohlgegründeten Tantz-Kunst . . .* (Leipzig: Chp. Heydlern, 1703); Meletaon [Johann Leonhard Rost], *Von der Nutzbarkeit des Tanzens. Wie viel selbiges zu einer Galanten und wohlanständigen Conduite bey einem jungen Menschen und Frauenzimmer beytrage; Auch wie man dadurch sowol die Kinder als erwachsene Leute von beederley Geschlechte zur Höflichkeit, Artigkeit und Freymüthigkeit anweisen solle* (Franckfurt und Leipzig: Joh. Albrecht, 1713); Gottfried Taubert, *Rechtschaffener Tanzmeister, oder gründliche Erklärung der Frantzösischen Tanz-Kunst*, vols 1–3. (Leipzig: Friedrich Lanckischens Erben, 1717). Although by a French author, still popular was Louis Bonin's *Neueste Art zur Galanten und Theatralischen Tantz-Kunst* (Franckfurt und Leipzig: Joh. Christoff Lochner, 1712).

21. Braun's and Gugerli's depiction of the dance configurations and their social functions in the court of Louis XIV provide a good narrative of how dances were used for social regulation and control of the nobility, Braun and Gugerli, *Macht des Tanzes*, 164–65. Whether the classical French dance can be reduced to this function only, as Braun and Gugerli seem to indicate, is debatable. Dances also made possible new forms of the expression of one's nature.

22. Saftien, *Ars Saltandi*, 365–66. See also, Curt Sachs's *Eine Weltgeschichte des Tanzes* (Berlin: Dietrich Reimer & Ernst Vohsen, 1933), 2.

23. Taubert also mentions the bourrée as a standard dance, *Rechtschaffener Tanzmeister*, 10.

24. According to Fink the Viennese court was one of those that nurtured the minuet, Fink, *Der Ball*, 117. Witzmann indicates, however, that during the era of Maria Theresia the court of Hapsburg preferred to German dances, Witzmann, *Ländler*, 25.

25. Johann Wolfgang von Goethe, *Werke*, vol. 9 (Munich: Deutscher Taschenbuch Verlag, 1974), 389.

26. In fifteenth-century Italian dancing, the compliments were standardized in view of their practical use, Saftien, *Ars Saltandi*, 108. For their characteristics by the early nineteenth century, see for instance, Ernst Christian Mädel, *Anfangsgründe der Tanzkunst oder genaueste Angabe zur Erlernung und Wiederholung aller jezzo üblichen Tänze, ohne Beihülfe eines Tanzmeisters* (Erfurt: Ernst Christian Mädel, 1801), 26, 33, 41–49. Normally the compliment was based upon a combination of positions two and three but a combination of one and four was also used, as Bartholomay points out in describing the compliment forward (*Vorkompliment*), Bartholomay, *Tanzkunst*, 265–74.

27. Pasch, *Beschreibung wahrer Tanz-Kunst*, 103.

28. One of the earliest (1782) defenses of the minuet against the perils of the waltz can be found in Carl Georg von Zangen, *Etwas über das Walzen, nebst einigen Gedichten und Anhang einiger Oden* (Wetzlar: Philipp Jacob Winkler, 1782), 7–12.

29. Salomo Jakob Wolf, *Beweis daß das Walzen eine Hauptquelle der Schwäche des Körpers und des Geistes unserer Generation sey. Deutschlands Söhnen und Töchtern angelegentlichst empfohlen.* Zweyte Auflage (Halle: Johann Christian Hendel, 1799), 19. See also Zangen, *Etwas über das Walzen*, 7–8. More moderate but still moralistic undertones can be found in Vieth, *Versuch einer Encyklopädie*, vol. 2, 289 and GutsMuths, *Gymnastik 1804*, 34.

30. Braun and Gugerli, *Macht des Tanzes*, 166–77; Witzmann, *Ländler*, 175–83.

31. Hentschke, *Allgemeine Tanzkunst*, 35.

32. Roller, *Systematisches Lehrbuch*, 19. For a nostalgic longing for the lost art of the minuet see Bartholomay, *Tanzkunst*, 74; Dietrich Alexander Valentin Ivensen, *Terpsichore, ein Taschenbuch für Freunde und Freundinnen des Tanzes in Liv-, Kur- und Estland* (Riga: Steffenhagen und Sohn, 1806), 21, 48; Christian Länger, *Terpsichore. Ein Taschenbuch der neuesten gesellschaftlichen Tänze, worin zugleich Anweisung gegeben wird, wie man 40 Touren und 76 Tänze ohne orchesigraphische Zeichnungen und ohne Lehrer erlernen kann. Zum Nutzen und Vergnügen für Freude der Tanzkunst* (Würzburg: Etlingersche Buch- und Kunsthandlung, 1824), 10; Mädel, *Anfangsgründe der Tanzkunst*, 13; Franz Xaver Nadler, *Kallischematik, oder Anleitung zu einem edlen Anstande und zur schönen, gefälligen Haltung des Körpers, . . .* (München: George Jaquet, 1834), 148–50; Gotthelf Tschütter, *Terpsichore. Ein Taschenbuch der neueren Tanzkunst für Anfänger und solche, die bereits einige Kenntnisse erlangt haben und sich darin vervollkommnen wollen* (Dresden; Leipzig: Arnold'sche Buchhandlung, 1828), XIII. For Schönwald, as for most of his collegues, the minuet was the queen of all dances, the only one which truly promoted bearing, Andreas Schönwald, *Grundregeln der Tanzkunst* (Freyburg: Herdersche Buchhandlung, 1812), 30. Cf. *Neuer Tanz- und Ball-Kalender für 1801* (Berlin: Johann Friedrich Unger, August von, 1800), 114. See also the complaints in the *Journal des Luxus und der Moden* about the disappearance of the minuet, "Eger," *Journal des Luxus und der Moden* (November 1799): 559. At the same time a physician from Hamburg, Rambach, tried to reintroduce the minuet as an optimal exercise which allowed gradual change between motion and immobility, Johann Jakob Rambach, *Versuch einer physisch-medizinischen Beschreibung von Hamburg* (Hamburg: Carl Ernst Bohm, 1801), 220. Cf. Johann Evangelist Wetzler, *Ueber den Einfluß des Tanzes auf die Gesundheit nebst Verhaltensregeln* (Landshut: Anton Weber'sche Buchhandlung, 1801), 10. Even in a social club, *Tunnel* of Leipzig, in the 1830s some members voiced their wish to return to the minuet, Walter Lange, *Der Tunnel 1831 bis 1931* (Leipzig: Verlag Deutsche Buchwerkstätten, 1931), 48.

33. Eduard David Helmke, *Neue Tanz- und Bildungsschule. Ein gründlicher Leitfaden für Eltern und Lehrer bei der Erziehung der Kinder und für die Erwachsene Jugend, um sich einen hohen Grad der feinen Bildung zu verschaffen und sich zu kunstfertigen und ausgezeichneten Tänzern zu bilden* (Leipzig: Christian Ernst Rollmann, 1829), 4. Cf. Schönwald, *Grundregeln der Tanzkunst*, IX.

34. Pasch, *Beschreibung wahrer Tanz-Kunst*, 42. Pasch uses the term *Geste* which signifies all the expressive movements of the body, in addition to steps. On the nineteenth-century nostalgia for *port de bras*, see Bartholomay, *Tanzkunst*, 32–34; August von Rosenhain, *Bemerkungen über das Tanzen; nebst einer gründlichen Anleitung zu den jetzt beliebtesten Tänzen. Besonders für seine Scholaren bearbeitet* (Schleswig: Königliches Staubstummen-Institut, 1821), 28; Franz Anton Roller, "Ueber die Bildung des Körpers zum Tanzen," in *Erstes Toilettengeschenk. Ein Jahrbuch für Damen* (Leipzig: Georg Voss, 1805), 63; Franz Anton Roller, "Versuch einer Theorie der Tanzkunst," in *Zweites Toilettengeschenk. Ein Jahrbuch für Damen* (Leipzig: Georg Voss, 1806), 120. Especially in the allemande, an old, solemn, and graceful dance in 4/4 time with characteristic flow to the arms and the figuration, Franz Anton Roller, "Die Allemande," in *Viertes Toilettengeschenk. Ein Jahrbuch für Damen* (Leipzig: Georg Voss, 1808), 54–58.

35. Vieth, *Versuch einer Encyklopädie*, vol. 2, 301, 335. See also Nadler, *Kallischematik*, 78; Helmke, *Neue Tanz- und Bildungsschule*, 27.

36. Hentschke, *Allgemeine Tanzkunst*, 5. Bartholomay, although conservative in his adherence to the classic French school of dancing, distinguishes between the *port de bras* in ballroom and ballet, Bartholomay, *Tanzkunst*, 34.

37. Nadler, *Kallischematik*, 37; Hentschke, *Allgemeine Tanzkunst*, 118. "Here the face has to express openness and cheerfulness. The look must be lively."

38. See Mädel, *Anfangsgründe der Tanzkunst*, 25, 33–34; Gourdoux-Daux, *Tanzkunst*, 25–26. On the extensive research on minuet choreography see Saftien, *Ars Saltandi*, 347–353 and the references given.

39. Mädel, *Anfangsgründe der Tanzkunst*, 143–44. Gourdoux-Daux identified in the waltz false positions, Gourdoux-Daux, *Tanzkunst*, 53.

40. Vieth, *Versuch einer Encyklopädie*, vol. 2, 342. Schönwald considered the waltz to be a dance without bearing, Schönwald, *Grundregeln der Tanzkunst*, IX. Gaulhofer wants to draw the conclusion that the new culture of dancing which replaced the minuet was atheoretical. In reference to the nineteenth-century ballroom dances he maintains that "the new dance figuration should have brought about its own independent theory. Yet it never materialized," Karl Gaulhofer, *Die Fußhaltung. Ein Beitrag zur Stilgeschichte der menschlichen Bewegung*, vol. 1 (Kassel: Rudolph'sche Verlagsanstalt, 1930), 146.

41. Witzmann, *Ländler*, 24. See also Braun and Gugerli, *Macht des Tanzes*, esp. chapters "Der Walzer wird König, und der Bürger sucht seine Verhaltensform" and "Der Wildling wird gezähmt: der Wiener Walzer im 'bürgerlichen' Jahrhundert."

42. As mentioned earlier, the emergence of an individual couple and the gradual merging of the audience and the performers did not necessarily entail a shift toward a more democratic and bourgeois culture of dancing. See also Witzmann, *Ländler*, 80–81; Eichberg, *Leistung*, 158, 185.

43. Tschütter, *Terpsichore*, 228; Helmke, *Neue Tanz- und Bildungsschule*, 87. Gourdoux-Daux, a French dancing master whose manual was translated into German in 1830, introduced two variations of the waltz—*la valse de change* and *la Russe*. The first one includes, in addition to a set number of eight couples, figures. *La Russe* was designed for two or three couples that dance certain figures, Gourdoux-Daux, *Tanzkunst*, 58–59. According to Fink, whose material comes mainly from South Germany and Austria, before the 1850s the number of waltzing couples was always limited in public dancing venues, Fink, *Der Ball*, 52.

44. Franz Anton Roller, "Wahrscheinliche Ursache des Verfalls der Tanzkunst als Privatvergnügen,""in *Toilettengeschenk. Ein Jahrbuch für Damen* (Leipzig: Georg Voss, 1807), 108; Roller, *Systematisches Lehrbuch*, 20. In the *Journal des Luxus und der Moden* 1802, a "Z." suggested that the local theaters should be in charge of promoting ballroom dancing, Z.,"Der Tanz, wie er ist, und seyn könnte," *Journal des Luxus und der Moden* (Januar 1802): 7.

45. Anonymous, "Vorwort des Herausgebers" in Hentschke, *Allgemeine Tanzkunst*, vii.

46. Z., "Tanz, wie er ist," 6.

47. Helmke gives an account of a widely publicized performance in 1812, Eduard David Helmke, *Almanach der neuesten Modetänze auf das Jahr 1833. Für Freunde und Freundinnen der höheren Tanzkunst* (Merseburg: Fr. Weidemann, 1835), 106–8.

48. Braun and Gugerli, *Macht des Tanzes*, 232–34, explain the enormous demand for courtesy literature and the rise of a specific discourse of bearing by the increased bourgeois awareness of etiquette after the Congress of Vienna.

49. Bartholomay, *Tanzkunst*, 74.

50. Schönwald, *Grundregeln der Tanzkunst*, 30; Roller, "Theorie der Tanzkunst," 121.

51. "Künstlich angebildet," August Hermann Niemeyer, "Anstand," in *Allgemeine Encyclopädie*, vol. 3, eds. Ersch and Gruber, 243. As Johann Christoph Adelung mentions in his *Grammatisch-Kritisches Wörterbuch der hochdeutschen Mundart*, vol. 1. (Leipzig: Breitkopf und Härtel, 1793), 377, the word *Anstand* was new to the German language at the end of the eighteenth century. For instance Zedler's *Universal-Lexikon*, vol. 1, 105, defined it as synonymous with *Stillstand* (standstill), which referred to the immobility of planets or physical objects or "for artisans also to know about the skills" (bey den Handwerckern bald von der Lehre und Schule zu verstehen). The motivation to introduce it as a concept of social behavior was the need to find a German equivalent for the French word *air*. It is exactly this meaning which Adelung gave to *Anstand*. "That which pleases, as far as this verb expresses the skillfulness in behavior, the relationship of behavior to innate perfections, which one has or, at least should have in respect to ones status, vocation, and the environment." (Dasjenige, was anstehet, so fern dieses Verbum das Schickliche in dem äußern Betragen ausdruckt, das Verhältnis des äußern Betragens mit den innern Vollkommenheiten, die man hat, oder doch vermöge seines Standes und Berufes, und der jedesmaligen Umstände haben sollte), Adelung, *Grammatisch-Kritisches Wörterbuch*, vol. 1, 377. Thus, *Anstand* was understood as a quality of behavior that could be derived from the social conventions and status qualities of the existing social order. It is, however, clear that Adelung's understanding, which very likely followed the common usage, was challenged by new qualities. Johann Christoph Friedrich GutsMuths (1793) extended the scope of this concept by speaking of "manly carriage" (*männlichem Anstand*) which was based on "physical power and dexterity" (*körperliche Kraft und Schmeidigkeit*), GutsMuths, *Gymnastik 1793*, 372. According to this definition, *Anstand* was now something powerful that belonged to the human (male) nature and transcended the conventional limitations of the old social order, whereas the other part was tightly bound to the very same order. This tension was reflected in the common usage of the word throughout the first decades of the nineteenth century. On the one hand, *Anstand* was correct only when it was spontaneously expressed. On the other hand the social aspect, meaning the plain conventions of the existing social order, became less and less important because the requirements of an *anständigen* conduct increased with the expectations of higher education (*Bildung*) which was connected with the upper class. See Niemeyer, "Anstand," 243.

52. "The genuine, noble carriage should not be an empty expression of public representation but it must be an expression of the inwardly, completely, intellectually cultivated human being," *Neues Conversations-Lexicon oder encyclopädisches Handwörterbuch für gebildete Stände. Herausgegeben von einer Gesellschaft rheinländischer Gelehrten*, vol. 1 (Köln; Bonn, 1824), 292.

53. Helmke, *Neue Tanz- und Bildungsschule*, 8.

54. Helmke, *Neue Tanz- und Bildungsschule*, 9.

55. Braun and Gugerli see Helmke as the bourgeois ideologue who rejected the etiquette of inequality and advocated an internalized sense of propriety, Braun and Gugerli, *Macht des Tanzes*, 233. It is true that this was his aim but the detailed prescriptions of behavior in the practical part of the book testify against this intention. In fact, Helmke's

practical prescriptions refute his theoretical plan for a humanistic, inward *Anstand.*

56. Helmke, *Neue Tanz- und Bildungsschule*, 12.

57. Schönwald, *Grundregeln der Tanzkunst*, 32–34.

58. Bartholomay, *Tanzkunst*, IV.

59. Christian Länger's *Terpsichore* (1824) gave an exhaustive account of écossaises. Louis Casorti described rarer dances, such as the *chaine* and galop, Louis Casorti, *Der instructive Tanzmeister für Herren und Damen, oder die Kunst, sich in kurzer Zeit durch bloßen Selbstunterricht* (Iimenau: Bernh. Fr. Voigt, 1826), esp. 35–100. A host of annuals, such as Becker's *Taschenbuch zum geselligen Vergnügen*, and women's journals, such as *Toilettengeschenck*, disseminated new dancing music for home consumption, musical soirees, and balls. See, for instance, A.H., "Kurze Uebersicht von neuen und interessanten Kompositionen für die musikalischen Leserinnen dieses Toilettengeschenks," in *Viertes Toilettengeschenk. Ein Jahrbuch für Damen* (Leipzig: Georg Voss, 1808), 61–63.

60. Franz Anton Roller, "Unser jetziger Tanz," in *Erstes Toilettengeschenk. Ein Jahrbuch für Damen* (Leipzig: Georg Voss, 1805), 69.

61. Marlies Prüsener, "Lesegesellschaften im 18. Jahrhundert," *Archiv für Geschichte des Buchwesens* 13 (1973): 411–14.

62. Martin Welke gives a considerably higher number. According to his estimation, there were some 1,000 reading societies during the late eighteenth and early nineteenth centuries, Martin Welke, "Gemeinsame Lektüre und frühe Formen von Gruppenbildungen im 17. Und 18. Jahrhundert. Zeitungslesen in Deutschland" in *Lesegesellschaften und bürgerliche Emanzipation. Ein europäischer Vergleich*, ed., Otto Dann (München, 1981), 45. But considering Prüsener's meticulous and conservative use of sources—she has included only those societies documented either in journals or archival records—a reliable number might be closer to her estimation. See Prüsener, "Lesegesellschaften," 376.

63. In Lothar Gall's large project on the city and bourgeoisie in Germany in the nineteenth century, the emphasis is predominantly on the forms of domination (*Herrschaft*), Lothar Gall, "Vom alten zum neuen Bürgertum. Die mitteleuropäische Stadt im Umbruch 1780–1820," in *Vom alten zum neuen Bürgertum. Die mitteleuropäische Stadt im Umbruch 1780–1820*, vol. 14, *Historische Zeitschrift. Beihefte (Neue Folge)*, ed. Lothar Gall (München: Oldenbourg, 1991) 6–8. Also Lothar Gall, "Die Bassermanns. Eine Mannheimer Bürgerfamilie zwischen Ancien Régime und moderner Welt," in *Bildungsbürgertum im 19. Jahrhundert*, vol. 3, *Lebensführung und ständische Vergesellschaftung*, ed. M. Rainer Lepsius (Stuttgart: Klett-Cotta, 1992) 104–12. Gall has elaborated on what Thomas Nipperdey indicated in his article, "Verein als soziale Struktur in Deutschland im späten 18 und frühen 19. Jahrhundert," in *Gesellschaft, Kultur, Theorie. Gesammelte Aufsätze zur neueren Geschichte* (Göttingen: Vandenhoeck & Ruprecht, 1976), see esp. 182–83. Gall see, associations as the vehicles of modernization. Yet, the instruments he uses are not sensitive to the questions that arise from "below." Trepp's depiction of the intricate social networking of women in Hamburg indicates a new approach. The social clubs imitated and formalized many of the practices that had been established on an informal level by reading circles, dinners, family circles, and private balls. See Trepp, *Sanfte Männlichkeit*, esp. 370–98. Cf. also Habermas, *Frauen und Männer*, esp. 137–71.

64. Herbert Freudenthal, *Vereine in Hamburg. Ein Beitrag zur Geschichte und Volkskunde der Geselligkeit* (Hamburg: Museum für Hamburgische Geschichte, 1968), 41.

65. On the formation of casinos and clubs from the reading societies see Prüsener, "Lesegesellschaften," 526–29. Prüsener dates the change from reading societies to social clubs in the last decade of the eighteenth century. As a criterion she uses the increasing number of women, Prüsener, "Lesegesellschaften," 513. This is not always adequate. In Berlin, for instance, several reading societies included women from the beginning, Deborah Hertz, *Jewish High Society in Old Regime Berlin* (New Haven: Yale University Press, 1988), 89–93. Also in Hamburg the famous reading society of Klopstock and Büsch gave women leading positions, Trepp, *Sanfte Männlichkeit*, 392. None of them, however, was particularly entertaining. We can therefore see these societies as imitating the intellectual flair of French salons. Hein's periodization is more accurate. He sees the early 1800s as the divide, Dieter Hein, "Soziale Konstituierungsfaktoren des Bürgertums," in *Stadt und Bürgertum im Übergang von der traditionalen zur modernen Gesellschaft*, vol. 16, *Historische Zeitschrift, Beiheft*, ed. Lothar Gall (München: R. Oldenbourg, 1993), 155–68.

66. Gall developed his argument of classless bourgeois society in "Liberalismus und bürgerliche Gesellschaft," 324–56. See also Gall,"Vom alten zum neuen Bürgertum," 10–17, in which he elaborates on his old thesis, specifying its scope to the increasing transgression of boundaries between the educated middle class and the traditional patrician groups and the subsequent dynamics of the German bourgeoisie during the nineteenth century. The associations (*Vereine*), according to Gall, were the sites of a bourgeois utopia.

67. I have not included Berlin in my sample for a variety of reasons. First, whereas Berlin's role as the center of the gymnastics movement was self-evident, it showed little if any leadership in support of moderate exercises, such as dancing and walking. In the contemporary commentaries Vienna occupies this position. Nor was Berlin a typical German city of reading societies and social clubs but a city of intellectual salons that only Vienna could match. On the salons of Berlin, see the exhausting narrative of Petra Wilhelmy, *Der Berliner Salon im 19. Jahrhundert (1780–1914)* (Berlin: Walter de Gruyter, 1989) and Hertz, *Jewish High Society*, analysis of the Jewish salons in the late eighteenth and the early nineteenth century. The wealth of recent scholarship on Berlin and its educated middle class allows it to be included in the comparison when appropriate.

68. Gall, "Vom alten zum neuen Bürgertum," 5, has suggested a typology as following: 1. Cities of commerce and trade (Frankfurt am Main, Cologne, Hamburg, Bremen); 2. Early industrial cities (*Frühindustrielle Gewerbestädte*) (Aachen, Heilbronn, Esslingen, Augsburg); 3. Industrial cities (Dortmund, Essen, Bocum); 4. Capitals (*Residenzstädte*) and administrative cities (Munich, Karlsruhe, Wiesbaden, Münster); 5. University towns (Göttingen, Heidelberg); 6. Traditional cities (Wetzlar, Konstanz, Würzburg, Nördlingen); 7. Cities with rapidly changing statuses (Mannheim). With certain modifications—I did not differentiate between types of commercial cities—I have adopted Gall's model.

69. Cf. Prüsener, "Lesegesellschaften," 412 and the map on 529–30.

70. Gerhard Tanzer, *Spectacle müssen seyn. Die Freizeit der Wiener im 18. Jahrhundert* (Vienna: Böhlau, 1992), 214–17.

71. The members of the Ludlamshöhle, including the poet Grillparzer among others, considered the main focus of their club to be on entertainment. Yet entertainment, especially with dancing music played by more than one instrument, was required to be registered with the police. See, Heindl, *Gehorsame Rebellen*, 288–89.

72. Tanzer has described an official politics of leisure that started in the Josephinian era and benefitted middle class more than any other by allowing it to enter gardens, theaters, and parks, which now became "public." Tanzer, *Spectacle,* 281–82.

73. Fink argues that the difference in carnival regulations, especially with regard to the masquerades, was dependent on the local denomination. There is, however, little evidence that religious background made a major difference in the nineteenth century. Her documentation pertains mainly to the late eighteenth century. Fink, *Der Ball,* 39.

74. Ingo Tornow, *Das Münchner Vereinswesen in der ersten Hälfte des 19. Jahrhunderts. Mit einem Ausblicke auf die zweite Jahrhunderthälfte* (Munich: UNI-Druck, 1977), 43–45, has traced the foundation of "Museum" to around 1803 and "Harmonie" around 1804. No exact evidence is available but the second, and first preserved editions of their statutes are from 1808 and 1806 respectively. See also Prüsener, "Lesegesellschaften," 533.

75. In Vienna, the invitations to aristocratic and high society homes became available to the haute bourgeoisie and wealthy travelers as a matter of custom by the end of the eighteenth century (*Gesellschaften zu geben*). These social centers were fixtures in the official address books and travel guides, Tanzer, *Spectacle,* 200. Cf. Heindl, *Gehorsame Rebellen,* 275–78. Hebenstreit mentions in his travel guide of 1840 about the balls and assemblies that "such are still quite common in Vienna and someone who has been recommended to an important home will have an easy access to them," Wilhelm Hebenstreit, *Der Fremde in Wien und der Wiener in der Heimath* (Wien: Leop. Grund, 1840), 140.

76. August Lewald, *Panorama von München,* vol. 1 (Stuttgart: Hallberg'sche Verlagsbuchhandlung, 1835), 87. Although Huber reported about the exclusive assemblies and salons of the Munich aristocrats and wealthy Jewish families, Huber, *München im Jahre 1819,* vol. 1, 319, the centers of social life were elsewhere. Among the artistic elite, such as Wilhelm von Kobell, the club had become the center of life. Paul Heyse was a guest of Kobell one evening. Yet Kobell thought it completely appropriate to leave his guest after a time in order to "go to my club," Georg Jacob Wolf, ed., *Ein Jahrhundert München 1800–1900. Zeitgenössische Bilder und Dokumente* (München: Hanfstaengl, 1919), 245.

77. *Staatsarchiv Hamburg.* Bibliothek A 507/54/1 "Verfassung und Gesetze der Harmonie. Revidirt im November 1815 (Hamburg: Hermann Restler, 1815)," 1. *Universitätsarchiv Tübingen.* 406/3. "Vorschlag zur Vereinigung der hier bestehenden einzelnen Lesegesellschaften und zur Errichtung eines allen Klassen hiesiger Gebildeten gemeinsamen Verbands für Umgang und Zeitlektüre." [12/30/1817].

78. In her close reading of the "private" sphere of upper middle class women in Hamburg Trepp has distinguished ten different forms of social networking and bonding, Trepp, *Sanfte Männlichkeit,* 372–94. After comparative research on other cities it could be possible to proceed toward a typology of social forms based on a gradually increasing level of formality and publicity. This suggests that the associations and social clubs were not only progenitors of public sphere, state, and political parties but also shaped private sphere.

79. "Miscellen aus München," *Journal des Luxus und der Moden* (März 1808): 211; "Skizzen zum neuesten Gemälde von München," *Journal des Luxus und der Moden* (März 1811): 159.

80. Buek, *Wegweiser durch Hamburg,* 220–21.

81. Ernst Kroker, *Die Gesellschaft Harmonie in Leipzig 1776 bis 1926. Zum hundertfünfzigjährigen Bestehen der Gesellschaft* (Leipzig: Teubner, 1926), 50–51.

82. Lange, *Der Tunnel*, 61.

83. *Universitätsbibliotek Tübingen*, 16 A 9129. "Statuten des Tanz-Sängerkränzchens der Sängerkranz-Mitglieder." According to Eifert, the local leader of the gymnastic movement, Wüst founded it in 1829, Max Eifert, *Geschichte und Beschreibung der Stadt Tübingen* (Tübingen: Ludwig Friedrich Fues, 1849), 219.

84. Schmidt, "Das Buschbad, bey Meißen," *Journal des Luxus und der Moden* (Februar 1799): 76.

85. One of the regular advertisements of the Blasibad announced on October 13, 1828, that "all my friends and clients can then . . . entertain themselves by dancing on Monday, the 20th," "Blasibad," in *Intelligenz-Blatt für die Oberamts-Bezirke Tübingen, Rottenburg, Horb und Herrenberg* 82 (10.13.1828): 436.

86. "Bruchstück einer Reise von Frankfurt nach Wisbaden, Langenschwalbach, Schlangenbad und Brückenau, nebst Nachrichten von diesen Bädern im Monat August 1808," *Journal des Luxus und der Moden* (September 1808): 629.

87. Fink, *Der Ball*, 95–190.

88. *Stadtarchiv Leipzig*. Kap. 35, Tanzgesellschaft im Gewandhaus, Nr. 3. "Beilagen zum Protokoll der Tanz-Gesellschaft im Gewandhause vom Jahr 1810 bis 1811." Fol. 62: Betr. der Kontinentalsperre.

89. *Stadtarchiv Leipzig*. Kap. 35, Tanzgesellschaft im Gewandhaus, Nr. 4. "Beilagen zum Protokoll der Tanz-Gesellschaft im Gewandhaus vom Juli 1817 bis 1818." Fol. 4: Brief an Mitglieder betr. dem Programm.

90. *Stadtarchiv Leipzig*. Kap. 35, Tanzgesellschaft im Gewandhaus, Nr. 4. "Beilagen zum Protokoll der Tanz-Gesellschaft im Gewandhaus vom Juli 1817 bis 1818." Fol. 8: Erster Ball, Sonntags, den 19. October, 1817. The letter is from October 17, 1817.

91. On Küstner and his activities at the city theater of Leipzig, see Fritz Hennenberg, *300 Jahre Leipziger Oper. Geschichte und Gegenwart* (Munich: Langen Müller, 1993), 29–36. Küstner left in 1828 Leipzig, landed first in Darmstadt, and later made a career as an efficient theater manager in Munich and Berlin.

92. According to the repertory of the city theater, there was a performance of Ferdinando Paër's oper *Il Sargino* on Sunday, November 30, the night the *Tanz-Gesellschaft* had its ball. See Oscar Fambach, ed., *Das Repertorium des Stadttheaters zu Leipzig 1817–1828* (Bonn: Bouvier Verlag Herbert Grundmann, 1980), 13. The identity of Mr. Stein is not clear; according to the World Biographical Index by K.G. Saur Publishing (World-Wide-Web version: http://www.biblio.tu-bs.de/acwww25u/wbi_en/), Eduard Franz Stein (1794-1828) is the most likely candidate.

93. *Stadtarchiv Leipzig*. Kap. 35, Tanzgesellschaft im Gewandhaus, Nr. 4. "Beilagen zum Protokoll der Tanz-Gesellschaft im Gewandhaus vom Juli 1817 bis 1818. Fol. 16–18: Küstner an das Directorium des Gewandhausballs. Ausschliessung einiger Schauspieler, 18. December, 1817." See also, *Stadtarchiv Leipzig*. Kap. 35, Tanzgesellschaft im Gewandhaus, Nr. 4. "Beilagen zum Protokoll der Tanz-Gesellschaft im Gewandhaus vom Juli 1817 bis 1818." Fol. 21–22: Die Vorsteher der Tanz-Gesellschaft auf dem Gewandhaus an die Herren Mitglieder des Theatervereins und des Inspections-Ausschusses, 24 December, 1817.

94. Only the part of the correspondence included in the papers of the *Tanz-Gesellschaft des Gewandhauses* has been preserved. Concerning von Haugk's letter see *Stadtarchiv Leipzig*. Kap. 35, Tanzgesellschaft im Gewandhaus, Nr. 4. "Beilagen zum Protokoll der Tanz-Gesellschaft im Gewandhaus vom Juli 1817 bis 1818." Fol. 16–18:

Küstner an das Directorium des Gewandhausballs. Ausschliessung einiger Schauspieler, 18. December, 1817.

95. *Stadtarchiv Leipzig*. Kap. 35, Tanzgesellschaft im Gewandhaus, Nr. 4. "Beilagen zum Protokoll der Tanz-Gesellschaft im Gewandhaus vom Juli 1817 bis 1818." Fol. 16–18. Concerning the elaboration on recognition see *Stadtarchiv Leipzig*. Kap. 35, Tanzgesellschaft im Gewandhaus, Nr. 4. "Beilagen zum Protokoll der Tanz-Gesellschaft im Gewandhaus vom Juli 1817 bis 1818. Fol. 19–20": Der Theaterverein und der Inspections-Ausschuß an die Tanz-Gesellschaft.

96. *Stadtarchiv Leipzig*. Kap. 35, Tanzgesellschaft im Gewandhaus, Nr. 4. "Beilagen zum Protokoll der Tanz-Gesellschaft im Gewandhaus vom Juli 1817 bis 1818." Fol. 21–22.

97. In fact, Küstner attended the New Year's ball and had said he would bring three guests. The documents do not tell whether they were actors. See *Stadtarchiv Leipzig*. Kap. 35, Tanzgesellschaft im Gewandhaus, Nr. 4. "Beilagen zum Protokoll der Tanz-Gesellschaft im Gewandhaus vom Juli 1817 bis 1818." Fol. 26–28: Anmeldung zum vierten Ball, 20 December, 1817.

98. Jean Charles [pseud. of Karl Johann Braun von Braunthal], *Wien und die Wiener. Ihr öffentliches und häusliches, geistiges und materielles Leben. Ein Wegweiser für Einheimische und Fremde* (Stuttgart: Metzler, 1840), 150. On the practice of invitation in Vienna, see Tanzer, *Spectacle*, 200. On "open homes" in Berlin see Hertz, *Jewish High Society*, 98. Trepp's observations suggest that invitations and "open homes" were common among bourgeois families in Hamburg as well, Trepp, *Sanfte Männlichkeit*, 380–90.

99. Introduction of visitors, regulation of attendance, and use of club facilities were key points of all bylaws. See *Universitätsarchiv Tübingen*. 406/3. "Vorschlag zur Vereinigung;" *Geseze des Museums zu Tübingen* (Tübingen: Schramm, 1822), 10; Lange, *Der Tunnel*, 33; *Museum für die Geschichte der Stadt Leipzig*. Blauer Kasten E 2/51–128. "Gesellschaft Erholung." Fol. 87: Gesetze der Erholung. Berathen und genehmigt in einer am 5. April 1832 gehaltenen Generalversammlung (Leipzig: Hirschfeld, 1832), 21. See also *Bayerisches Hauptstaatsarchiv*. Staatsarchiv München, RA 21208. "Die Gesellschaft des Museums in München betr. De anno 1819–1846." Nr. 11: Verfassung des Museums unter dem besonderen Schutze Seiner königlichen Majestät von Baiern. Neue mit dem Beschlüssen der bisherigen General-Versammlungen vermehrte Auflage (München, 1808), 8.

100. The question of women as visitors was more complex and will be discussed later.

101. *Geseze des Museums (Tübingen)*, 10.

102. *Stadtarchiv München*. Vereine 338, Fol. 10/a: "Allgemeine Bestimmungen für die Gesellschaft des Frohsinnes zu München. 3. Aufl. (Munich: Rösl, 1834)," 20 and *Stadtarchiv München*. Vereine 336, Fol. 15/a: "Statuten der Privat-Gesellschaft zur kleinen Erheiterung in München 1841."

103. Friedrich Johann Lorenz Meyer, *Skizzen zu einem Gemälde von Hamburg*, vol. 1 (Hamburg: Friedrich Hermann Nestler, 1801), 139.

104. Lewald, *Panorama von München*, 99.

105. § 11 of the bylaws allowed each member, in addition to wife and children, three resident guests, and also foreigners. See *Stadtarchiv Leipzig*. Kap 35, Tanzgesellschaft im Gewandhaus, Nr. 1. "Beylagen zum Protocollbuch der Freytägigen Tanz-Gesellschaft pro An. 1787–1788." Fol. 1–4: Satzung und Protocoll. In the 1811 bylaws this article was liberalized to allow any number of guests, *Stadtarchiv Leipzig*. Kap. 35, Tanzgesellschaft im Gewandhaus, Nr. 3. "Beilagen zum Protokoll der Tanz-Gesellschaft im Gewandhause

vom Jahr 1810 bis 1811." Fol. 45–47: Entwurf der neuen Satzungen.

106. Fambach, *Das Repertorium*, 228; Wilhelm Kosch, *Deutsches Theater-Lexikon. Biographisches und bibliographisches Handbuch*, vol. 1 (Klagenfurt: Ferd. Kleinmayr, 1953), 536.

107. A woman's name appears independently on the attendance lists for the first time on September 30, 1817. Pauline Dufour-Ferouce was now included as an ordinary member, *Stadtarchiv Leipzig*. Kap. 35, Tanzgesellschaft im Gewandhaus, Nr. 4. "Beilagen zum Protokoll der Tanz-Gesellschaft im Gewandhaus vom Juli 1817 bis 1818." Fol. 11–12: Zweiter Ball.

108. Trepp, *Sanfte Männlichkeit*, 370–98; Habermas, *Frauen und Männer*, 396–400.

109. Meyer called them "weiberausschliessenden Männerklubs," Meyer, *Skizzen*, vol. 1, 140.

110. *Gesetze der Gesellschaft Harmonie 1845. Berathen und genehmigt in einer am 15. März 1845 gehaltenen Generalversammlung* (Leipzig: Wilhelm Vogel, 1845), 5.

111. *Stadtarchiv München*. Vereine 338, Nr. 10/a: "Bestimmungen des Frohsinnes (1834)," p 11. Compare similar regulations in the club Terpsichore *Stadtarchiv München*. Vereine 338, 24/b: "Satzungen der Privat-Gesellschaft Terpsichore in München. 1840," 4 and Museum, see *Bayerisches Hauptstaatsarchiv*, Staatsarchiv München, RA 21208: "Die Gesellschaft des Museums in München betr. De anno 1819–1846," Nr. 11: "Satzungen der unter besonderem Schutze Sr. königlichen Majestät von Bayern bestehenden Gesellschaft des Museums in der Haupt- und Residenzstadt München. Dritte nach den Beschlüssen der General Versammlungen von 1808 bis 1825 vermehrte, und durch ein Allerhöchstes Rescript vom 16. November 1825 allergnädigst genehmigte Auflage (München, 1825)," 24–25.

112. *Stadtarchiv München*. Vereine 338, Nr. 10/a: "Bestimmungen des Frohsinnes (1834)," p 11.

113. Meyer, *Skizzen*, vol. 1, 142. Friedrich Daniel Ernst Schleiermacher, "Versuch einer Theorie des geselligen Betragens." (*Berlinisches Archiv der Zeit und ihres Geschmacks* 5, Teilband 1, Berlin 1799), in *Kritische Gesamtausgabe. Erste Abteilung. Schriften und Entwürfe*, vol. 2 (Berlin; New York: Walter de Gruyter, 1984), 178.

114. Ilse Makowski, *Emanzipation oder "Harmonie"—zur Geschichte der gleichnahmigen Mannheimer Lesegesellschaft in der ersten Hälfte des 19. Jahrhunderts* (München: Saur, 1988), 46–61.

115. Helmut Janson, "45 Lesegesellschaften um 1800 bis heute," in *Harmonie-Almanach* (Bonn: Stein-Verlag, 1963), 90. Quoted in Makowski, *Emanzipation*, 46. On Casino, its competitor, Museum, and their fusion into Harmonie, see Dieter Hein's excellent "Bürgertum in Karlsruhe und Mannheim 1780–1820," in *Vom alten zum neuen Bürgertum. Die mitteleuropäische Stadt im Umbruch 1780–1820*, vol. 14, *Historische Zeitschrift. Beihefte (Neue Folge)*, ed. Lothar Gall (Munich: Oldenbourg, 1991), 485–94. Cf. Friedrich Walter, *Mannheim in Vergangenheit und Gegenwart*, vol. 2, *Geschichte Mannheims vom Übergang an Baden (1802) bis zur Gründung des Reiches* (Frankfurt am Main: Weidlich, 1907), 87.

116. Makowski, *Emanzipation*, 51. See also Hein, "Bürgertum in Karlsruhe und Mannheim," 490–91. Hein emphasizes the conversational nature of Museum but does not go into women's participation.

117. Makowski, *Emanzipation*, 57–58.

118. *Universitätsbibliotek Tübingen*. 16 A 9129. "Statuten des Tanz-Sängerkränzchens der Sängerkranz-Mitglieder," 2. "The dancing assemblies (*Tanzkränzchen*) take place every three months. The directors of the club can increase the number during the winter and proportionately decrease it during the summer months if there is need." Cf. Eifert, *Geschichte*, 219.

119. The Festschrift explains the goals briefly. "On February 3, 1836 in the Badischen Hof, the first ball of the Casino-Club took place. Subsequent balls were held shortly after this at short intervals," *90 Jahre Casino-Gesellschaft Mannheim e. V. Als Festgabe unseren Mitgliedern und Freunden zum 90jährigen Jubiläum gewidmet* (Mannheim, 1925), 11.

120. *Stadtarchiv München*. Vereine 338, 24/b: "Satzungen der Terpsichore (1840)," 3.

121. *Bayerisches Hauptstaatsarchiv*, Staatsarchiv München, RA 21208: "Die Gesellschaft des Museums in München betr. De anno 1819–1846," Nr. 11: Satzungen des Museums (1825), 24–25.

122. *Stadtarchiv München*. Vereine 338, 24/b: "Satzungen der Terpsichore (1840)," 4.

123. The bylaws of 1810, which followed the old guidelines, did not explicitly ban women or confine membership to men. They were written in such a way, however, as to assume that members would operate as families. See, for instance, §8, which defined the terms of guests. A guest was understood as somebody not belonging to the family, which could always attend. See *Stadtarchiv Leipzig*. Kap. 35, Tanzgesellschaft im Gewandhaus, Nr. 3. "Beilagen zum Protokoll der Tanz-Gesellschaft im Gewandhause vom Jahr 1810 bis 1811." Fol. 49–51: Satzungen.

124. Kroker, *Harmonie*, 46.

125. "Bekenner der Mosaischen Religion," *Museum für die Geschichte der Stadt Leipzig*. Blauer Kasten E 2/14–24. "Verein Erheiterung, Gesetze, Programme, Tafellieder, 1836–1872," Fol. 38: Gesetze der Gesellschaft Erheiterung in Leipzig. Genehmigt in der am 8. April 1832 gehaltenen ausserordentlichen Conferenz (Leipzig: Breitkopf und Härtel, 1832).

126. Lewald, *Panorama von München*, 91.

127. Gabriel Merkel, *Briefe über Hamburg und Lübeck* (Leipzig: Hartknoch, 1801), 290, uses here a local invective, "*de Aastug, de Juden*" which was normally said to children and servants. See, *Hamburgisches Wörterbuch*, vol. 1 (Neumünster: Karl Wachholtz Verlag, 1985), 19.

128. Merkel, *Briefe über Hamburg*, 290–91. In Hamburg, the Jewish and non-Jewish communities had hardly any social contacts, although their commercial connections were very intertwined. In this respect, the aristocratic and feudal society of Berlin was much more inclusive than republican Hamburg, as Arno Herzig has shown in his "Die Juden in Hamburg 1780–1860," in *Die Geschichte der Juden in Hamburg*, vol. 2, *Die Juden in Hamburg 1590 bis 1990*, ed. Arno Herzig (Hamburg: Dölling, 1991) 62.

129. According to Ralf Zerback, "Unter der Kuratel des Staates. Die Stadt zwischen dem Gemeindeedikt von 1818 und der Gemeindeordnung von 1869," in Richard Bauer, *Geschichte der Stadt München* (München: Beck, 1992), 292, the Jewish community in Munich, small as it was, was gradually integrating with the bourgeois society. This observation calls for a further exploration of the routes available for Jewish integration. On the influence of Jewish merchants, *Messejuden*, on Leipzig see Adolf Diamant's compilation *Chronik der Juden in Leipzig* (Chemnitz: Verlag Heimatland Sachsen, 1993), esp. 4–90.

During the 1830s, Jewish merchants attained equal rights with Christian merchants to use the public shops, *Gewölbe*. Juridical equality of Jews in Saxony was guaranteed in the laws of 1849 and 1851. See also Josef Reinhold's instructive and well-documented "Jüdischer Messebesuch und Wiederansiedlung von Juden in Leipzig im 18. und frühen 19. Jahrhundert," in *Judaica Lipsensia. Zur Geschichte der Juden in Leipzig*, ed. Manfred Unger (Leipzig: Edition Leipzig, 1994), 12–26. In Hamburg, relations between the lower class and the Jewish community were tense, leading in 1819 to the so-called "Hepp-Hepp-riots," attacks against Jewish merchants. As Raoul Wenzel Michalski shows in his "Die Hamburger Presse und die 'Judenfrage' 1819–1849," in *Die Hamburger Juden in der Emanzipationsphase (1780–1870)*, ed. Peter Freimark and Arno Herzig (Hamburg: Hans Christians Verlag, 1989), 159, the Jews were treated as spoilers of non-Jewish business (*Geschäftsverderber*). On the "Hepp-Hepp-riots in general, see Stefan Rohrbacher, *Gewalt im Biedermeier. Antijüdische Ausschreitungen in Vormärz und Revolution (1815–1848/49)* (Frankfurt am Main: Campus, 1993), 94–156.

130. On Varnhagen and Hertz see Hertz's *Jewish High Society*, esp. 75–119 and Wilhelmy, *Berliner Salon*, on the classical period of salons in Berlin between c. 1800–1820, esp. 67–113. On Fanny von Arnstein, see Hilde Spiel, *Fanny von Arnstein. Daughter of the Enlightenment 1758–1818* (New York: Berg, 1991) and William O. McCagg, *A History of Habsburg Jews, 1670–1918* (Bloomington and Indianapolis: Indiana University Press, 1989), 60–63, and Felix Czeike, *Geschichte der Stadt Wien* (Vienna: Molden, 1981), 182. In addition to Berlin, Vienna, and other major cities, the salons soon found an audience in eminent spas, such as Pyrmont. See Reinhold Kuhnert, *Urbanität auf dem Lande. Badereisen nach Pyrmont im 18. Jahrhundert* (Göttingen: Vandenhoeck & Ruprecht, 1984), 196–97. On Ems, see Hermann Sommer, *Zur Kur nach Ems. Ein Beitrag zur Geschichte der Badereise von 1830 bis 1914* (Stuttgart: Steiner, 1999), 32–33. On Jewish visits to spas in the late nineteenth century, see also Marion Kaplan, *The Making of the Jewish Middle Class. Women, Family, and Identity in Imperial Germany* (Oxford: Oxford University Press, 1991), 124–26.

131. Herzig, "Die Juden in Hamburg 1780–1860," 62–63.

132. Jacob Toury's stimulating analysis of autobiographies in his *Soziale und politische Geschichte der Juden in Deutschland 1847–1871. Zwischen Revolution, Reaktion und Emanzipation* (Düsseldorf: Droste Verlag, 1977), 119–38, provides important starting points for delving into the emotionally and socially ambivalent and complicated relationships between Jews and gentiles in the Vormärz. See also Kaplan, *The Making*, 126–34, on Jewish-gentile relationships in Imperial Germany.

133. Lewald, *Panorama von München*, 90. See also Huber, *München*, 319.

134. Lange, *Der Tunnel*, 47. The Saxonian decrees of 1791 had attempted to abolish discrimination against Jewish merchants in Leipzig. Although the city council attacked these measures, the emancipation of Jews remained on the agenda and accentuated in the 1830s. See, Reinhold, "Jüdischer Messebesuch," 21, 25. Systematic research on the acceptance of Jews in gentile clubs during the Vormärz is still lacking.

135. The bylaws of Concordia mention nothing about its Jewish connection, *Stadtarchiv München*. Vereine 338, 8/a: "Statuten der Privat-Gesellschaft Concordia." See also Tornow, *Münchner Vereinswesen*, 50.

136. Walter, *Geschichte Mannheims*, 243.

137. Toury, *Soziale*, 127.

138. Freudenthal, *Vereine in Hamburg*, 64; cf. Herzig, "Die Juden in Hamburg 1780–1860," 65. Although the Jewish associations and clubs since the Reichsgründung have been well researched, see Erika Hirsch, *Jüdisches Vereinsleben in Hamburg bis zum ersten Weltkrieg: jüdisches Selbstverständnis zwischen Antisemitismus und Assimilation* (Frankfurt am Main; New York: P. Lang, 1996), the associational life of German Jews after the seventeenth century is in need of thorough empirical investigation.

139. Monika Richarz, "Einleitung," in *Jüdisches Leben in Deutschland. Selbstzeugnisse zur Sozialgeschichte 1780–1871* (Augsburg: Deutsche Verlags-Anstalt, 1976), 57.

140. *Stadtarchiv Leipzig*. Kap 35, Tanzgesellschaft im Gewandhaus, Nr. 1."Beylagen zum Protocollbuch der Freytägigen Tanz-Gesellschaft pro An. 1787–1788." Fol. 1–4.

141. *Stadtarchiv Leipzig*. Kap. 35, Tanzgesellschaft im Gewandhaus, Nr. 4. "Beilagen zum Protokoll der Tanz-Gesellschaft im Gewandhaus vom Juli 1817 bis 1818." Fol. 4: Brief an Mitglieder betr. dem Programm.

142. *Stadtarchiv Leipzig*. Kap 35, Tanzgesellschaft im Gewandhaus, Nr. 1."Beylagen zum Protocollbuch der Freytägigen Tanz-Gesellschaft pro An. 1787–1788." Fol. 7–20: Verzeichnisse und Teilnehmerliste der Tanz-Gesellschaft-Tage.

143. Ludwig Bechstein and O. Kleinknecht, *Leipzig* (Schweinfurt: Kleinknecht und Schäfer's Kunstverlag, 1844), 51. See also *Ganz Leipzig für Acht Großchen. Neuer und vollständiger Wegweiser für Fremde und Einheimische. Mit Plan von Leipzig und Karte des Laufes der Leipzig-Dresdner Eisenbahn* (Leipzig: Weber, 1838), 58.

144. *Vorschläge zu einigen provisorischen Einrichtungen in der Gesellschaft der Harmonie* (Leipzig, 1829), 1. Cf. *Gesetze der Gesellschaft Harmonie (1845)*, 5.

145. *Staatsarchiv Hamburg*. Bibliothek A 507/54/1."Verfassung und Gesetze der Harmonie," 10.

146. *Bayerisches Hauptstaatsarchiv*. Staatsarchiv München RA 21208: "Die Gesellschaft des Museums in München betr. De anno 1819–1846." Nr. 11: Verfassung des Museums (1808), 6.

147. *Stadtarchiv München*. Vereine 338, Nr. 10/a: "Bestimmungen des Frohsinnes (1834)," 3 and *Stadtarchiv München*. Vereine 338, 14/a: "Statuten der Gesellschaft des Kaufmanns-Casino." On the social diversification of social clubs see Michael Sobania's studies on Aachen and Karlsruhe, "Vereinsleben und Formen bürgerlicher Assoziationen im 19. Jahrhundert," in *Bürgerkultur im 19. Jahrhundert. Bildung, Kunst und Lebenswelt*, ed. Dieter Hein and Andreas Schulz (Munich: Beck, 1996), 179–80.

148. *Universitätsarchiv Tübingen*. 406/3. "Vorschlag zur Vereinigung," Fol. 2–3.

149. *Universitätsarchiv Tübingen*. 406/3. "Vorschlag zur Vereinigung," Fol. 4–7.

150. Some of the dancing clubs, such as the Kasino im Elbpavillon in Hamburg, were affiliated with a hotel or restaurant and were required to use the services of the owner, see H. [Ant. Joh. Heinr.] Meyer, *Hamburg und Altona nebst Umgegend. topographisch-statistisch-historisches Handbuch für Einheimische und Fremde*. Mit einem neuen Plan der Stadt nebst Wall-Anlagen (Hamburg: Schuberth & Niemeyer, 1836), 278. Several clubs had a contract with a local proprietor. See, for instance, *Universitätsbibliotek Tübingen*. 16 A 9129. "Statuten des Tanz-Sängerkränzchens der Sängerkranz-Mitglieder." See also *Stadtarchiv Leipzig*. Kap. 35, Gesellschaft Tunnel, Nr. 1. "Acta: Die Angelegenheiten des Tunnels betreffend. 23. Juni 1845–1846." Fol. 41: Angebot eines Lokals. In the case of the Tanz-Gesellschaft im Gewandhaus, the contract was especially liberal allowing the

members to use outside services to provide dinner. See the remarks on "eigene Küche," for instance, "Beilagen zum Protokoll der Tanz-Gesellschaft im Gewandhaus vom Juli 1817 bis 1818. 8. Erster Ball." Stadtarchiv Leipzig. Kap. 35, Tanzgesellschaft im Gewandhaus, Nr. 4 Leipzig.

151. That the seating order was an important instrument of social representation and bonding is indicated by some evidence in the papers of the Tanz-Gesellschaft im Gewandhaus and the Tunnel. The Tanz-Gesellschaft circulated a subscription list before every ball. The attending members signed the list and also indicated where they wanted to be seated and with whom. Most of the attendees preferred a family table, but some chose to be seated with their friends. Heinrich Küstner wished to share a table with one Gruner at the ball on November 30, 1817, as reported in *Stadtarchiv Leipzig*. Kap. 35, Tanzgesellschaft im Gewandhaus, Nr. 4 Leipzig. "Beilagen zum Protokoll der Tanz-Gesellschaft im Gewandhaus vom Juli 1817 bis 1818." Fol. 13. Dritter Ball, whereas at the subsequent ball Mr. Dufour-Jansen preferred to be seated with Mr. Mayer and his family, see *Stadtarchiv Leipzig*. Kap. 35, Tanzgesellschaft im Gewandhaus, Nr. 4 Leipzig. "Beilagen zum Protokoll der Tanz-Gesellschaft im Gewandhaus vom Juli 1817 bis 1818." Fol. 26. Vierter Ball. The importance accorded to seating is indicated even more clearly in the papers of the Tunnel. We can see in the floor plan of a ball given sometime between 1845 and 1846 that the main room, the so-called "Neuer-Saal" of the Hotel de Pologne, see Lange, *Der Tunnel*, 35, was reserved for distinguished members. The prominent publisher and cultural trailblazer Karl Herrlosssohn, for instance, was seated with his own family and entourage at table number eight (8), which was located at the second focal point of the elliptically arranged room, *Stadtarchiv Leipzig*. Kap. 35, Gesellschaft Tunnel, Nr. 1. "Acta: die Angelegenheiten des Tunnels betreffend. 23. Juni 1845–1846." Fol. 98, 100: Sitzungsordnung.

152. The papers of dancing clubs include surprisingly few documents on dancing programs. The Tunnel of Leipzig was not an exception. But among the preserved documents we find those from such extraordinary events as the visit of Johann Strauss Sr., November 18, 1845. The program started with a polonaise and continued with a waltz, a galop, and a française. After intermission, the orchestra played two waltzes, a polka, two françaises, two galops, three waltzes, and finished the program with a *cotillon*. See *Stadtarchiv Leipzig*. Kap. 35, Gesellschaft Tunnel, Nr. 1. "Acta: die Angelegenheiten des Tunnels betreffend. 23. Juni 1845–1846." Fol. 50: Tanz-Ordnung im Tunnel am 18. November 1845, Concert im Tunnel am 18. November 1845. While Strauss' visit might have occasioned an exceptional program, a more typical program can be found in the "Tanz-Ordnung" of the carnival masquerades of January 17, 1846. The ball started with a polonaise and continued with a polka, a galop, a française, two waltzes (presumably after intermission), a *cotillon*, two polkas, and two galops, *Stadtarchiv Leipzig*. Kap. 35, Gesellschaft Tunnel, Nr. 1. "Acta: die Angelegenheiten des Tunnels betreffend. 23. Juni 1845–1846." Fol. 63: Von Concordia betr. der gemeinsamen Tanzveranstaltung. Exactly the same program was danced in the carnival masquerade of February 28, 1846. See *Stadtarchiv Leipzig*. Kap. 35, Gesellschaft Tunnel, Nr. 1. "Acta: die Angelegenheiten des Tunnels betreffend. 23. Juni 1845–1846." Fol. 73: Concordia-Maskenball.

153. Roller, *Systematisches Lehrbuch*, 252.

154. Roller, *Systematisches Lehrbuch*, 308.

155. After 1808, it was soon dethroned by the famous Apollo-Saal.

156. On Mehlgrube see Tanzer, *Spectacle,* 229 and Hans Pemmer, *Alt-Wiener Gast- und Vergnügunsstätten.* (Wien: Manuskript, 1969). [Wiener Stadt- und Landesarchiv, Bibliothek B 1372 1–3], 152.

157. Tanzer, *Spectacle,* 231. Indications of the increasing aversion of the aristocracy to public balls were recorded by Franz August von Kurländer in his "Briefe an eine Dame über den diesjährigen Fasching in Wien," *Zeitung für die elegante Welt* 85 (1832): 673. He identified a public ball with cholera: "We were worried at the end of last year that the rampages of cholera would also influence the dancing events. This conclusion was justified because these two extremes are united at some points: warming up and cooling off, tea and ice, healthy and unhealthy air, aggressive motion, even cramps can happen in both. All these features characterize both extremes and are even part of them."

158. Adolf Schmidl, *Wien, wie es ist. Ein Gemälde der Kaiserstadt und ihrer nächsten Umgebungen in Beziehung auf Topographie, Statistik und geselliges Leben, mit besonderer Berücksichtigung wissenschaftlicher Anstalten und Sammlungen* (Wien: Carl Gerold, 1833), 284; *Wien wie es ist. Fortsetzung der Sitten- und Charaktergemälde von London und Madrid.* (Leipzig: Magazin für Industrie und Literatur, 1827), 189; *Kritik über den Apollosaal nebst einigen rezensirenden Bemerkungen über die bereits erschienenen Schilderungen desselben* (Wien, 1808), 11; Josef Richter, *Der wiederaufgelebte Eipeldauer. Mit Noten von einem Wiener.* Heft 3 (1809) (Wien: Rehm, 1799–1821), 6. See also Witzmann, *Ländler,* 5 and Tanzer, *Spectacle,* 231.

159. *Wien wie es ist,* 180.

160. "Ueber Pyrmont 1798," *Journal des Luxus und der Moden* (February 1799): 75.

161. "Ueber Pyrmont. Mlle Kirchgeßner. Feten in Pyrmont," *Journal des Luxus und der Moden* (November 1803): 612. As Fuhs, *Mondäne Orte,* 60–67, correctly points out, Pyrmont was one of the aristocratic spas, different in terms of etiquette and conduct from its bourgeois competition, such as the spa of Driburg. On the spirit of aristocratic distinction in Pyrmont, see also Kuhnert, *Urbanität auf dem Lande,* 146–62.

162. "Gesundbrunnen in Liebenstein," *Journal des Luxus und der Moden* (October 1799): 507.

163. "Ueber das Seebad zu Doberan am heiligen Damme an der Ostsee," *Journal des Luxus und der Moden* (März 1799): 144.

164. "[E]in Fremdartiges Vornehmthun," "Aus den Taunusbädern, Ende Julius" I, *Zeitung für die elegante Welt* 166 (1827): 1327. In 1841, an anonymous commentator remarked on the same lack of social bonding, "Correspondenz aus Ems," *Zeitung für die elegante Welt* 219 (1841): 876.

165. "Aus Karlsbad. Ende Julius," *Zeitung für die elegante Welt* 164 (1833): 656. Cf. "Aus Karlsbad. Ende Julius," *Zeitung für die elegante Welt* 165 (1833): 660.

166. Ferdinand Gustav Kühne, "Bade-Leiden und Freuden. Ein Capriccio," *Zeitung für die elegante Welt* 251 (1835): 1003. Kühne was also highly critical of what he considered to be an excessive refinement of lifestyle. "One is nowhere else more confused [than at a spa], nowhere else more anxious about dressing, nowhere else more servile to the laws of the so-called distinguished manners (*Ton*)," Ferdinand Gustav Kühne, "Bade-Leiden und Freuden. Ein Capriccio," *Zeitung für die elegante Welt* 252 (1835): 1006

167. "Correspondenz aus Teplitz," *Zeitung für die elegante Welt* 133 (1842): 532. See also the anonymous description of the spa of Ems around 1841, "Correspondenz aus Ems I," 875. On the spa of Radeberg, see "Das Augustusbad bei Radeberg," *Journal des Luxus und der Moden* (October 1805): 681.

168. "Leben in München. Februar 1817," *Journal des Luxus und der Moden* (März 1817): 201.

169. Bartholomay, *Tanzkunst*, 246.

170. Helmke, *Neue Tanz- und Bildungsschule*, 90.

171. Pemmer, *Alt-Wiener*, 152.

172. Helmke, *Neue Tanz- und Bildungsschule*, 90.

173. See the detailed discussion on membership in the chapter "Inside the Ballroom Doors."

174. Although in some programs, such as in Leipzig during Strauss's 1845 visit, a cotillion was placed as the last dance, the waltz was more popularly used for this purpose.

175. *Universitätsarchiv Tübingen*. 406/202: "Organisation von Bällen der Museumsgesellschaft." Fol. 15. Rechtfertigung wegen des unanständigen Betragens auf dem letzten Ball. 24. Juli 1826. See the description of this conflict in Alf-Rüdiger Schmucker and Sebastian Kolb, *Die Museumsgesellschaft Tübingen—ein Mittelpunkt kultureller Geselligkeit* (Tübingen: Museumsgesellschaft Tübingen, 1992), 34–5. The transcription and translation of the original document is mine.

176. Helmke, *Neue Tanz- und Bildungsschule*, 97.

177. Casorti, *Instructiver Tanzmeister*, 25; P. Lahire, *Das non plus ultra der Tanzkunst. Eine gründliche Anweisung, nach welcher Jeder in sehr kurzer Zeit ohne Tanzlehrer der geschickteste Tänzer werden kann*. 2nd ed. (Nordhausen: Ernst Friedrich Fürst, 1842), 43.

178. Eduard David Helmke, *Die Kunst, sich durch Selbstunterricht in kurzer Zeit zum feinen Weltmann und sehr geschickten Tänzer zu bilden* (Merseburg: Sonntagsche Buchhandlung, 1831), 83; Mädel, *Anfangsgründe der Tanzkunst*, 53–54.

179. Corporal punishment and disciplining belonged to the traditional paternal rights of the husband. In the Prussian Civil Code (Das Allgemeine Landrecht) of 1794 this was, in effect, preserved into the nineteenth century, as Reinhart Koselleck shows in his *Preußen zwischen Reform*, 641–42.

180. The semantics of Bartholomay's account shows clearly what a passive role women played in a formal ball setting. A lady did not sign her own name, and she actually did not give her card but "let it be given." "Wo das Vorherengagiren der Damen gebräuchlich ist, da ist auch, um Irrungen vorzubeugen, der Gebrauch eingeführt, daß sowohl die Herren, wie auch die Damen mit eigends dazu verfertigen, alle Tänze, die den Abend wahrscheinlich getanzt werden, bezeichnenden Karten sich versehen, oder damit versehen lassen. Hat man von einer Dame die Zusage zu einem Tanze erhalten, so läßt man, sofern es nicht der nächste ist, sich von ihr ihre Karte geben und zeichnet darauf neben dem Tanze, zu dem man sie aufgefordert hat, seinen Namen und daher den ihrigen auf die eigene Karte. Auf diese Weise kann kein Irrthum entstehen und man kann zugleich aus der Karte der Dame sehen, welchen Tanz sie noch frei und welchen sie nicht mehr frei hat," Bartholomay, *Tanzkunst*, 252. On the elaborate art of invitation cards, see also Fink, *Der Ball*, 54. By the middle of the nineteenth century, dancing invitations had developed into dance diaries. The diary of an unknown aristocratic lady from the 1840s and 1850s gives an insight into the way invitations and social bonding were calculated. A copy of this kind of diary is owned by Mrs. Homering from the Reuß-Museum, Mannheim.

181. *Bayerische Staatsbibliothek*, Handschriften, CGM 6054: "Harmonie, Museum, Landwirtschaftlicher Verein." Tanzordnung 7ten Jänner 1809, [Unpaginated]. Cf. Bartholomay, *Tanzkunst*, 252.

182. *Neue vollständige Tanzschule für die elegante Welt oder faßliche und umfassende Anleitung zum gesellschaftlichen und theatralischen Tanz: Zum Selbstunterricht sowohl wie auch zum Handbuch für den Tanzlehrer bestimmt*. Nach den neuerschienen Werken eines Blasis, 1. Ballett-Tänzers am Coventgarden-Theater zu London, eines Blanchard u.a. bearbeitet (Ilmenau: Bernhard Fr., 1830), 32.

183. Honneth, *The Struggle for Recognition*, 95–128.

184. Honneth's theory of social recognition is about the formation of political identities. Although Honneth borrows from Hegel, he pays less attention to the rhetorical underpinnings of Hegel's notion of recognition. For Honneth the body has a negative function. It can be only violated or defended, whereas the positive function of the body as a vehicle of social recognition plays no role in his theory. See Honneth, *The Struggle for Recognition*, 132–34.

185. Kuhnert, *Urbanität auf dem Lande*, 149.

186. Pasch, *Beschreibung wahrer Tanz-Kunst*, 107.

187. Ivensen, *Terpsichore*, 22; Franz Anton Roller, "Körperliche Bildung oder Erziehung der Jugend," in *Drittes Toilettengeschenk. Ein Jahrbuch für Damen* (Leipzig: Georg Voss, 1807), 103.

188. Schleiermacher, "Versuch," 165.

189. Schleiermacher, "Versuch," 170. Although it is justifiable to see in Schleiermacher's text a piece of moral theory whose point of reference would be in Kant's and Fichte's ethical thinking, I agree with Peter Seibert's *Der Literarische Salon. Literatur und Geselligkeit zwischen Aufklärung und Vormärz* (Stuttgart: Verlag J.B. Metzler, 1993), 313–23. The life in Schleiermacher's salon, Seibert argues, was comparable to an artistic performance that existed for its own sake. Bernd Oberdorf's *Geselligkeit und Realisierung von Sittlichkeit. Die Theorieentwicklung Friedrich Schleiermachers bis 1799* (Berlin: Walter de Gruyter, 1995), 503–7, a profound interpretation of Schleiermacher's early thinking, locates the articles "Versuch einer Theorie" in ethics, which is possible but misses obviously the point that Schleiermacher himself wanted to make, namely the aesthetic nature of pure sociability.

190. Schleiermacher, "Versuch," 169.

191. See Seibert, *Der literarische Salon*, 310–12, and Wilhelmy, *Berliner Salon*, 89.

192. Schleiermacher, "Versuch," 182.

# Chapter Six

# Walking

In Goethe's *Faust*, there is this scene, "Before the City Gate." People of all kinds are walking out. We see a group of apprentices wandering out of the city and bickering over the destinations and their relative merits: whether it is the beauty of the route, quality of beer or bloom of girls. Further away, we notice two servant girls wandering, too, and teasing each other over their lovers, while two students have noticed the girls themselves. But two bourgeois girls watching the students are not happy at all that so handsome men can "chase after these silly maids." And so the panorama of walking citizens opens in front of us. Burghers, beggars, soldiers, and old women join the slowly moving stream of strolling people. Wagner and Faust, navigating among the strollers, find their way up to the hill and enjoy the colorful view down to the village and its cheering crowds, though Wagner does not fully like what he sees:

> To take a walk with you, good sir,
> Is a great honor and reward,
> But I myself should never so far err,
> For the uncouth I always have abhorred.
> This fiddling, bowling, loud delight—
> I hate these noises of the throng;
> They rage as if plagued by an evil sprite
> And call it joy and call it song.

After having said this Wagner finds himself joining a wildly dancing group of peasants.[1] Goethe, who obviously used his own walking experience from Tübingen while visiting his publisher, Cotta, in 1797, captured in masterful strokes the social meanings and internal tensions of walking.[2] While all seemed to enjoy, the source of their pleasure was not at all clear, whether it was the destination, the route, the beauty of nature, erotic excitement, or the sudden discovery of peasants dancing and cheering wildly.

Walking has a dual nature. It is physical motion and at the same time social interaction. Walking is an important means of transportation; pedestrians carry their shopping bags and children, push their strollers or wheelchairs, walk their dogs. I will not take on utilitarian walking. My attention is directed toward a type of walking that is not at all considered fundamental. In fact, the point of departure is the moment when walking started to spread as an end in itself, when it left behind its instrumental nature and became a source of pleasure, walking for its own sake, the kind of walking that Faust and Wagner experienced. Why and how walking for pleasure became so popular among the German educated middle class? In the current scholarship, walking for pleasure has been discovered as an artistic configuration that influenced and was keenly depicted in classic European painting.[3] Furthermore, a wealth of literary studies has seen walking or promenading as a poetic symbol, as a parable of meditation, melancholy, grief, longing, and the sublime perception of nature.[4] Yet only recently have the social history of walking received the attention it rightly deserves. Katharina Oxenius's study on the transformation of walking in Paris and Gudrun König's detailed analysis of promenading in Württemberg between 1780 and 1870 have opened new venues in understanding the educated and cultivated classes through their walking practices. König considers walking culture as part of the ideology of nature and an expression of romantic escapism.[5] Oxenius has discovered something different. In Paris, the representational aristocratic promenader of the eighteenth century was replaced by a more relaxed and "natural" walker and, later, by a new kind of social figure whom Walter Benjamin described as saunterer, *flâneur*.[6] Yet we do not find the *flâneur* wandering in the sublime environment of wild nature. The *flâneur* was an urban figure of sidewalks and shop windows. Although the longing for solitude and flirting with the unknown and danger played a part in inviting the literary heros and heroines to walk, walking in the mainstream culture was and remained a form of social interaction.

To fully appreciate the differences between the metropolitan culture of Paris and the parochial habits of Tübingen, Mannheim, or Leipzig and also to fully understand how the changes in walking culture influenced the everyday life of the educated middle class we have to add two important strokes to Oxenius's and König's picture. First, we have to understand how, in the beginning of the nineteenth century, an independent discourse on walking emerged. Second, when walking was changing alongside the changes of walking environment it seems that "nature" cannot provide a satisfactory starting point for the understanding of this environment. Being a powerful poetic figuration itself, "nature" simply duplicates the assumed distinction between civilization and non-civilization, without explaining it. Walking did not take place in the nebulous realm of an idealized nature but in and on such concrete environments as parks, promenades, boulevards, sidewalks, spas, city walls, and forests. By concentrating on the changes of city structure and the spas, I attempt to describe the specific conditions of walking for pleasure in the beginning of the nineteenth century. After these clarifications we can consider the different modes of walking, promenading, and their changes; we can see the place of walking culture in cultivated conduct, the institutions which perpetuated it, and, finally, the increasing challenge of gymnastics to classical walking.

## Learning to Walk

In old sciences, walking occupied two separate but closely connected contexts—dietetics and dancing. Christian Jahn, a dietitian, recommended in 1757: "Of all kinds of exercise walking in an open field is the easiest motion. It is also very healthy and recommendable if it is taken moderately after a meal. That kind of motion does not harm the body but is beneficial."[7] Doctors regularly prescribed walking as therapy, especially when a patient was a fragile scholar, because walking was, as Samuel André Tissot pointed out, a moderate exercise.[8] It was an ideal instrument to preserve and restore the balance between the body and its environment.

Whereas the relationship between walking and dietetics was instrumental, dancing had a more methodical kinship to walking. Walking (*Gang*) was an essential component of classical dancing. Signifying not only the simplest motion of the human body but also an elementary form of self-representation, the instruction of walking was assigned to the dancing masters. Villaume maintained in 1787 that, "in fact, it is the duty and the most important part of the art of a dancing master to teach young people to stand and walk."[9] Vieth was even more enthusiastic about the magic power of the dancing master.

> The teacher of this art completely re-creates the body of his student. . . . He is wry and clumsy, has hollow knees, his feet show straight forward, his belly is bulging, arms hanging, and shoulders tensed. But under the guidance of the dancing master he will show up in few months with an upright body in charming positions. He can perform all his movements with an ease and express himself with decency and acceptance in the high society.[10]

At the center of this enthusiasm for dancing was the belief that the methodically regulated dancing step could be transferred to walking, on the promenades, sidewalks, and pathways of German cities and spas. The Bavarian court dancer Franz Xaver Nadler claimed that "all human motion consists of five postures and they are also the basis of the carriage in walking, standing, and dancing, without exception."[11] According to leading dancing masters, these postures could be transferred to walking but only if one "straightens in all steps first the foot and then puts down the ball of the foot bending it outwards."[12] This kinetic invention had a great advantage over the stepping with a flat and straight foot. By allowing the walker to bend his body to the front as well as to the sides without losing his balance it was especially useful for the performance of compliments.[13]

The continuing and increasing interest in the dietetic order of life and the insistent promotion of the classical code of motion by dancing masters explains some of the social uses of walking in the first half of the nineteenth century. Yet these factors fail to provide a sufficient understanding of why walking for pleasure started to gain momentum. Doctors had prescribed walk as therapy since ancient Greece and dancing masters had exerted their power over aristocratic and patrician walkers for centuries. Yet, after the 1770s, observations of increasing love for strolling in public became prevalent. We have to turn our attention, therefore, to a new component that found its place in walking. It is difficult to describe this new component in one word. We can find traces of it in the new valorization of nature that König and Kurt Wölfel have seen gaining ground in the accounts of solitary walking. Goethe's Werther, wandering in a friendly yet ever-changing nature, was the classical figure of these accounts. Somewhat later, Anton Reiser, the protagonist of Karl Philipp Moritz's *Bildungsroman*, followed the same lonely path of a solitary walker.[14] What these accounts omitted was the other side, walking as collective action. Walking was not only solitary wandering in nature but also strolling on the sidewalks, promenades, and boulevards, as the mature Goethe so well depicted in *Faust*.[15] A promenade was an ensemble of different classes, an effort in public interaction and experience, an expression of what Habermas has called a representative public sphere in which agents represent themselves as the embodiments of authority.[16] In Paris in the parks of the Tuilerie and Palais-Royal, it was the nobility and the educated bourgeoisie that dominated this public sphere.[17] It is, however, misleading to maintain that the representational aspect of walking would have been exclusively—especially in Germany—a demonstration of aristocratic and patrician power and bourgeois subordination to this power. Contemporary observations suggest that the late eighteenth century discovered walking as a source of aesthetic gratification that was guided by customs and habits of perception yet, at the same time, inspired by a sense of freedom and even playfulness. This was obvious in solitary walking in nature. Yet it seemed possible in the distanced perception of the strolling crowds as well.

How was this new quality inserted into walking? In 1793, Jean Paul, an avid walker and wanderer, characterized in his *Die unsichtbare Loge* walking from a perspective that on one hand, anticipated the emerging lifestyle of the educated middle class, and on the other hand pointed toward possible escapes from it. He divided walkers into four groups. The first were the promenaders whose motivation for walking derived from vanity and fashion and who wanted to display their emotions, cloths or walking style. Then came the dietetic walkers, persons with weight problems and scholars who did not particularly enjoy walking but did it for digestion or nice weather. The third group in Jean Paul's theory were the aesthetic walkers who behaved like landscape painters and made constant observations of their walking environment. The best were the theological or metaphysical walkers who, in addition to their aesthetic interest, "not only walk with the eyes but also with the heart."[18] Indicating his growing desire to see walking as a unique and separate activity void of utilitarian use, Jean Paul's adversaries were obvious: the (aristocratic) promenaders and the dietetic walkers.

Yet theology was not the only justification for walking as an autonomous practice. Karl Gottlob Schelle, a Saxonian writer and a disciple of Christian Garve, saw walking "as an agreeable game," during which "the mind's awareness should not be tense."[19] The playful experience of walking had, according to Schelle, an immediate impact on one's health but it was also meaningful as non-instrumental and disinterested activity. It produced a social experience of and in nature, aesthetic gratification.[20] Unlike Jean Paul, whose aversion to promenading and the culture of vanity was manifest, Schelle took a positive stand toward promenading. For him, walking was both a meditation on sublime nature and what he called "disinterested liking of human beings."[21] Walking in nature was, according to Schelle, concentration and, consequently, a solitary undertaking on which conversation would have mainly a disruptive impact.[22] It served the broadening of one's mind. Although an important part of walking experience, solitary walking in nature was a one-sided strategy that needed a counterbalance. The walker had to overcome his melancholic mind-set, return to the city, find his or her ways to the promenades, and mix with the crowd. But how could one avoid the aristocratic culture of vanity, objectionable to Schelle as well?[23] His answer was as simple as it was opaque: one should keep a distance from the social being of the walkers and only find one's gratification in the variety of their appearances. That is to say, one should be nonchalant and detached from the surrounding fellow promenaders. This same idea we see in Schleiermacher's proposal of an ideal form of social life that he outlined in the "Theory of Sociability."[24] According to Schleiermacher, a successful social life was possible only if the participants cultivated the social form, i.e., conversation, as an end in itself. They should treat the others in conversation aesthetically, i.e., playfully, and conversation as art. Schelle transferred this idea to walking and social promenading; they became for him ends in themselves, autonomous sources of pleasure.

After the 1770s, German writers had become increasingly aware of the unique characteristics of walking for pleasure. By 1800, we can distinguish two major approaches they took. The first one, certainly noticed in the scholarship, saw in walking an escape from cities and a new mode of perceiving nature. Yet a revived valorization of social promenading complemented and challenged this Romantic view. Although they shared an aesthetic vision of walking as an autonomous activity, they had dramatically different preferences. Whereas the ideology of walking in nature took its distance from the cities, the followers of Schelle affirmed the actual changes in the urban landscape.[25] Contrary to the Romantic interpretation of nature, it was the cities and the promenades that became the dominant environments of walking for pleasure during the first half of the nineteenth century.

## Space

Walking as an end in itself is of urban origin. As Schelle remarked, "the peasant lives in nature, he is always wandering among its phenomena, and, yet, experiences next to nothing of them." Only the one who moved between the country and the city was capable of experiencing nature in the manner that made a walker.[26] The key to understanding walking in the beginning of the nineteenth century, it seems, is not the improved means of transportation, the increasing number of country villas, nor the growing desire to see and witness unspoiled nature. The key to the culture of walking was the changing physical appearance and structure of German cities. Between 1750 and 1850, German cities went through a dramatic architectural transformation, whose most important aspect was the leveling of the fortifications that occupied a considerable piece of land around the city centers. After depicting the main stages of this massive landscaping, I turn to two components that directed the ways the land was used—the ideology of beautification and the influence of spas as a paradigm of a balanced environment. Finally, I take the first step in describing how walking was shaped by these spatial circumstances and was endowed with a specific temporal structure.

The correct question to start with is not why the German cities were encircled by walls. Almost all of them were. The appropriate question is why the fairly thin stone and brick walls of medieval cities were so often replaced by gigantic fortifications. Mannheim was encircled by a system of walls, moats, and glacis that was more than 250 meters wide. In Hamburg the fortifications were no less impressive. When the Dutch engineer, Johan van Valckenburgh finished the final great improvement of the defense system in 1625, moats of 69 meters width, two walls, and glacis of 70 to 90 meters enveloped the old Hanseatic city.[27] Equally well fortified were Leipzig, Vienna, and Munich. Tübingen was a former district fortification (*Landesfestung*) but its role as a key defense system had already seriously declined by the end of the seventeenth century. The castle, Hohentübingen, was well fortified but the city was regularly and easily captured by enemy troops; it lacked the extensive glacis and moats of a normal Baroque fortification. Cities equipped with the new defense system were seemingly well prepared to stand against a siege, artillery attacks, and random offences of mercenaries or bandits, so common during the Thirty Years War.[28] As a result of these military considerations, several German cities received their peculiar compact structure and shape.

In the scholarship on walking, the palpable presence of city walls has been noted for its negative impact because only their leveling, as König argues, brought about the decisive turn to an animated bourgeois culture of walking.[29] As much as this conclusion is correct in emphasizing the novelty of the new walking culture after 1800, it fails to pay due attention to the fact that in many cities the massive defense facilities were excellent walking and recreational areas. Munich is a good example. Even before the new fortifications were completed in the 1660s, the

Bavarian court had allowed dignitaries to take over main portions of the wall and bastions for their private gardens.[30] In Vienna, where the defense systems were not razed until the 1850s, the bastion between Burgtor and Carolinentor as well as the glacis remained central locations for promenading.[31] Unlike the muddy and often crowded streets within the city, the walls and glacis made relatively dry and organized walking paths. Moreover, in cities like Hamburg which were located on a large plain, the high and broad earthwork provided rare opportunities to enjoy a panorama over the city, the river, and the Alster lagoon.[32] We can now see that the excessive militarization of German cities after the late sixteenth century systematically enclosed substantial areas for walking. But if this consequence was, by and large, unintentional, so were the effects of the leveling of the walls.

By 1800, most of the German cities were dismantling their fortifications. As in their construction, military concerns were, once again, predominant. Already by the end of the seventeenth century, artillery had improved so much that the walls and bastions were in need of reinforcement. In Hamburg, the city council reacted to the imminent threat by building new walls and bastions between 1679 and 1686 which were even higher than the fortifications of Valckenburgh.[33] But in few decades, these walls also became obsolete against an increasingly powerful artillery. Decisive were the experiences of the Seven Years War (1756–63) when some small cities were forced to dismantle their fortifications. Larger cities confronted the unhappy choice of substantially upgrading their defense systems—and thus obviously overwhelming their financial resources—or completely leveling their walls.[34] The task was daunting. Napoleon calculated that a city like Hamburg needed 25,000 men to defend it for two months. Even in the case of success, the price could be severe destruction. "At the end of the eighteenth century," Bocklitz mentions of Hamburg, "military defense of this city virtually meant its demolition."[35] For other cities, lacking the financial resources of Hamburg, the decision to raze the city walls was inevitably even more difficult.

The leveling of fortifications in German cities was a long, complicated, tortuous, and, above all, an expensive venture. In Leipzig, the first steps were taken as early as 1701, when mayor Franz Romanus, decided to drain the moats and turn the outer walls into gardens.[36] Yet only after the Seven Years' War did the arguments against fortified cities become so compelling that some cities took more drastic measures. Leipzig was one of those cities that decided to dismantle the fortifications.[37] After 1778, mayor Carl Wilhelm Müller expedited the opening of the city. Then began a process during which gradually, over several decades, the constraining walls were destroyed, bastions dismantled, the massive gates torn down, and the former moats filled.[38] Most of the other cities hesitated. With no large-scale wars in sight and the frightening economic costs of leveling mounting, the resolution was lacking in several major cities. Mannheim, for instance, was so weakened by the severe economic down-turn after the court moved to Munich in 1778, that the massive fortifications remained completely intact. Then the war came and hesitation turned to regress. Mannheim is a case in point. In 1795, the Austrian troops destroyed its fortifications completely and much of the city. Until the end of the war it was repeatedly under siege, sacked, and ravaged by different troops.[39] Munich's experience was less detrimental. Although previously neglecting the reparation and preservation of its bastions and walls, the city authorities started to renovate them after 1792 so that four years later they could be used successfully against the rapidly advancing French troops. Understanding the temporary nature of their victory, the city council decided in 1801 to dismantle and transform the defenses to civilian purposes.[40] Hamburg, plagued by the stinginess of its council, postponed the leveling of the walls until it was too late. First, when the Russians occupied the city in 1813 in order to halt the advancing French troops their commander, general Friedrich Karl von Tettenborn, ordered the renovation of the already partly dismantled defenses. However, after a few months the Russians surrendered without serious fighting and the French Marshall Devoust took over the city and ordered the completion of the renovation of the walls and bastions.[41] These military lessons confirmed what had become a reality after the Seven Years War.

After the War of Liberation, the main wave of wall razing started. In Hamburg, the committee for dismantling the fortifications started its work in 1819. By 1828, it had virtually finished its work, only some minor operations continued into the 1830s.[42] In Mannheim, because of the war and the lack of money, the leveling, which had already started in 1799, continued until 1821.[43] Yet, in 1838, a local journal still complained about the remnants of the wall. "This shapeless heap of stone . . . stands like a remnant of an earlier time period. It stands as a troublemaker hostile to the advancing beautification of which this city can be so proud."[44] The demolition of the massive defenses was in reality a complicated and traumatic experience. In Munich, for instance, the first decisive measures were taken in 1802 when the leveling of the fortifications between the Karlstorrondell and the Maximiliansplatz started. Yet the final touches to this area were made as late as 1900.[45] It took almost as long to tear down the wall in the eastern part of the city, in the Anger- und Graggenauviertel. It was finally accomplished in 1897, mainly through private initiatives.[46] While the majority of the cities seem to have started the leveling of walls during the first two decades of the nineteenth century and essentially finished it during the 1830s, they were occupied with the residuals of demolition and leveling almost throughout the century. And then in some very rare cases, the defenses remained untouched until the middle of the nineteenth century. Vienna is the most distinguished example of these latecomers. Not until 1857, with the establishment of the City Expansion Commission, did the serious dismantling of walls, extensive glacis, and defenses start, creating the famous Ringstraße of Vienna.[47]

To understand the momentum which the razing of city walls gained between 1800 and 1830 we have to turn to the causes of this development. The considerable delay in Vienna shows how important military considerations still were in the middle of the nineteenth century in justifying the preservation or dismantling of fortifications. Only a few months before the establishment of the City Expansion Commission, some of the military leaders considered the leveling inadmissable.[48]

But Vienna was an exception that confirmed the rule, imposed by a variety of indigenous pressures that significantly expedited dismantling. In several cities, the population growth was accelerating during the first decades of the nineteenth century. Moreover, the educated middle class was increasingly receptive to the new ideology of beautification.

In Munich, as Reinhard Bauer and Ernst Piper have noticed, the leveling of the city walls was significantly influenced by the increasing demographic pressure for expansion.[49] The relationship between the swelling population and the leveling of the city walls was unmistakable; the city was expanding rapidly and the growing population was crying for housing. Whereas the census of 1781 gave a population of only slightly over 37,000,[50] forty years later the population exceeded 60,000 and only ten years later, in 1834, Munich almost reached 90,000.[51] A somewhat similar pattern can be found in Vienna, in which c. 175,000 people lived in 1754.[52] During the following thirty-six years only a modest growth of 18% was reached, whereas between 1790 and 1830 the population suddenly increased more than 50% to over 300,000.[53] Leipzig also grew at the same rate, although its population had declined after the Seven Years' War. By 1840, it had reached a level of 50,000 people.[54] The northern metropolis, Hamburg, was growing briskly as well. The population of 120,500 around 1811 had reached c. 171,000 by 1850.[55] Tübingen and Mannheim deviated from this general pattern. Tübingen remained a small university town whose demographic fluctuations were closely tied to the incoming students. Mannheim stagnated because of the economic downturn after Karl Theodor's move to Munich. Only around 1860, did the city reach the same population level it had in 1777.[56] From a merely demographic point of view the equation between the fortifications and the growing population seemed easy to solve—the huge areas discovered were to be used for housing. As the examples of Leipzig, Munich, Hamburg, and later the Ringstraße of Vienna show, this was one answer but not the only one.[57] In reality, large, if not the main parts of the former fortifications were transformed into parks and promenades.

How could we understand this, to some extent, unexpected outcome? An important factor in influencing the social and political preferences of municipal decision-makers was the ideology of beautification that started to make inroads into the public discourse toward the end of the eighteenth century.[58] In 1775, Johann Peter Willebrand published his *Grundriß einer schönen Stadt* (The Outlines of a Beautiful City), which introduced the central ideas of beautification in Germany. In addition to architectural changes, he recommended more recreational and dietetic use of fortifications. They should be transformed into parks and promenades by decorating the walkways, planting trees and bushes.[59] Even more influential was Christian Hirschfeld's *Theorie der Gartenkunst*, published in five volumes between 1779 and 1785. It laid out the principles of beautification that remained dominant until the late nineteenth century. The ideology of beautification was, as König has demonstrated, by and large embraced by the Dismantling Commissions, which were founded in several cities after 1800 to control the leveling of city walls and the planning of land use to satisfy predominantly pedestrian needs.[60] Yet it is important to notice that these measures were not unprecedented. Not only were the fortifications used for walking purposes, but the enclosed inner cities also saw efforts to create promenades long before the destruction of walls seriously started. In particular, the authorities of Leipzig were inventive in using fortifications for promenading without tearing down the structure itself. Beginning with the famous Bürgerpromenade by the Barfußpförtchen, in 1725, a number of extensive walking areas were created within the city walls.[61] In Hamburg, Jungfernstieg, and in Vienna the Graben all signified early public spaces for promenading—places to see and to be seen.[62]

Although the ideology of beautification did not create walking for pleasure, it definitely had an impact on its popularity by encouraging the leveling of city walls and, consequently, development of green areas for leisurely walking. In Leipzig important steps were taken in the 1780s. In the area between the Hallesche Tor and Grimmaische Tor, most of the moats were filled and part of them incorporated as ponds in the new landscape garden which notably changed the nature of walking in and around the city. The filling of moats between the Ranstädter Thor and Barfußpförtchen began in 1798.[63] Yet the city and the new parks remained separated by the wall until the 1820s. Through new gates, especially the Georgenpförtchen, citizens had an improved access to these new areas and to the surroundings of the city.[64] Leipzig had become the classical city of promenades, a favorite of the walking philosopher, Karl Gottlob Schelle.[65]

The epitome of the beautification movement was the landscape garden and its most famous example was the Englische Garten in Munich.[66] Originally a military garden in the shape of a bastion, the Englische Garten was founded in 1789 by the decree of the Elector Karl Theodor: "not only to benefit and entertain the army but to use as a public promenade for civilians as well as military persons."[67] Count Rumford, an ennobled American protegee of the Elector and an untiring father of this project, wanted to see his venture full of "pleasure houses, ballrooms, restaurants, entertainments."[68] Friedrich Ludwig Sckell, the former royal gardner from Mannheim, realized these plans in a full-fledged public park during the early nineteenth century.[69] As a space for walking and promenading the landscape garden was perfect. It seemed to go beyond the boundaries of a promenade, which provided only a limited and regulated space with little variation. At the same time, it avoided the irregularities and aggravations of an untouched forest. Yet the residents of Munich did not immediately embrace this new creation. Several city descriptions complain how the people used this lavish space as simply a cultivated obstacle between the city and the surrounding villages, the popular destinations of Sunday walks.[70] Obviously the urban space alone did not encompass the walking experience. It also needed spaces for practice and imitation.[71]

What defined the conditions of walking in major cities was not always valid in smaller cities and towns. In an economically weak Mannheim the walls and their demolition had a limited and delayed impact on promenading. In fact, the extensive area left by the leveled walls was initially used as farmland.[72] Only in 1808, did the work start on the Schloßgarten, which was adjacent to the fortification area. It was inaugurated in 1811 and became soon a popular resort for all city-dwellers.[73] In Tübingen, the creation of parks and promenades was even less related to the leveling of walls, which never occupied the extensive space that the elaborate defense systems of Mannheim or Leipzig did. Yet the beautification movement played a dominant role here as well. In 1818, the proposal by Groß, the police commissioner of Tübingen, to create a promenade on the Wöhrd, the delta of Neckar immediately outside the city wall, was still treated as unnecessary and useless. However, the city council became increasingly aware of the urban environment.[74] During the 1830s, most of the towers of the city wall were torn down and new gates were added to the wall, making the access to Wöhrd and other surrounding areas easier than ever. The university professors in particular were concerned with the beautification. As a result, representatives of the university and the city council convened in 1842 for the initial meetings to establish a private association to "beautify the surroundings of Tübingen."[75] In a series of meetings the members, being principally in agreement over the beautification—the gardeners of the university and city were in charge of this part—addressed the conflict of interest which this new project necessarily implied. The city community, staunchly represented by the council, had traditional rights to use Wöhrd for its livelihood, like pasturing sheep, goats, and geese. University professors, students, and other persons of the educated class who saw their needs and wishes best served through promenades and places for "games and gymnastic exercise" contested these rights.[76] The committee did not succeed in a sweeping renovation of Wöhrd. In fact no Beautification Association was founded in Tübingen until 1862 because the interests of the city council were irreconcilable with the cultivated ideology of beautification.[77]

If the city environment gave conflicting messages regarding the beautification and creation of walkways and promenades, the ideology of beautification could always be reinforced by turning to its paradigmatic manifestation to spas. A standard spa consisted of one or several springs, a central promenade, dining room and ballrooms, lodgings, and a network of walkways leading up to the nearby mountains or to the seashore. Like the Jungfernstieg in Hamburg, the Bürgerpromenade in Leipzig or the Graben in Vienna, the central promenade also came first in the spas. Apart from the attraction of the springs, it was a social gathering point. Aristocratic women played here an specially crucial role in setting the tone and the type of fashion. In Pyrmont the Große Allee was the center, crowded by aristocrats and dignitaries:

> The Große Allee becomes increasingly lively toward the middle of July until it reaches its high point on Golden Sunday. Afterward the number of guests decreases rapidly and soon one can see the residents of the city of Pyrmont, without any fear of the pomp of foreigners, on the Boulevard playing the dominant role. In August, a new spa season starts but the first one by far exceeds this one in glitter.[78]

However, from 1800 on there was a rising number of complaints against the aristocratic setting of the tone. Pyrmont and Carlsbad, to mention the most renowned spas, were famous for their spirit of distinction cultivated by the nobility and royal families.[79] The Napoleonic Wars provided some temporary alleviation from these social constraints by making the aristocrats wary of traveling to and through possibly hostile regions.[80] A more permanent relief was found, however, in the creation and enhancing of walking paths that, by taking the promenader nearly into the wilderness, created an opportunity for less regulated and socially controlled strolling. As the reporter of the Ronnenburger Bad explains, there must be "well-preserved walkways" which "wind through the forest and . . . up to a hill from an enclosed meadow." This would create an atmosphere conducive for aesthetic wandering and socializing.[81] Carlsbad and Pyrmont both improved their pathways, often through private donations and initiatives, so that the fatigue and sweat caused by the previously uneven walking paths did not bother the visitor anymore.[82] These walking experiences, gently imposed through dietetic regimens and the social guidance of the aristocracy, were a significant part of middle class life not only because the number of visitors rose in the bigger spas to several thousand per year but also because of the length of spa-visits—many guests spent more than two weeks of their summer in this setting.[83] In the early nineteenth century, a visit to a spa, was a popular activity of middle class men and women, an activity that possessed a permanent place in their annual schedules.

## Time

Whereas the traces of walking space can be discovered in the structure of cities and spas, the time schedules of walking were contained in daily, weekly, and annual routines, almost too trivial to be conceptually addressed. Yet routines are by definition trivial. They necessarily exclude those who either consciously resist any routines or whose routine is to maximize the time spent for one particular practice. Walking was a routine practice. Whereas Friedrich Vischer, a professor of aesthetics at the University of Tübingen, went for a stroll regardless of the weather or season, for average walkers the seasonal changes set the limits for their desires to combine sociability with the enjoyment of nature.[84] Prater, the social stage of Vienna, opened the walking season on April 1.[85] The high points of the season were the so-called Prater rides (*Praterfahrten*) on Easter Monday and May First, when tens of thousands of residents flocked to this park: dignitaries in their carriages, young aristocrats on horseback, and the rest as pedestrians.[86] Schmidl's claim that the season was over by the middle of June is not completely accurate.[87] What was over, was the hierarchical self-presentation of the nobility and the bourgeois dignitaries who now retreated to their villas in the countryside. For the lower class and an increasing number of upper class people who remained in the city, the high point of the year was the rowdy festival on Brigittenau around mid-

July, the so-called Brigittakirchtag. Other cities, though unable to match Vienna in its elaborate display of promenading, followed the same seasonal rhythm. Spring and early fall—e.g., in Hamburg— were the seasons for walking.[88] Toward the end of June the time on summer villas, countryside, and spas began, with their respective daily and weekly schedules.[89]

The annual schedule, the seasonal changes in walking, were distributed equally. The norms applied to everyone who wanted to be counted as a city-dweller and subscribed to social promenading. The differences, however, were emerging in weekly and daily schedules. We know, for instance from Munich, that the Society (*die schöne Welt*) promenaded in the Hofgarten during the summertime on Sundays and holidays "especially after the Theatiner Mass that took place at 11 a.m."[90] Their servants, however, met already at 7 a.m. on the same day by the Chinesischer Turm in the Englische Garten.[91] Yet they shared the same weekly schedule: Sunday was the primary day for promenading. Koch informs us that in Vienna the closest promenades, Graben, the bastion between the Burgtor and Carolinentors, and the adjacent glacis were regularly used for strolling even on weekdays.[92] Robert von Mohl and Friedrich Vischer, p'ofessors from Tübingen, also had a daily walking tour, either on Wöhrd or on the surrounding hills.[93] Yet Sunday was the primary day. It was the day to go to Prater, to take one's family to Schwabing or to lead it to Tivoli (Leipzig), have a glas of beer or two and invite one's wife to "a pleasant, peaceful waltz."[94]

More important than the allocation of weekly time for walking—the limited amount of leisure did not provide much leeway—was the changing structure of daily time spent for walking. Once the city walls were razed, the traditional closing of the gates did not restrict the accessibility of promenades. In 1801, one who wished to visit a good French restaurant in Hamburg, still had to leave early enough to "take a walk on the earthwork before the City Gates closed."[95]

Table 6.1. Robert von Mohl's Daily Schedule, Mohl, *Lebenserinnerungen*, 149

| *Time* | *Activity* |
|---|---|
| 4 am | Waking up and breakfast |
| | Work |
| 12 pm | Brunch and rest |
| | Walk |
| | Work |
| 6 pm | Lunch |
| | Visits to families and *Museumsgesellschaft* |
| | Walk |

But Robert von Mohl's daily schedule from the 1840s (Table 6.1.) did not show these constraints because most of the city walls in Tübingen were already demolished and a late night walk was possible. In scholastic life, walking was the peripatetic moment of the day. In Munich, Schelling, Thiersch, and Görres, the academic notables of the city, regularly strolled in the Hofgarten.[96] Mohl's first walk, however, might not have fulfilled this intellectual function but was, rather, a dietetic device of improving digestion before the second working period of the day. The second one, right before going to bed, had the same dietetic function but it also tells that von Mohl was a nobleman who was quite aware of his divided duties as a scholar and a man of the world.[97] A man of the world, on the other hand, would borrow his habits of social walking from spas and even more likely so if he liked spas and health resorts as much as von Mohl did. His private library included more than 100 titles on baths and spas in Württemberg.[98] Besides their spatial organization spas provided a peculiar time schedule that encouraged and even prescribed promenading, providing time for the planning of company and destinations. The first walk normally took place in the morning, after the bath or water-drinking, and the second one in the afternoon before lunch. Several guests also liked walking right before dinner.[99] This timing created an optimal space for socializing.

The spatial and temporal coordinates of walking culture are now visible. Rudimentary facilities for walking for pleasure, emerging since the early eighteenth century in progressive German cities, received a new impetus after the walls started to crumble and the ideology of beautification established new standards. This ideology and the example of spas enforced and reproduced the temporal structure of walking as routine and ritual. The space and time, increasingly available for walking after the turn of the nineteenth century, could be used in different ways. German educated middle class adopted several modes of walking each of which had its own characteristics.

## The Modes of Walking

Unlike instrumental walking, i.e. walking for transportation or walking to restore one's health or improve one's physical condition, promenading was a routine, a ritual in which only the appearance counted. In the scholarship this ostentatious mode of walking has been often seen as an expression of aristocratic and bourgeois self-presentation. Self-presentation, later combined with the worship of nature, remained, according to Oxenius and König, an important function of walking culture in the nineteenth century.[100] Yet walking as self-presentation was not only an arbitrary expression of one's vanity but a means of seeking and receiving social recognition. It included how one perceived others and the ways one wanted to be perceived by others. For a dignitary in the early eighteenth century, the perception of others amounted to the reinforcement of one's power and social status. This was, often, also the way one wanted to be perceived by others. In the early nineteenth century, the leveling of city walls opened the outskirts for walkers and in the spas the same centrifugal forces, enhanced by the improved walkways, carried the guests toward the surrounding mountains, hills, and forests. How did this expansion of walking space influence walking as an act of social recognition?

Karl Johann Braun von Braunthal, alias Jean Charles, described in 1840 the public performance which took place every spring on the Prater. Moving in three lines, one in luxurious carriages, followed by a column of riders, and the third one walking, the Society and city dwellers of Vienna were engaged in what Braun called "a huge masquerade, an enormous outdoors ball, at which only horses danced, but the laws of absurd luxury were as tyrannic as at any assembly among mirrors and girandolas."[101] But unlike a masquerade, which always had a component of surprise, this one had a strict unwritten and untouchable choreography. The ladies of the royal, noble, and patrician families were in the center. Competing for the view, they were sitting in carriages, seemingly unmoved by the riding chevaliers. All this was carefully recorded by the middle class audience strolling on the parallel walkways. In the background they could hear the cheering, crying, and singing from the Würstelprater, the Prater of the townspeople.[102] This massive public display of Vienna as a social promenade was not a vanishing phenomenon. Since 1766, when Joseph II opened the Prater for the public, the number of attending promenaders was consistently in the several tens of thousands.[103] We cannot find anything comparable elsewhere in Germany. Strolling on the Bürgerpromenade in Leipzig, the Jungfernstieg in Hamburg, let alone on the Wöhrd in Tübingen, did not carry the meaning of a public demonstration of one's cultural domination. One obvious explanation for this difference is the lack of space in the promenades of Leipzig, Munich, Mannheim, and Hamburg, and if carriages were used when a trip was undertaken to Gohlis near Leipzig, Wandsbek near Hamburg or Bogenhausen und Harlaching near Munich, they were used for transportation to the targeted destinations, not for self-presentation as such.[104]

Promenading by walking was different from rigid social demonstration a la Vienna. According to Bartholf Senff, it was "a great ball to which everyone had an access without being introduced. No promenade committee can be seen here; rather each participant makes himself comfortable without being bored by speeches."[105] It was this seemingly disorganized idea of being together without any ostensibly defined leadership that endowed promenading with an appearance of egalitarianism. Yet promenaders were not necessarily looking for similarity and familiar features. Schelle saw in a promenader a character who was animated by the desire for aesthetic playfulness.[106] Pleasant play would be directed toward nature as well as other human beings which could either be in the background or participating in promenading themselves. A promenader was a curious person. The competition of fashion and extravagance, fine-tuned in the spa promenades, characterized walking on Jungfernstieg and the Bürgerpromenade in Leipzig. It was a place where "first comes the coattail, then the skirt, then the money, and only then love."[107] It was a place for contest of taste but also a place for mutuality.

While displaying the ball-like setting of a status contest, the spa promenade and its urban imitations also allowed for a variety of other, less competitive forms of walking. The Sunday walk was one of these. Like any form of walking, the Sunday walk was not an invention of the early nineteenth century. Yet the rapidly expanding walking space now made it a popular exercise among the middle class. In Munich, the Society set out for a promenade to the Hofgarten after the mass, *Theatiner-Messe* which was given at 11 am, while the middle-class man waited until late afternoon before he and his whole family took a walk. Josephine Kaulbach's family first attended the morning service and on the way back often visited relatives and friends. After lunch the mother and children went to the churchyard to see the family graves. After a while, the father came and led the whole family to a grand promenade. Without entering it, they passed the Hofgarten, went through the Englische Garten, and reached their destination in the village of Schwabing after an hour and a half. The father had his beer, a cold buffet was eaten, and the children had their buns or cakes. By dinnertime they were back at home.[108] The Sunday walk was not only an ostentatious performance, especially not for the middle class. It generally had a destination. In Hamburg, as Rambach writes, city-dwellers left the city on Sundays for Altona, Wandsbeck, Harvestehude, and other nearby resorts where several popular restaurants were located.[109] In Leipzig one of these casual destinations was Tivoli, located at a convenient distance in the southern vicinities of the city. The Wenck family used to go there on Sundays. After some walking the parents had a cup of coffee and the children got their cakes. When the family finally reached Tivoli, the father had his beer and mother received her share of dancing.

> Finally, when a delightful and peaceful waltz started, father remembered abruptly his Sunday duty. He carefully placed his cigar on the table, conspicuously cleared his throat and offered his hand to mother with a grand gesture. Soon they both whirled on the smooth floor while the marital offsprings admired their performance. [After the dance] father took his breath for a moment, look around in order to find the exit, and took his red silky handkerchief, and led with manly honor his beaming better half back to the garden—and the children triumphantly followed.[110]

Absolute satisfaction was thus reached in this family exercise.

Sunday walk was a family affair that was sometimes accompanied by close relatives and friends. Yet from the 1810s on the documents begin to tell about more contractual and associational forms of walking. Rich social clubs could now afford summer residences. The *Journal des Luxus und der Moden* reports in 1811 that the Harmonie, the second most important society in Munich, had purchased a new summer house in Schönfelder Forst, near the Englische Garten. Its location was convenient for social life and the members were particularly delighted at having "an overview of this [Englische Garten] and the residents of Munich promenading within." The Museum, the most prominent social club in the city, had tried to do the same for several years.[111] In Leipzig, there were no difficulties in finding a garden lot. Immediately outside the city wall there were several large private gardens which provided good locations for associational life. In the 1830s, the Tunnel rented a garden with baths, promenades, and a greenhouse from one of its members, Wilhelm Gerhard, whereas the Glocke, another carnival club, organized successful "promenades to Eythra, Lütschena, Grasdorf."[112] These informal social walks were paralleled by academic promenades, which belonged to the professorial lifestyle. Traditionally academic walking, unlike the students' wandering, was peripatetic, meditative, and often solitary. Robert von Mohl, who had been a professor of political science since 1824 at the University of Tübingen, was still treated in the 1840s as "a dandy and playboy," a person who had challenged the social boundaries of a respectable academic, when he actively engaged in conversational walks to neighboring towns and villages.[113] But for a student like Eduard Zeller in Tübingen, walking was a part of an ordinary lifestyle.[114]

More than anything else it was the spas that encouraged social walking and walking groups. Whereas neither the extensive families nor the solid and familiar associations were available to provide structure for walks, the walker had to engage in social bonding and calculation if he or she wanted to make his or her strolling a gratifying experience. Although solitary walking was at least a theoretical option, the spa guests, according to several reports, did not like walking alone. Sociability was considered a necessary virtue of a good walker. And a good walker was the one who could engage good company. How could one engage appropriate company for a walk? Regardless of the constant complaints about the spirit of distinction that the noble and royal families nurtured at German spas there were no categorically exclusive prescriptions for bonding. Congeniality was important. Although the dietetic rhythm of spas provided opportunities for socializing, conversation, and bonding throughout the day, early meetings at the springs were especially suitable for joining a walking group. In Töplitz, especially famous for its discrimination against commoners, one important reason for the lack of communication and socializing, besides the class divisions, was the fact that people did not meet each other by the well.[115] The well, the very reason for the existence of a spa, was the social arena that set the daily schedule and program. Naturally, lunch could also prove opportune for social networking, but very often seating followed social ranking and excluded or made difficult to find the most exciting and pleasant partner: the one across the social divide. Furthermore, in an average daily schedule the first walk took place before the lunch.[116]

After the group was composed, the walk could begin. Whereas in the last decades of the eighteenth century the endeavor required a substantial amount of sweating, the paths became increasingly comfortable during the first decade of the nineteenth century. In the summer of 1801 Carlsbad had already received a new path to Hirschsprung. The hilltop, which only recently could be reached "by going through bushes and rocks with sweat on the brow and wounded hands," was now equipped with a "gently winding, broad and a park-style path." At the same time the "delightful scene" which earlier rewarded all the efforts was now replaced by a view over "the beautiful Egerthal, and in the scenic Erzgebirge."[117] The relief from physical pain and effort was paralleled by the change from the sublime to the pastoral. The agreeable aesthetic experience, evoked through a walk, amounted to the most comfortable socializing a visitor to the Ronneburger Bad could dream of: "I am not always alone. Friends walk with me; we play and joke, and arrange our outings. At the resting-place we give small lectures and tell many different anecdotes."[118] In spas lacking the prestige and abundance of wealthy donors, which considerably contributed to the beautification of Carlsbad, a pastoral walking experience could still be cultivated. A summer guest in Liebenstein, in 1805, was reminded of the limits of reason and enlightenment in a rural church which he visited on his walk on the road "leading by the idyllic amiable cottages that the Duke built along the street for the diligent cutlers."[119] Naturally this park-like transformation of spas was not agreeable for everybody, as comments, for instance from Wilbad in Württemberg, indicate in 1814.[120] Yet the average walking experience fully embraced these improvements; it was in accordance with the perception of a tamed and agreeable nature and it definitely corresponded to the mode of walking, to its configuration as leisurely physical motion.

The ultimate limit of classical walking was its relationship to the countryside and uncultivated forest. The park-like venues to the hilltop were not only for the sake of comfort, they also made it possible to retain the measured step of dancing so fundamental for the conduct of walking. When Schelle warned against letting the walk degenerate into sport, he meant that sport and the aesthetic experience were incompatible. But he also implied that for an aesthetic attitude only a paved surface could be used and it was also important because the physical figuration of walking, the classical dancing step, was the prerequisite of walking as a social practice. A minuet step and appropriate greeting were not conceivable when a rough terrain, rocks, branches, and shrubs were absorbing a walker's energy and attention.

## Between Moderate and Vigorous Exercise

In this chapter, we have followed the transition of walking from a dietetic practice into an aesthetic activity for its own sake. In occidental tradition, walking was one of those exercises that any good dietetic prescription offered as a remedy against physical disorders and unbalances. In the eighteenth century, shaped by the dancing step, walking had established itself as a form of self-presentation. The final years of the eighteenth century witnessed a turn to walking-in-nature when the beautification and restructuring of cities provided uncomplicated access to the surroundings and the newly created public parks and landscape gardens. As the accounts of the contemporaries testify, neither dietetic, representational, nor walking for pleasure vanished in the early years of the nineteenth century. The reasons for this continuity were threefold. The very design of the increasing number of promenades and boulevards in German cities helped all these modes of walking to flourish. The constantly increasing popularity of spas and their enhanced promenades and walkways also contributed to the continuity of walking culture. Finally, all these modes of walking—dietetic, presentative, and walking for pleasure—shared a certain sense of caution. They were moderate exercises.

The casually used notion "moderate" (*mäßig*) carried several interrelated notions, such as *gemäßigt* (temperate), *mittelmäßig* (mediocre), and *mild* (mild). Its philosophical background was in Aristotle's ethical concept of the golden mean. Whereas Aristotle had formulated the doctrine of the golden mean as a strategy in dealing with moral judgements by avoiding extreme conclusions, the late eighteenth-century writers made it a practical guideline of action. In particular, the advocates of *Philanthropismus*, Basedow, Campe, Trapp, and Villaume, established moderation as the rationale of their educational program by associating it with two maxims. First, one should avoid extreme measures and methods in education and, instead, take a position in the "middle" whenever possible. This commonsense understanding of moderate education was combined with the requirement for a balanced education that would occupy a student's faculties evenly.[121] An excellent tool for moderation the members of the *Philanthropismus* found in dietetics, which promoted the avoidance of any excessive and vigorous actions in life. For Hufeland "the greatest secret for longevity lies in the moderation (*Mittelton*) in everything, the *aurea mediocritas* (golden mean). It is embedded in the moderateness (*Mittelmäßigkeit*) of a class, of the climate, health, temperament, diet, etc."[122]

In the ideology of moderation walking held a prominent position. It was considered the most favorable exercise, because it was, as Johann Nepomuk Feiler maintained in 1821, "the most moderate, relaxed, and thus healthiest exercise," which "most people treat instinctively as their necessary means of recreation and strengthening of the body."[123] Christian Jahn discouraged his patients from engaging in vigorous exercises, such as dancing, running, and ball games because these might have negative effects on those who had thick blood, a fiery temperament, and a choleric mindset.[124] Johann Wendt considered dancing acceptable after a meal, "provided that the passion of joy is accompanied in every respect with a sense of moderation."[125] In fact, much of the criticism of the new dances so common among the dietitians and dancing masters in the early nineteenth century, was directed against their excessive nature. Only the minuet was considered balanced and modest and thus fully in accordance with moderation.[126]

Schelle found that dietetic moderation had an aesthetic influence on walking. Walking was an exercise and simultaneously an experience of a balance between nature and culture, between the wilderness and the city. They both were necessary, Schelle argued, for a full pedestrian experience: nature invited to meditation, while the city and promenades gratified the senses.[127] Aesthetically, the kind of moderate walking that Schelle and his contemporaries preferred had much in common with lunchtime music (*Tafelmusik*), a centuries-old practice of court society and ceremonial dining. For Kant, not especially a music lover, all music was, more or less, lunchtime music, when he saw the purpose of the tones in "the furtherance of the vital processes in the body, the affect that agitates the intestines and the diaphragm, in a word the feeling of health."[128] In the same manner, Schelle could argue, a walker went through a stream of sensations, the perception of which "enhances bodily health, contributes to the recovery of the mind from strenuous labor."[129]

The kinship of dancing and walking was close. Not only were they moderate exercises but they also shared a common configuration: dancing provided the norm for good walking and a proper walking step. This relationship became a liability when an increasing number of critics of dancing and promenading shared GutsMuths's observation that the steps that determined good dancing and walking were always measured and, in fact, came close to regimentation and subordination.[130] From the 1770s on, when walking for pleasure started to find a permanent place in the canon of cultivated practices, its critics were determined to find less regimented forms of walking. They found them in hiking and wandering. The origins of hiking are not quite clear. Probably they went back to military exercise and to the virtue of a soldier's endurance and resistance against the hardships of a long march. Yet this seems to be only partially true, since, as Karl Gaulhofer has shown, the military posture of the seventeenth and eighteenth centuries was a modification of the classical dancing posture.[131] The other part of the explanation is pedagogical. Basedow and his supporters, especially Salzmann and GutsMuths, had adopted hiking for educational purposes, to harden the body. The first records of educational hiking go back to the Schnepfenthal *Philanthropinum* where GutsMuths organized long hiking tours to the Thuringian forests, and during the 1790s developed a theory of gymnastic walking. For GutsMuths, nature was a training field that, as an enemy of the human spirit and body, taught a boy how "his mind learns to carry burdens."[132] In his early efforts, GutsMuths was less interested in the method of walking than in its educational and dietetic impact. But unlike some of the older educators, such as Villaume, who took the dancing step as an ideal, GutsMuths soon became convinced that the direct use of a dancing *pas* in everyday walking was artificial and ludicrous.[133]

For dancing masters the important requirement for a proper walking step had been that the ball of the foot comes first and then the heel. GutsMuths, as much as he criticized the bad and artificial influence of dancing masters on German walking habits, still wanted to adhere to this requirement. It was Jahn who rejected the dancing step and required his gymnasts to step with flat foot:

> Proper carriage while walking [. . .] consists of a natural carriage of the whole body, especially the head. No contrived and affected motions are allowed; a light yet solid step on an even foot, without giving any preference to either side. The knee must be straightened in every step on the ground. The feet must point slightly towards sides but they shall not move back and forth. The arms can

> move slightly but not gyrate. Motion starts with the lower arm rather than with the upper one. The walking step should be neither dragging nor hopping, it should not wobble nor rock but be straight and solid. Bones and knees should not rub each other. The length of the step is in proportion with the length of the body and especially the legs, so that the body can stay balanced at every step.[134]

Jahn primarily considered one's carriage, but all these regulations had an important bearing on the ways of controlling one's body, especially the torso. Whereas the dancer was able to shift the balance from one foot to another instantly, the hiker could accomplish this only with considerable efforts if at all. Consequently, bows, so important for dancing and the art of complimenting, had to be reduced or removed from a hiker's repertoire.[135] This was the configurational basis for the egalitarian rules of behavior so much cherished by Jahn and his followers. It indicated the democratic spirit and seeming abolition of all asymmetric relationships within the *Turner* community. Furthermore, it pointed at the rupture between classical walking and hiking that materialized in the ways of social recognition.

The configurational rift between moderate walking and vigorous, gymnastic walking, so much desired by Jahn, materialized only partially during the three decades after the Wars of Liberation. While gymnastic guidelines and regulations continued to promote flat foot hiking, individual gymnasts were commonly found in engaging in dancing, and hiking tours often were more like nature walks.[136] We also find educators who merged the two configurations: Roller, the dance master of Shulpforte, advocated Jahn's gymnastics and Werner promoted classical, dancing-like exercise as gymnastics. And some adamant walkers simultaneously cherished gymnastic hiking. Friedrich Vischer propagated walking from the time he was a young lecturer in Tübingen in the 1830s. As an eminent member of the committee which was set up to beautify Tübingen, he called for a major overhaul of the city surroundings. The beautification of Wöhrd as a park and walking area was particularly close to his heart. Yet Vischer's inclination to traditional walking changed in the 1840s when he started to argue that walking was not just an aesthetic endeavor but primarily an instrument for hardening scholars' bodies, for leading them out of their studies and letting them get fresh air.[137] In effect, his program was not much different from the *Turner* movement. What is obvious in Vischer's proposal is the lack of attention to the social dimension of walking, to walking as a form of social self-presentation. Vischer's aesthetic walking was geared toward solitary strolling in nature or a peripatetic walking with a few chosen friends.[138] For this purpose, the dancing step was not necessary, or even beneficial.

What happened to walking between 1770 and 1850? Walking had evidently gone through a transformation. This transformation was encouraged by the increase of space and change of spatial arrangements in cities and spas. By the 1850s, most major cities had replaced their fortifications with parks and promenades. Those Germans who had the appropriate means for leisure found ways to reserve time in their daily and annual schedules for an activity that was becoming the most popular pastime. The question was how to find the most adequate and desirable way of walking. And, as the rapid increase of various programs, concepts, and proposals, suggest, the answer was an affirmation of all forms of walking. A dietetic walker and a gymnastic hiker could turn into a sociable stroller or peripatetic wanderer. Yet, something had changed. He or she did not walk because it was a necessity or prescribed by class and status but because walking in all its configurations had become an end in itself, an aesthetic activity.

## Notes

1. Johann Wolfgang von Goethe, "Faust," in *Sämtliche Werke*, vol. 7/1 (Frankfurt am Main: Deutscher Klassiker Verlag, 1994), 48–59.

2. Martin Kazmaier, *Tübinger Spaziergänge* (Pfullingen: Neske, 1977), 13–15.

3. Also Sabine Krebber, *Der Spaziergang in der Kunst. Eine Untersuchung des Motivs in der Kunst des 18. Und 19. Jahrhunderts* (Frankfurt am Main: Lang, 1990), locates walking in nature, although several of her pictures show people strolling in an urban environment.

4. On Rousseau's influence on the ideology of the solitary promenade in eighteenth-century poetry see Angelika Wellmann, *Der Spaziergang. Stationen eines poetischen Codes* (Würzburg: Königshausen & Neumann, 1991), 80–81, 88–90. Thomas Koebner, "Versuch über den literarischen Spaziergang," in *Das achtzehnte Jahrhundert. Facetten einer Epoche. Festschrift für Rainer Gruenter*, ed. Wolfgang Adam (Heidelberg, 1988), 39–40 distinguishes between the lonely promenader (*Spaziergänger*) and the socially interested *flâneur*. For him the lonely promenader emerges as the progenitor of a romantic figure. On the romantic conceptualization of walking as the solitary contemplation of nature see Kurt Wölfel, "Andeutende Materialien zu einer Poetik des Spaziergangs. Von Kafkas Frühwerk zu Goethes 'Werther,'" in *Zur Geschichtlichkeit der Moderne in Theorie und Deutung. Ulrich Fülleborn zum 60. Geburtstag*, eds. Theo Elm and Gerd Hemmerich (Munich: Wilhelm Fink Verlag, 1982), esp. 73–86. Markus Fauser does not subscribe to this romantic interpretation of walking. His contribution is the rediscovery of Karl Gottlob Schelle's classical treatise on walking as a conjunction of social act and solitary contemplation. See Markus Fauser, "Promenade als Kunstwerk. Karl Gottlob Schelles Theorie des Spaziergangs," in Karl Gottlob Schelle, *Die Spatziergänge oder die Kunst spatzierenzugehen* (Leipzig, 1802) (Hildesheim; Zürich; New York: Olms-Weidemann, 1990), 285-312.

5. It is, perhaps, not a mere accident that the town that provided such compelling materials for Goethe's walking scene, Tübingen, is also the academic environment of these two studies on walking culture. See König, *Kulturgeschichte des Spazierganges*, esp. 13–15.

6. Katharina Oxenius, *Vom Promenieren zum Spazieren. Zur Kulturgeschichte des Pariser Parks* (Tübingen: Tübinger Vereinigung für Volkskunde, 1992), esp. 55–92. Oxenius does not address Benjamin's idea in detail. As I will show later, Benjamin's idea of a *flâneur* cannot be reduced to a promenader who merely wants to "satisfy the desire of watching and pleasure," Oxenius, *Vom Promenieren zum Spazieren*, 95. The *flâneur* is, in fact, held hostage by the objects of his or her desire. See Walter Benjamin, *Charles Baudelaire. A Lyric Poet in the Era of High Capitalism* (London: Verso, 1983), 55. König does not consider the commercial aspect of autopoetic walking as relevant. For her the

*flâneur* is a rebel, König, *Kulturgeschichte des Spaziergangs*, 13. See also Tanzer, *Spectacle*, 262, who sees in Vienna an organic continuity between aristocratic promenading and bourgeois walking. On the relationship between strolling and hiking see the chapters in Wolfgang Albrecht and Hans-Joachim Kertscher, *Wanderzwang—Wanderlust. Formen der Raum- und Sozialerfahrung zwischen der Afklärung und Frühindustrialisierung* (Tübingen: Max Niemeyer Verlag, 1999).

7. Jahn, *Norma Diaetetica*, 163. See also Wedel[ius], *Diæta Literatorum*, 19; Krüger, *Diät oder Lebensordnung*, 408.

8. Tissot, *Gesundheit der Gelehrten*, 95. Although Tissot was aware of its limitations. He also recommended more vigorous exercise to boost blood circulation.

9. Villaume, *Bildung des Körpers*, 245.

10. Vieth, *Versuch einer Encyklopädie*. Vol. 2, 287.

11. Nadler, *Kallischematik*, 58.

12. "Streckt bei jedem Schritte erst den Fuß voraus und drückt die Spitze auswärts nieder," Helmke, *Neue Tanz- und Bildungsschule*, 29–30. Cf. Roller, *Systematisches Lehrbuch*, 51–52; Schönwald, *Grundregeln der Tanzkunst*, 2–3; Bartholomay, *Tanzkunst*, 40–44; Hentschke, *Allgemeine Tanzkunst*, 118–19.

13. Bartholomay suggested in bowing the maximum "opening of the feet," Bartholomay, *Tanzkunst*, 61. See also Roller who emphasized the social use of this technique, Roller, *Systematisches Lehrbuch*, 53. Above all, the technique designed for men, since women's greetings were mainly curtseys.

14. König, *Kulturgeschichte des Spaziergangs*, esp. 13–15; Wölfel, "Andeutende Materialien," 77–85.

15. It is interesting to note that this famous scene is preceded by another, truly melancholic and solitary scene, in which Faust goes through his spiritual and intellectual agony. The promenade that now follows thus overcomes emotionally the anomalies of melancholic solitude. This rather antiromantic solution shows, in addition to Goethe's impeccable sense for dialectics, the complexities of walking as both solitary and social action. See Goethe, "Faust," 48–59. Schiller's elegy of walking (*Spaziergang*) starts in nature, makes the solitary, meditative and observing journey through villages and cities, and returns to nature. Schiller had more influence on the perception of walking—as a solitary action in nature—than on the walking itself. See Friedrich Schiller, "Der Spaziergang," in *Schillers Werke. Nationalausgabe*, vol. 2/1 (Weimar: Hermann Böhlaus Nachfolger, 1983), 308–14.

16. Habermas uses the term, *repräsentative Öffentlichkeit*. Jürgen Habermas, *Strukturwandel der Öffentlichkeit. Untersuchungen zu einer Kategorie der bürgerlichen Gesellschaft* (Neuwied: Luchterhand,1965), 14–24.

17. Oxenius, *Vom Promenieren zum Spazieren*, 14. Wilhelm von Humboldt was especially fascinated by the Palais-Royale during his visit to Paris in 1789, see Wilhelm von Humboldt, *Wilhelm von Humboldt. Sein Leben und Wirken, dargestellt in Briefen, Tagebüchern und Dokumenten seiner Zeit*, ed. Rudolf Freese (Berlin: Verlag der Nation, 1955), 303–4.

18. Jean Paul, *Werke in drei Bänden*, vol. 1, ed. Norbert Miller (Munich: Hanser Verlag, 1969), 304–5.

19. Karl Gottlob Schelle, *Die Spatziergänge oder die Kunst spatzierenzugehen* (Leipzig, 1802). Reprint. (Hildesheim; Zürich; New York: Olms-Weidemann, 1990), 43.

20. Schelle, *Spatziergänge*, 44.

21. "[E]in uninteressirtes Wohlgefallen an Menschen," Schelle, *Spatziergänge*, 93.

22. Schelle, *Spatziergänge*, 72.

23. Schelle, *Spatziergänge*, 65–66.

24. The prescriptive code of Schleiermacher's social world implied that the participants were exclusively interested in the social aspect of these circles; they should be disinterested in the social benefits of conversations. In other words, they had to be socially disinterested in order to be interesting for socializing. See Schleiermacher, "Versuch," 165–72.

25. Although König correctly notes the importance of Schelle as a writer and also his opposition to Rousseau's ideology of nature, she fails to shift her attention from nature to the city as the dominant environment of autopoetic walking, König, *Kulturgeschichte des Spaziergangs*, esp. 35–36.

26. Schelle, *Spatziergänge*, 121.

27. Friedmann, *Alt-Mannheim*, 50. On Hamburg see Bocklitz's detailed but insufficiently documented presentation (it does not give source references), Bocklitz, "Hamburgische Festungsanlagen," esp. 125–29.

28. The fortification of Hamburg was so successful that none of the troops which approached the city during the Thirty-Years War had courage to test its defense. See Bocklitz, "Hamburgische Festungsanlagen," 138. On the fortification and castle, Hohentübingen, see Erwin Haas, *Die Sieben Württembergischen Landesfestungen* (Reutlingen: Verlag Harwalik, 1996), esp. the picture on page 127 and pages 146–57.

29. König, *Kulturgeschichte des Spaziergangs*, 38. Peter Grobe, *Die Entfestigung Münchens* (Munich: Oppermann, 1970), correctly emphasizes the non-military uses of fortifications. Willebrand also saw the importance of earthworks as promenading areas. In fact, it was a significant feature of a beautiful city to have well-planted and decorated earthworks, Johann Peter Willebrand, *Grundriß einer schönen Stadt, in Absicht ihrer Anlage und Einrichtung*, vol. 1 (Hamburg: Bohnsche Buchhandlung, 1775), 166–67.

30. Grobe, *Entfestigung Münchens*, 15.

31. Friedrich Koch, *Der wohlunterrichtete Fremdenführer in der kaiserl. königl. Haupt- und Residenzstadt Wien und ihren nahen Umgebungen* (Wien: Singer et Goering, 1844), 376. See also Tanzer, *Spectacle*, 258–263.

32. See especially the "chronicler" of Hamburg, Meyer, and his detailed description of the earthwork (*Wall*) by the turn of the nineteenth century in, Meyer, *Skizzen*, 14–23. See also Willebrand, who especially emphasized the advantages of earthworks in providing a real panorama to the surroundings of a city, Willebrand, *Grundriß einer schönen Stadt*. Vol. 1, 167.

33. Bocklitz, "Hamburgische Festungsanlagen," 145.

34. Kneschke, *Leipzig*, 22.

35. Bocklitz, "Hamburgische Festungsanlagen," 148.

36. Lutz Heydick, *Leipzig. Historischer Führer zu Stadt und Land* (Leipzig: Urania, 1990), 39. Kneschke gives the year 1702 as the starting point of Leipzig's beautification, *Leipzig*, 22.

37. Kneschke, *Leipzig*, 22.

38. As Kneschke shows, *Leipzig*, 463, the city council was occupied with the leveling of the walls as late as in the 1850s.

39. Karl Hauck, *Geschichte der Stadt Mannheim zur Zeit ihres Ueberganges an Baden* (Leipzig: Breitkopf & Härtel, 1899), 87. See also Friedmann, *Alt-Mannheim*, 45.

40. Peter Grobe's, *Die Entfestigung Münchens* provides the most comprehensive and detailed account of the dismantling of fortifications in Germany. My account follows the outlines of his presentation, although some corrections to the picture are necessary regarding its periodization and social consequences, Grobe, *Entfestigung Münchens*, 21–28.

41. See, for instance, Bocklitz, "Hamburgische Festungsanlagen," 149–51.

42. Evi Jung-Köhler, *Verlust und Chance. Hamburg 1842. Stadtmodernisierung beim Wiederaufbau nach dem grossen Brand* (Hamburg: Verein für Hamburgische Geschichte, 1991), 14. Cf. Bocklitz, "Hamburgische Festungsanlagen," 151–52.

43. Friedmann, *Alt-Mannheim*, 47. According to Walter, *Geschichte Mannheims*, 6, prince Karl Friedrich announced the complete demolition of the fortifications as late as 1803, showing so common indecisiveness for razing the walls.

44. Walter, *Geschichte Mannheims*, 244.

45. Grobe, *Entfestigung Münchens*, 35.

46. Grobe, *Entfestigung Münchens*, 40–46.

47. On the restructuring of Vienna after 1857 there is ample literature. I have used Carl E. Schorske's *Fin-de-siècle Vienna: politics and culture* (New York: Knopf, 1980), esp. 24–44. Schorske, however, pays no attention to the ways parks and streets shaped the area.

48. Schorske, *Fin-de-Siècle Vienna*, 29.

49. Reinhard Bauer and Ernst Piper, *München. Die Geschichte einer Stadt* (München/-Zürich: Pier, 1993), 147. This pressure worked only in conjunction with the declining military importance of the fortifications.

50. Manfred Peter Heimers, "Die Strukturen einer barocken Residenzstadt—München zwischen Dreißigjährigem Krieg und dem Vorabend der Französischen Revolution," in *Geschichte der Stadt München*, ed. Richard Bauer (Munich: Beck, 1992), 211.

51. Bauer and Piper, *München*, 159.

52. Czeike, *Geschichte der Stadt Wien*, 115.

53. Czeike, *Geschichte der Stadt Wien*, 134, 174.

54. Heydick, *Leipzig*, 60. See also Kneschke, *Leipzig*, 459 and, especially on the declining population after the Seven Years War, Hartmut Zwahr, "Leipzig im Übergang zur bürgerlichen Gesellschaft (1763–1871)," in *Neues Leipzigisches Geschicht-Buch* (Leipzig: Fachbuchverlag, 1990), 132.

55. Jung-Köhler, *Verlust und Chance*, 13.

56. On Mannheim's demographic development, I rely on Hein's "Bürgertum in Karlsruhe und Mannheim," 455.

57. Annelore Franke, *Leipzig um die Wende vom 18. zum 19. Jahrhundert* (Leipzig: Offprint, s.a.), 154. In Vienna the public monumental buildings dominated the new Ringstrasse district, see, for instance, Elisabeth Springer, *Geschichte und Kulturleben der Wiener Ringstrasse* (Wiesbaden: Franz Steiner Verlag, 1979), esp. 200–42.

58. For a contemporary overview of the beautification of European cities see "Verschönerungen der Städte unsers Zeitalters," *Journal des Luxus und der Moden* (July 1810): 404–7.

59. Willebrand, *Grundriß einer schönen Stadt*, vol. 1, esp. 164–80. On the beautification see König, *Kulturgeschichte des Spaziergangs*, esp. 38–40. Grobe too narrowly defines beautification as the increasing number of monumental buildings which gradually filled the empty space created and left by the fortifications, Grobe, *Entfestigung Münchens*, 16.

60. See König, *Kulturgeschichte des Spaziergangs*, esp. chapter on "Städtisches Grün" that details the development of walking facilities in four cities in Württemberg, Tübingen, Stuttgart, Ulm, and Wildbad.

61. Kneschke, *Leipzig*, 54.

62. Graben, a former marketplace, evolved as one of the centers of social promenading by the middle of the eighteenth century. On Graben see esp. Tanzer, *Spectacle*, 264. Hans Pemmer's careful depiction, "Der Graben und seine Bewohner," in *Jahrbuch des Vereins für Geschichte der Stadt Wien* 14 (1958): 114–32, is dated. More than the social organization of Graben Pemmer concentrates on the buildings, individual residents, and their particular histories. Further on Graben see Koch, *Fremdenführer*, 376; Schmidl, *Wien*, XI; *Wien wie es ist*, 17. Jungfernstieg has received, if possible, even less scholarly attention. See the contemporary remarks in Z., "Erster Spazziergang in und um Altona," *Hamburg und Altona* I (1801): 273–74. Also Merkel, *Briefe*, 256 and Rambach, *Physisch-medizinische Beschreibung*, 223.

63. Kneschke, *Leipzig*, 54–55.

64. The leveling of the city wall itself is not quite clear. The map "Statistische Tabelle von der Stadt Leipzig (1788)," in *"Leipziger Stadtpläne." Verzeichnis der in Leipziger Institutionen verfügbarer Karten und Pläne*, ed. Heike Boden, Alice Hecht, Thomas Nabert (Leipzig: Klingenberg, 1994) shows the city enclosed by a unified wall. Because the entrance fee (*Torgeld*) was not abolished until 1824, it is likely that the wall was substantially preserved until then, with some of the gates.

65. Schelle, *Spatziergänge*, 89.

66. In Leipzig the park between the Hallesches Tor and Grimmaisches Tor was also created as a landscape garden.

67. Bauer and Piper, *München*, 143.

68. Theodor Dombart, *Der Englische Garten zu München. Geschichte seiner Entstehung und seines Ausbaues zur großstädtischen Parkanlage* (Munich: Hornung Verlag, 1972), 40.

69. Dombart, *Englischer Garten*, 152.

70. Lewald, *Panorama von München*, 56–57; Wolf, *Jahrhundert München*, 142.

71. On Wörlitz, the first extensive landscape garden in Germany, see Erhard Hirsch's "'Zierde und Inbegriff des XVIII. Jahrhundert'. Der Dessau-Wörlitzer Kulturkreis im Spiegel der zeitgenössischen Urteile," in *Philanthropismus und Dessauer Aufklärung. Studien über den Philanthropismus und die Dessauer Aufklärung. Vorträge zur Kulturgeschichte des Dessau-Wörlitzer Kulturkreises.* Wissenschaftliche Beiträge der Martin-Luther-Universität Halle-Wittenberg 1970/3 (A 8) Halle (Saale). (Halle: Martin-Luther Universität Halle, 1970), esp. 129–134. Cf. also König, *Kulturgeschichte des Spaziergangs*, 32.

72. Friedmann, *Alt-Mannheim*, 50.

73. Friedmann, *Alt-Mannheim*, 50. Cf. Walter, *Geschichte Mannheims*, 80–84.

74. *Stadtarchiv Tübingen*. A 70/3330: "Verschönerung des Wöhrds." Fol. 1. "Plan." 05/05/1818. König, who provides a thorough account of walking in Tübingen, has omitted Groß's proposal. See König, *Kulturgeschichte des Spaziergangs*, 141. She does not recognize any improvement of walkways in the city until 1819, when the boulevards to Rottenburg and the so-called Platanen-Allee on Wöhrd were founded. See also Eifert, *Geschichte*, 215.

75. *Stadtarchiv Tübingen*. A 70/3330: "Verschönerung des Wöhrds." Fol. 2. "Der Privat-Verein für die Verschönerung der Umgegend von Tübingen." 05/28/1842. For the university the signers were Professors Hepp (president), and Fallati, for the city mayor Bierer, councilmen Memminger and Wolff. As for the leveling of the walls see Eifert, *Geschichte*, 214.

76. Kazmaier, *Tübinger Spaziergänge*, 41.

77. König, *Kulturgeschichte des Spaziergangs*, 305–7.

78. "Pyrmont im Sommer 1812," *Journal des Luxus und der Moden* (September 1812): 625. Kuhnert, *Urbanität auf dem Lande*, does not pay attention to the social function of the Main Boulevard. Fuhs, *Mondäne Orte*, 55, notices its commercial aspect.

79. "Pyrmont," *Journal des Luxus und der Moden* (September 1801): 492; "Ueber Warmbrunn," *Journal des Luxus und der Moden* (October 1803): 541; "Karlsbad, im August 1804," *Journal des Luxus und der Moden* (September 1804): 441; "Erinnerungen an Karlsbad, Eger und Töplitz," *Journal des Luxus und der Moden* (October 1804): 494; "Pyrmont im Sommer 1806 (Aus dem Brief einer Dame)," *Journal des Luxus und der Moden* (October 1806): 646.

80. "Bade- und Reise-Epoque. Wanderung durch die Bäder von Driburg, Pirmont und Geismar 1807," *Journal des Luxus und der Moden* (September 1807): 585.

81. "Das Ronneburger Bad im Herzogthum Altenburg," *Journal des Luxus und der Moden* (October 1812): 670.

82. "Scene aus dem Carlsbad im Jahr 1802, in einem Briefe," *Journal des Luxus und der Moden* (November 1802): 621–22; "Pyrmont 1812," 628. See also "Neue Anlagen in Karlsbad," *Journal des Luxus und der Moden* (January 1801): 11–12. "Follow me now to the Hirschsprung. Do you remember how often we climbed up with our faces sweating, wounds on our hands and faces, with wounded legs, through bushes and rocks on those steep paths and by abysses. And this all we did to see the delightful scene over the Calsbad far below us, and to enjoy the view to several distant landmarks."

83. Kühne, "Bade-Leiden," 1001–1007, 1011, provides a highly critical, even ironic, but well-informed insight into the spa culture of the early nineteenth century.

84. Kazmaier, *Tübinger Spaziergänge*, 51.

85. Schmidl, *Wien*, 286.

86. Koch, *Fremdenführer*, 382. On the social setting on the main boulevard of the Prater see also Hans Pemmer and Nini Lackner, *Der Prater* (Wien: Jugend und Volk, 1974), 147.

87. Schmidl, *Wien*, 288.

88. L., "Oeffentliche Spaziergänge," *Hamburg und Altona* I (1801): 14.

89. For Hamburg, see Rambach, Physisch-medizinische Beschreibung , 223.

90. Friedrich Wilhelm Bruckbräu, *Neuestes Taschenbuch der Haupt- und Residenzstadt München* (Munich: Lindauer, 1828), 100.

91. Wolf, *Jahrhundert München*, 142.

92. Koch, *Fremdenführer*, 376.

93. Mohl, *Lebenserinnerungen*, 149; Kazmaier, *Tübinger Spaziergänge*, 51.

94. Lippold, *Erinnerungen*, 23–24.

95. Z., "Zweiter Spazziergang in und um Altona," *Hamburg und Altona* I (1801): 313.

96. Lewald, *Panorama von München*, 60–61.

97. Mohl, *Lebenserinnerungen*, 140.

98. Mohl, Lebenserinnerungen, 150.

99. S., Fr.W., "Ueber Sichersreut in Franken," *Journal des Luxus und der Moden* (December 1798): 680; "Seebad zu Doberan," 144; "Gesundbrunnen in Liebenstein," 504.

100. In Paris, Oxenius, *Vom Promenieren zum Spazieren*, 87, identifies the children as the new subjects—and objects—of self-presentation in the beginning of the nineteenth century. Oxenius's observations are limited to parks and do not consider strolling on sidewalks. Tanzer, *Spectacle*, 262, provides further support to this thesis. König, *Kulturgeschichte des Spaziergangs*, 208, sees especially the spas as the classical places for self-presentation for all classes.

101. Charles, *Wien*, 51.

102. On the social setting of the Prater-Promenade see Schmidl, *Wien*, 287; Koch, *Fremdenführer*, 382; Hebenstreit, *Fremde in Wien*, 131.See also the remarks of Josef Richter, *Der wiederaufgelebte Eipeldauer. Mit Noten von einem Wiener* 36 (1804–1805): 24, 38.

103. Hebenstreit, *Fremde in Wien*, 131; Schmidl, *Wien*, 287. The figures vary between 10,000 and 30,000, see Pemmer, *Prater*, 27 and the rather moderate estimation of Bertrand Michael Buchmann, *Der Prater. Die Geschichte des unteren Werd* (Wien; Hamburg: Zsolnay, 1979), 69. On special occasions there were visitors numbering in even several hundreds of thousands, as at the wedding ceremony of Franz Joseph and Elisabeth of Bavaria, when over 200,000 people attended, see Buchmann, *Prater*, 71.

104. Santo Domingo [Eduard Lehmann], *Hamburg, wie es ist* (Leipzig: Reclam, 1838), 215. In Munich self-presentation in the carriage might have played some role see Huber, *München*, 338–39, who tells how "all classes either in carriages, on horse or by walking visit daily" the Englische Garten.

105. Senff, *Buntes Leipzig*, vol. 2, 11.

106. "In the context of promenading the attention of the mind should not be tense. Rather than being earnest it should be an agreeable game," Schelle, *Spatziergänge*, 43.

107. Senff, *Buntes Leipzig*, vol. 2, 18. Concerning Hamburg cf. Rambach, *Physisch-medizinische Beschreibung*, 223.

108. Wolf, *Jahrhundert München*, 65.

109. Rambach, Physisch-medizinische Beschreibung , 223.

110. Lippold, *Erinnerungen*, 23–24.

111. "Skizzen zum neuesten Gemälde von München," *Journal des Luxus und der Moden* (Julius 1811): 467.

112. Lange, *Der Tunnel*, 35; *Geschichtliche Rückblicke auf das Glockenleben 1837–1937. Zur Erinnerung an das 100jährige Jublefest zusammengestellt als Festgabe* (S.l., s.a.) [Museum für Geschichte der Stadt Leipzig, Sig.: I M 319], 7.

113. "Stutzer und Lebemann," Mohl, *Lebenserinnerungen*, 140, 181.

114. Eduard Zeller, *Erinnerungen eines Neunzigjährigen* (Stuttgart: Uhland'sche Buchdruckerei, 1908), 81.

115. "Schilderung der Sächsischen und Böhmischen Bäder Radeberg, Schandau, Sieshübel und Töplitz im Sommer 1804," *Journal des Luxus und der Moden* (August 1804): 405. The reporter tells about the Carlsbad: "In the morning people socialize there [by the spring] without any consideration for rank and order. There one can already make arrangements for the afternoon recreation as happened often during my visit. Here, by the spring, the lover of beautiful, wild nature, the indefatigable walker can already make appointments with kindred spirits,""Carlsbad und Töplitz," *Journal des Luxus und der Moden* (November 1798): 628.

116. On a daily spa schedule see, for instance, B. & H., "Landeck," *Journal des Luxus und der Moden* (Januar 1798): 20; "Lauchstädt," *Journal des Luxus und der Moden* (Januar 1798): 28; "Pyrmont im Jahr 1797. Mein Vermächtniß für das Moden-Journal," *Journal des Luxus und der Moden* (September 1798): 508. On Carlsbad see, "Carlsbad und Töplitz," 628. See also S., Fr.W., "Ueber Sichersreut," 680. On Doberan see, "Seebad zu Doberan," 144. On Liebenstein see, "Gesundbrunnen in Liebenstein," 504 and E.A.L. von Teubern, "Das Bad zu Liebenstein im Sachsen-Meiningischen im Sommer 1804," *Journal des Luxus und der Moden* (September 1804): 448.

117. "Neue Anlagen in Karlsbad," 11–12. König, *Kulturgeschichte des Spaziergangs*, 222, uses the same depiction to argue for a romantic turn in the walking culture. Yet the environment which the promenadors encountered on their walkways was predefined in civilizational terms: it was tamed.

118. "Ronneburger Bad 1812," 670.

119. "Liebenstein und Brückenau," *Journal des Luxus und der Moden* (August 1805): 551.

120. "Die Würtembergischen Bäder und Gesundbrunnen," *Journal des Luxus und der Moden* (September 1814): 585.

121. See especially Villaume's famous chapter on "Ob und in wie fern bei der Erziehung die Vollkommenheit des einzelnen Menschen seiner Brauchbarkeit aufzuopfern sey?" in *Allgemeine Revision des gesammten Schul- und Erziehungswesens*, vol. 3, ed. Joachim Heinrich Campe (Hamburg: Carl Ernst Bohn, 1985), 470–84, 570–77, in which he argues that moderation is more useful and thus more virtuous than one-sided perfection. In other words, he argued for a mediocre habitus. See also the comments on educational practices in Dessau, "Einige der allgemeinen Pflichten," *Philanthropisches Lesebuch* 2 (1778): 126.

122. Hufeland, *Makrobiotik*, 81 and esp. 106–11. On the early dietetic notions of moderation see, for instance, Wedel[ius], *Diæta Literatorum*, 19 and Jahn, *Norma Diaetetica*, 164.

123. Feiler, *Handbuch der Diätetik*, 215. This same statement can be found already in Wedel, *Diæta Literatorum*, 19. Cf. also Christian Friedrich Ludwig Wildberg, *Handbuch der Diaetetik für Menschen im gesunden Zustande* (Leipzig: Cnobloch, 1828), 285.

124. Jahn, *Norma Diaetetica*, 164.

125. Johann Wendt, *Ueber den Tanz als Vergnügen und Schädlichkeit. Ein Beytrag zur Diätetik*. Zweyte Auflage (Breslau: August Schall, 1804), 16.

126. See, Ivensen, *Terpsichore,* 34 and the complaints from the Pyrmont spa, "Pyrmont im Jahr 1797," 508–9. For Wolf, the notorious critic of the waltz, the minuet was acceptable because of its moderateness, *Beweis daß das Walzen,* 17.

127. Schelle, *Spatziergänge*, 64.

128. Immanuel Kant, *Critique of Judgment*, trans. Werner S. Pluhar, (Indianapolis: Hackett, 1987), 194, 203. On lunchtime music, see Werner Friedrich Kümmel's excellent article "Tafelmusik aus medizin- und musikhistorischer Sicht," in *Ernährung und Ernährungslehre im 19. Jahrhundert*, ed. Edith Heischkel-Artelt (Göttingen: Vandenhoeck & Ruprecht, 1976), 386–407. According to Kümmel, the effect of lunchtime music was dietetic, signifying the overarching function of this music but also its subordinate status. On the long tradition of musical therapy and its revival in the eighteenth century, see Lesky, "Van Swietens Hypochondrie," 182–83.

129. Schelle, *Spatziergänge*, 43–44. The humanist, Ficino, had described both walking and music as excellent remedies against the corruptive influence of black bile on a scholar's health. See Kümmel, "Homo litteratus," 77.

130. GutsMuths, *Gymnastik 1793*, 371.

131. Gaulhofer, *Die Fußhaltung*, 50. Gaulhofer calls this posture which lays the stress on the toes and keeps the feet open, "dancing master posture" (*Tanzmeisterstellung*).

132. GutsMuths, *Gymnastik 1793*, 263. Although the programs of the Dessau *Philanthropinum*, emphasized educational hiking, in reality traditional walking, *Spazieren*, remained dominant. On Dessau see, "Von den täglichen Aufsicht," *Philanthropisches Archiv* 3 (1776): 115–17; "Einige der allgemeinen Pflichten," 120. On the Pädagogium Regium in Halle see Ernst Christian Trapp, "Ueber das Hallische Erzihungsinstitut," *Pädagogische Unterhandlungen* 5 (1783): 58.

133. In the first, 1793 edition of *Gymnastik*, GutsMuths distinguished between the "measured dancing steps" and "natural, relaxed fashion of walking," GutsMuths, *Gymnastik 1793*, 371. He, however, did not specify what kind of configuration and style of stepping would be natural, i.e., what kind of foot position conveyed the impression of a relaxed and vigorous man. In the second, 1804 edition, he was even more explicitly in favor of the traditional step: "It is always a sign of a peculiar slackness and weakness when the foot touches the ground bent, the heel first and later the ball of the foot," GutsMuths, *Gymnastik 1804*, 186.

134. Jahn, *Die deutsche Turnkunst (1816)*, 4. Vieth also considered that "walking on a flat foot is the most natural way and the least exhausting." It was, however, important that the heel touched the ground slightly before the toes, Vieth, *Versuch einer Encyklopädie*, vol. 2, 147, 150. This walking is completely separated from the motion which the dancing master is supposed to cultivate; walking as *Gehen* is for him a physical performance in order to move and hike.

135. Not the performance and the movement of torso but the firmness of step was Jahn's purpose; he recommended uneven terraine, Jahn, *Die deutsche Turnkunst 1928*, 4–6.

136. See a more detailed discussion in Chapter 4, esp. in the section on "Gymnastics in Context."

137. Kazmaier, *Tübinger Spaziergänge*, 46–47. On Vischer's acitivites for the beautification of the Wöhrd, see König, *Kulturgeschichte des Spaziergangs*, 299–302. On Vischer's positive view of gymnastics, especially its military form, see Fritz Schlawe, *Friedrich Theodor Vischer* (Stuttgart: J.B. Metzlersche Buchhandlung, 1959), 195. Vischer, a left wing liberal, saw gymnastics as a vehicle of mobilizing people, to make it a militaristic subject of power. For this purpose Jahn's gymnastics was for him less adequate than the traditional exercises, dancing, riding, and especially fencing. They should be elevated to a higher level of significance, to military exercise, "of which fencing is a regular part." See, especially Vischer's article, "Das akademische Leben und die Gymnastik. Ein frommer Wunsch." It was published in 1845 in Schwelger's *Jahrbücher der Gegenwart*, Friedrich Theodor Vischer, "Das akademische Leben und die Gymnastik. Ein frommer Wunsch," in *Kritische Gänge*, vol. 3 (Berlin: Meyer & Jessen, 1920), 385–401.

138. See, for instance, his letter to Strauß, Tübingen, March 15, 1850 in Theodor Friedrich Vischer, *Briefwechsel zwischen Strauß und Vischer*, vol. 1 (Stuttgart: Klett Verlag, 1952), 248, in which Vischer mentions Dr. Baur, Wohl, and Schwelger as his regular walking companions.

*Part Three*

# The Crises of the 1830s

# Chapter Seven

# Cholera

The first three decades of the nineteenth century ushered in two changes that were important for the educated middle class and its conduct of the body. During the militaristic fervor of the Napoleonic Wars, the tribal activities of gymnastics challenged the pattern of moderate—dietetic—exercise that had evolved in aristocratic circles and were then adopted by the bourgeoisie. The same period saw a turn of the tide after authorities suppressed the gymnastics movement and re-established political equilibrium. At the same time, the rapidly expanding network of social clubs, spas, and urban parks and promenades re-emphasized moderate bodily exercise, especially dancing and promenading, as the exercises of choice for the rising educated middle class. During the 1830s, a series of events left the political and physical equilibriums seemingly unchallenged yet ultimately undermined them. The first of these was cholera, which throughout the century spread the fear of sudden death, even to those who saw themselves beyond its reach. The battle against cholera, which started as a battle of medical doctors against a disease, soon turned into laymen's self-defense against an overwhelming force of nature. Because no effective medical therapy against cholera was developed until the 1890s, the only means available were preventive measures that dietetic literature had recommended for centuries. But who determined the extent and quality of dietetic prevention? At stake was whether and how much state authorities were entitled to intervene in the bodily conduct of the individual, particularly a cultivated person. In Germany, the battle against cholera effectively prolonged the dietetic strategy of life, the defense of bodily autonomy against increasing pressures from state authorities.

## Cholera Spreads

Georg Wilhelm Friedrich Hegel celebrated his sixty-second birthday on August 27, 1831. Tivoli, an entertainment district on the outskirts of Berlin, was an unusual place for a man of such stature to celebrate this event.[1] However, Hegel had a good reason for this arrangement. Cholera was approaching, and all who could had left the city or kept their visits to a minimum. News of *cholera asiatica* had rapidly spread since September 1830, when the disease broke out in Moscow. Russian troops quelling civil uprisings brought it to Poland in early 1831. In May, it appeared in Prussia, first in Danzig and two months later in Königsberg. By late July and early August, educated Berliners were certain that sooner or later the disease would reach the capital, despite extraordinary protective measures such as control of travel and *cordons sanitaires*. And they were right. Two days after Hegel's birthday gathering, cholera felled its first victim in the Prussian capital.[2]

Hegel withdrew to his garden, spending time studying, discussing politics with friends, playing chess with his two sons, and taking short walks. His life was quite comfortable and his withdrawal from the city—not from his social class—seemed propitious. By the second week of November, cholera was clearly on the decline. Hegel had kept his distance from the city and the university almost three months and was growing increasingly impatient, for his self-imposed isolation had disrupted the fulfilment of professorial duties. Moreover, the law professor Eduard Gans, a liberal disciple and increasingly popular colleague of his, was about to start his lectures. The dean of Prussian and German philosophers felt he was losing ground and decided that he must start his lectures, too.[3] What happened next is not completely clear. We know that at 5 p.m. on Friday, November 11, Hegel entered the auditorium to continue his lectures on the history of philosophy and the philosophy of rights. According to Johann Jacoby and David Friedrich Strauß, who both attended these lectures, his sunken, almost cadaverous appearance foreshadowed an inevitable death, but by the same token, substantiated the enormous strength of Hegel's spirit, which regardless of physical pain thundered "titanic thoughts" and displayed "the appearance of pure mind."[4]

Marie Hegel, his wife, saw events differently. According to her, Hegel gave his lectures with his old vigor and liveliness. Therefore the events on Sunday came for her as a total surprise. After his breakfast at 11 a.m. in high spirits, Hegel developed a severe stomachache and nausea. The doctor came at 2 p.m. but provided little help. Hegel felt nauseated and anxious throughout the rest of the day and the following night. The next morning, Monday, November 14—the anniversary of the day Leibniz had died—Hegel awoke peaceful but exhausted. By 3 p.m. he had broken out in a cold sweat and his skin became ice cold. Soon after that, he had difficulty breathing. He then entered a soft, deep sleep. Georg Friedrich Wilhelm Hegel had passed away.[5] For Marie Hegel it was the death of a saint. "Would you have recognized," she asked Christiane Hegel, the philosopher's sister, "symptoms of cholera in any of this?"[6] Yet the medical diagnosis was clear: cholera combined with an apoplectic fit.[7]

The final days of Hegel, besides offering a vivid image to stem our philosophical curiosity, provide an insight into the workings of cholera and, more important for this discussion, how it was perceived by the educated middle class. Yet cholera also was a public threat. Although the epidemic was in decline, Hegel was not its last victim in Prussia. After an interruption after January 1832, the disease broke out anew the following summer. At the same time cholera ravaged Hamburg as well as Lübeck, and, to a lesser extent, Prussian cities south of Berlin, such as Halle and Magdeburg. The Hapsburg Empire was hit much harder than Prussia. In Hungary, more than 150,000 and in Galicia almost 100,000 died, while the death toll for the Empire climbed to more than 250,000 casualties in 1831 and more than 100,000 in the subsequent epidemic of 1832.[8] After spreading to England, France, Spain, and Italy, cholera returned to Germany in August 1836, with Bavaria as its epicenter. Between October 1836 and January 1837, 1,061 people died from this disease.[9] After 1837, cholera disappeared almost entirely from Europe, only to return in 1847 and reappear every decade after that. Until the 1890s, it regularly swept the continent, claiming hundreds of thousands of victims.

## The State Intervenes

In spite of its cataclysmic power, cholera's social ramifications call for anything but a straightforward explanation.[10] During its early appearances in the 1830s and 1840s, cholera was more often than not intertwined with political and social upheavals. In addition, the first epidemic overlaps a change in medical epistemology that drew public attention to the disease as it slowly approached from Southern Asia and as its effects became known. However, the medical profession was anything but unified in explaining the nature and dissemination of cholera. All these factors made the disease into a powerful social phenomenon, transforming social structures and intellectual conventions virtually overnight.

The traditional and more or less effective prophylaxis against epidemics, especially plagues, was isolation. Both *cordons sanitaires* for communities and individual quarantines were used. Cholera seemed to provide exceptionally good opportunities for enacting these methods in a most rigorous and effective way. Soon after it turned into an epidemic in India in 1817, news of its pathology and proliferation started to trickle into Germany. Throughout the 1820s, the medical profession sporadically discussed its etiology and possible therapies. When the disease hit Orenburg, a large region in Southern Russia, in 1829, physicians and medical authorities became alarmed. In the late fall of 1829, the Prussian government sent Karl Ignaz Lorinser, a district physician from Oppeln in Silesia, to investigate the effects and spread of cholera, which in the meanwhile had reached the border of Galicia and Siebenbürgen.[11] During his expeditions in Russia and

Austria, Lorinser collected extensive materials and kept a systematic diary on instances of the disease and the legislative and practical measures that the Russian and Austrian governments had taken to prevent its spread. He was skeptical about the possibilities of protecting the population through state intervention and especially critical of the extensive system of isolation that the Russian and especially the Austrian governments had initiated.[12] Despite its having sent him to find out what other governments had done to stem the disease, Lorinser's observations were ignored by the Prussian government.

A decision already had been reached in Berlin while Lorinser was in the midst of his travel in Russia and Austria. Four established physicians, Johann Christoph Albers, Hermann Quincke, Edmund Dann, and Ernst Barchewitz, were sent to Russia to report on the progress of cholera and the efficacy of preventive measures.[13] The king and his government based their decision on these reports and on the recommendations of a cholera committee, created by the Minister of Education, Karl Sigmund von Altenstein in the late fall of 1830. The tone of the authorities was clear: cholera was contagious and could be defeated only through decisive measures, *cordons sanitaires*, and incarceration. As a consequence, the leading principalities of the Germanic Confederation, the absolutist monarchies of Prussia and Austria, opted for state intervention in protecting their territories and populations against the devastating epidemic. Barbara Dettke has analyzed in detail the steps taken by the Prussian government to stop the advance of cholera at its borders.[14] Whereas Austria, with its long eastern border, had proposed protective measures by the fall of 1830, Prussian authorities decided to wait. Throughout the spring, the advance of the disease was carefully followed, mainly via monitoring reports from observers in Russia. In April, officials were surprised and alarmed by an outbreak of the disease in Warsaw, though observers had reported earlier that cholera already had disappeared in Russia. Following the example of Austria, which had established *cordons sanitaires* at its borders in January 1831, the Prussian government sealed its borders, at the beginning of May 1831, using three lines of military and civilian guards. Entrance was allowed only by permit for those who came from "clean" areas.[15] In addition, imported goods and even mail were subject to careful controls.

If preventive measures against an invasion of cholera from outside the borders resembled a military blockade, measures within the country were, if possible, even more severe. In Berlin they were spelled in the *Verordnung über das Verfahren bei der Annäherung und dem Ausbruche der Cholera in Berlin*, which the highest cholera authorities, general Ernst Ludwig von Tippelskirch, the military commander of Berlin, and Magnus Friedrich von Bassewitz, the highest civilian officer in Brandenburg (*Regierungspräsident*) had signed on August 23, 1831. It was based on the decree of June 28, 1831. The *Verordnung* defined the organizational structure of cholera prevention in Berlin and determined the measures authorities and private citizens should undertake in case cholera approached and broke out—which had happened already. In the city of Berlin, overall control was in the hands of a central cholera authority headed by the police commander. The members were representatives of different city authorities and medical doctors.[16] Interestingly, this authoritarian and interventionist structure, which followed the Austrian model, was cushioned by local committees in charge of prevention at the grassroots level.[17] Although they also were headed by a local police commander, the body of these committees was to consist of "appropriate residents of the electoral district for city council."[18] This two-pronged (and incipiently democratic) approach also was incorporated in the guidelines for prophylactic measures. It was built into both the Prussian and Austrian regulations as a combination of control and dietetic care. The poor, and especially their hygienic standards, had to be overseen; those suspected of being infected were to be incarcerated, and lack of moderation (*Unmäßigkeit*) should be fought.[19] All these factors were considered critical in preventing the spread of the disease.

Once cholera broke out, the central and local authorities were ordered to intervene in a most drastic manner. All gatherings were forbidden. The diseased were to be transported to cholera hospitals or isolated in their homes, along with those in the same household (and in some cases, even in the same building). Moreover, the decree ordered the contaminated building carefully guarded, roped off from the street and other buildings, and a sign with the word "cholera" to be displayed upon its wall. In some cases, the building was to be locked and the key kept by the local cholera committee.[20] Even the pets living with the cholera patient were to be isolated or killed.[21] Finally, in case of death, the corpse was to be delivered to a special graveyard at night, after an examination by a cholera doctor.[22]

Intrusive as they were, the public measures were augmented by recommendations on individual conduct. In the Austrian instructions, these were considered especially important. The authorities were convinced that an individual's predisposition facilitated the spread of cholera, as much as the contagious nature of the disease. Whereas a collective health policy was considered the only efficient counter to the contagion, an individual could regulate his or her own predisposition. One part of individual conduct was related to measures against contagion, which was best avoided by hygiene and disinfection. The cholera committee of Berlin, for instance, described in detail how contaminated items and persons should be disinfected, what chemicals should be used—chloride and vinegar—and how the fumigation should be effected as a measure against polluted air and objects. Instructions directly related to the transmission of contagion was, however, separate from a host of recommendations about one's general lifestyle. A list of dietetic proscriptions advised the avoidance of harmful food and drink, irregular lifestyles and melancholic affects, cold weather and filthy air, while recommending regular physical exercise and sleep. All excess, on the grounds of overburdening one's body and mind, was especially warned against. As § 17 of the Austrian regulations stated: "all strenuous and continuing work, soldiers' and messengers' rapid marching, an unstable lifestyle, and nightly wandering should be entirely avoided."[23] Above all, one should keep calm and preserve normality as much as possible.[24] This was an almost classic dietetic rule. It had its advocates in

Berlin, where Hufeland was its most famous, although not the most unwavering, promoter. His approval of *cordons sanitaires* was tentative and he was not at all clear about the transmission of cholera.[25] The dietetic conviction was particularly strong among the Viennese medical profession, which under the control of the leading doctor, *Protomedicus* Joseph Andreas von Stifft had taken a radical turn toward Hippocratic medicine. Its leading proponent, Johann Valentin von Hildenbrand, aggressively promoted a version of environmental medicine in which the seasons, location, and weather affected the proportions of bodily humors in the individual.[26] Hildenbrand's views, which rejected contagion as an explanation, were crucial because as the professor of internal medicine at the University of Vienna he was in charge of the censorship of cholera literature.[27]

Few areas in Germany had tangible experience with cholera. Prussia, a paradigmatic case for state intervention that rested on administrative regulation to counter the spread of cholera, was one of the few principalities of the Germanic Confederation that had a concrete experience of the epidemic. The first wave of cholera in 1831-32 was limited to the eastern and northeastern part of the Confederation. Among the areas affected were Austria, the eastern territories of Prussia, Hamburg, Lübeck, and the region of Lüneburg in Hannover; some cases in Mecklenburg, Holstein, and the Saxonian Duchies also were reported. Most of the Germanic Confederation remained free of cholera during the first wave. Not until 1832, when cholera spread from France and the Netherlands to Hesse (Kassel), Rhineland (Mühlheim, Aachen) and from Bohemia all the way to the eastern corner of Bavaria (Landshut), it experienced the disease.[28] Because of this advantage, Prussian doctors dominated the cholera discourse that inundated the medical public with books, journals, reports, and pamphlets. The absence of advice from Austrian doctors, under the strict control of Stifft and his emissaries, was all the more striking.[29]

In Leipzig, which saw no cholera during the first wave, medical doctors actively participated in the debate over cholera. Justus Radius published his *Allgemeine Cholera-Zeitung* here, which catalogued news and theoretical contributions related to cholera from all over Germany and Europe.[30] Even in Tübingen, which was hundreds of miles from the areas at risk, prominent physicians such as Ferdinand Gmelin and Friedrich Schnurrer worked intensively on the topic.[31] Cholera was not known only by actual victims, but, above all, through public discussions on effective prophylactic measures against it. From late 1830 through 1832, these discussions occupied the German educated public and influenced the conduct of life, regardless of whether a city or district was struck by cholera. Cholera was the subject of daily discourse and, more concretely, in the measures that governments took to defend their territories against the approaching epidemic.

And governments were alarmed indeed. Following the example of Russian, Austrian, and, later, Prussian legislation, most minor principalities and city councils made preparations for the approaching epidemic. Baden, for instance, introduced military cordons at its borders in 1831 and held them successfully through 1832.[32] But the crucial months of delay had taught an important lesson, especially in the western principalities. Unlike the regulations of Austria and Prussia, domestic measures taken in minor principalities emphasized personal conduct and tranquility of mind. The harsh practices of hospitalization and individual quarantine were mentioned only incidentally in their decrees. For instance, the Bavarian orders for the prevention of cholera of May 3, 1832, explicitly stated "that one should also avoid, whenever possible, all institutions which cause fear and unrest and all regulations which restrict mobility in the country."[33] In Mannheim, which first saw cholera only in 1849, the authorities in 1832 recommended "protection against cold and humidity, preservation of moderation, . . . cleanliness . . . avoidance of all fear of this disease. The disease could be prevented by an appropriate diet and conduct of life" because it was only conditionally contagious.[34] This important point in the definition of cholera implied a hierarchy of preventive measures: Above all one should pay attention to personal predisposition.

Personal prophylaxis was also an important principle in the recommendations given to the city council of Leipzig by a committee under the leadership of Johann Christian August Clarus, professor of medicine at the University of Leipzig and director of the Clinic at the Jakobspital. In principle, Clarus and his colleagues endorsed the measures so far undertaken by the city authorities. In terms of legislation, much had been accomplished: eleven governmental decrees or orders and eight municipal decrees regarding the prevention of cholera. The physicians wanted to shift public attention to special improvements in prophylactic arrangements. First of all, they called for the opening of a private hospital "in which foreigners, students, shop clerks, and other persons who do not belong to public hospitals and yet lack adequate care in their homes, can be accepted for a low fee."[35] The special needs of the educated middle class, including those of its poorer segments, required recognition in their own right and treatment targeted to their members.

Hamburg, which in the summer of 1831 had adopted *cordons sanitaires*, soon reversed its policies. For a city dependent on free traffic and transportation of goods, the overly restrictive measures, readily adopted by Prussia and Austria, would have been damaging in the long run. In the fall of 1831, Hamburg significantly modified its cholera regulations, turning to a more liberal treatment of both the victims and the general population. Johann Carl Georg Fricke, a member of the cholera committee, summarized the initial regulations and measures in his report of November 6, 1831: Major gatherings should be avoided; contaminated buildings should be marked with a "Cholera" sign; two cholera hospitals should be established with 200 beds in each; however, only those who requested to be transported to a hospital should be taken there if circumstances and medical examination allowed.[36] After the outbreak of disease, an addenda of October 10, 1831 made crucial adjustments to these regulations. The requirement of a cholera sign was dropped and the sanction of special graveyards for cholera casualties was changed to a voluntary basis. Only upon the particular wish of the family could a cholera victim be buried in the special graveyard.[37] The relaxation of cholera countermeasures show that the economic interests of the commercial bourgeoisie outweighed the mortal threat of cholera to the population.[38] Making a virtue of necessity, the city council assumed a laissez-faire attitude toward cholera, leaving the treatment and prophylaxis to private intiative and the consequences to private responsibility.

In November 1831, after the first wave of cholera started to decline, the non-interventionist policies gained in popularity in other principalities as well. In Austria, the government had tried to prevent panic among the population by avoiding the use of the word "cholera." Once this proved unsuccessful in 1831, a new strategy was chosen during the next epidemic, in the following summer. The government ordered the authorities to avoid unbearable aggravations in imposing regulations on behavior of the population.[39] In Prussia, a new decree was released on January 31, 1832, when the disease had virtually vanished, only to return again the following summer. Although differences from the previous decree (from that of May 1831) were insignificant—both incarceration and military cordons were accepted as legitimate tools of prevention—the shift in tone was remarkable in its psychology. Not surprisingly, this shift was aimed at the group whose loyalty and cooperation were of special importance—the educated middle class. Marie Hegel fought for her rights to bury her husband "in the graveyard where Solger and Fichte rest" at an honorable time, at 3 pm—and not as the regulations required, at night.[40] Her request was accepted. The new regulations declared the special graveyards optional.[41] Moreover, the harsh regulations on quarantines and isolation were made more lenient. Private doctors were allowed to attend the stricken if they could pay for medical attention and it required on the permission of the head of the family for an infected person to be transported to a hospital. If transportation was necessary, it should not be "dangerous for the diseased and should be as inconspicuous as possible."[42] The new regulations removed much of the symbolic threat of cholera policies toward the educated middle class, its self-conception, and forms of social recognition.

## Defending Bodily Autonomy

Beyond the symbolic politics of cholera, there were a host of other factors that pushed governmental policies in a more lenient direction. In Leipzig, the committee under Clarus had recognized the political potential of cholera. Worried by how the approaching epidemic was intertwined with social tensions among the population, Clarus and his colleagues claimed that

> a certain hectic tension, an elevated susceptibility for passionate stimulation seems to be spreading around nowadays. It might have its physical origin in the peculiar disposition of the neural system. Yet it is only waiting for an external impulse to burst into the flames of fanaticism. The deeper, moral reason for this phenomenon is an egotism and self-centeredness that misguided public opinion has promoted. It worships only self-made idols.[43]

With the possibility of social insurrection, the price of governmental intervention would have been too high. In Leipzig, where the memory of the September uprising of 1830 was still fresh, this analysis was quite accurate.[44] What in Leipzig was only a possibility became a reality in Königsberg. Soon after the disease broke out in Königsberg, on June 22-23, 1831, the authorities tried to impose severe restrictions and control. This triggered outrage, which developed into open revolt among the population on July 26 and 27.[45] Pushed by the daily pressure of cordoning and control, the crowd became highly suspicious about the medical explanation of cholera. As was often the case with ordinary plagues and other epidemics, its energies were turned against the doctors. They were accused of poisoning the population.[46] The government's prohibition of ordinary funerals for cholera victims added to the social unrest. Only after intervention by local artillery troops, allied with student volunteers, was the rebellious crowd suppressed. This can partially be explained, as Clarus did in Leipzig, by referring to the "hectic tension," i.e., the revolutionary atmosphere among the population. Such revolts, however, came primarily from the underclass. The question remains: How did the educated middle class, the cultivated class position itself in this bodily confrontation?

At stake were the symbolic sensibilities that the educated middle class attached to what Marie Hegel called that "disgusting word" cholera.[47] Dettke, Evans, and Delaporte have pointed out that cholera was regarded as a disease of the lower class, and this perception created rifts between state authority and the loyalty of the educated middle class.[48] But there also was something more profound at stake, which reveals itself when we place the cholera discourse in the wider context of the cultivated conduct of life. It was no accident that the men who played such a prominent role in reinvigorating dietetic ideology at the beginning of the nineteenth century, Hufeland and Burdach, were at the center of the cholera debate. Flanked by Lorinser, they argued against the active policies of Prussian and Austrian authorities that reinforced repressive state intervention.

As Lorinser, after returning from his expedition to Austria and Russia in 1829–30, submitted his report to the Prussian ministry of education—the medical issues belonged to its jurisdiction—he was convinced that cholera could not be defeated by military cordons and isolation policies. This conclusion derived from the miasmatic theory of cholera. According to it, cholera was an atmospheric disease whose spread was encouraged by specific qualities of local climates, which meant that the disease lived everywhere and there was no perfect—or even effective—protection against it. The individual could decrease only his personal predisposition to cholera and, in case of actual illness, survive by strengthening his body by following the rules of dietetics. The opposing theory relied on the idea of contagion, in which cholera was spread through physical contact. Thus it implied the possibility of effective protection: If all physical contact with the diseased were avoided, infection would be impossible. The senior officials at the Prussian department of education who refused to accept Lorinser's report, led by the director of the medical section, Rust, were defiant advocates of contagionism and, consequently, of all public prophylaxes, especially military cordons and quarantine of the diseased.[49] All over Europe, scientific battle lines were drawn parallel to crucial differences in practical health policies. In general—with some local variations—those in favor of miasmism emphasized private dietetics, whereas the advocates of contagionism supported state intervention.[50] This was the situation in Prussia and in most German principalities during the summer of 1831, when the first crucial steps for cholera prevention were taken.

The relationship of miasmism and contagionism was anomalous. The advocates of both theories could show conclusive evidence refuting their opponents. According to the miasmatic theory, cholera should have remained endemic to India but, as contagionists pointed out, it advanced to areas with a completely different climate and atmosphere: northern Europe, Russia, and Scandinavia. By the end of 1831, the advocates of miasmism could show equally strong evidence against contagionism. Despite all the *cordons sanitaires* and isolation of the diseased, neither the Austrian nor the Prussian government could halt the progress of cholera. Without admitting the logical reason for this anomaly, namely the impotence of any known medical prophylaxis and therapy in facing such an overwhelming epidemic, the medical profession took a stand that was quite natural, and definitely safe for its reputation. It did not want to appropriate a field that it could not manage by its own methods. After 1832, the responsibility for prophylaxis shifted to cultivated individuals who were supposed to make use of their dietetic knowledge as best they could. How was this shift possible? In the dominant interpretations of cholera the shift in power from governmental health policy to private dietetics has been explained as the victory of miasmism.[51] Undoubtedly miasmic theories ruled in England, France, and Hamburg even before the outbreak of cholera, and in the rest of Europe after the first wave was over. But in Germany the small print of the cholera debate reveals a more complex story than a simple scientific controversy between two theoretical positions.

When the German debate on the causes of cholera reached its high point, during the spring of 1832, Hufeland, though known to be leaning toward the miasmatic camp, tried to calm the antagonists by acting as a mediator between them. He argued that all doctors were basically contagionists. The point of difference was whether there were an infectious relationship between the contagium and the diseased, and whether it were disseminated through personal, miasmatic or miasmatic-personal contagion.[52] For Hufeland the result was a combination of both explanations: "Cholera [is] a new, foreign disease that has been transported from Asia to Europe. It is conditionally contagious but cannot be blocked off through quarantine. Its origin is always the same, its cause is always transmission (*Übertragung*), but not only personal transmission."[53] In Lorinser we find the same caveat: Despite his support for miasmism, he never had any doubt that there was some kind of contagion that transmitted the disease.[54] There were contagionists who tried to refute all this, but even they found common ground with the miasmatists. It was most often located in the description of the contamination;

whether the disease was thought to be caused by miasma or contagium, a personal predisposition was always included as one factor of its materialization. Even the first, resoundingly contagionist, instructions from Prussian authorities did not forget to mention this.[55] A case in point were the general instructions in Leipzig, provided by Clarus and his colleagues, which described a set of rules that decreased one's predisposition to the disease. First, strict order and cleanliness in one's environment and life were required. But this rule, a recommendation to harden one's body, were complemented through dietetic recommendations of moderation: warm clothing, moderation in eating and drinking, and moderate physical exercise should be accompanied by sociability, music, and dancing. Finally, one should, "walk . . . or ride on a horse or in a carriage . . . at least an hour a day. During the current season, choose the early hours, from 8 to 9 in the morning and 3 to 5 in the afternoon. Avoid humid and damp places, swamps, and areas of putrid vapors and the proximity of hospitals."[56] This program was propagated as a universal prophylaxis against cholera, specially after the first negative experiences of *cordons sanitaires* and quarantines. With an eye to the lower class, which was showing signs of restlessness, Clarus required that each class should be able to think of the common good. Regardless of its mortal impact on society, cholera now appeared as an effective means of restoring the lost sense of community, *Gemeinsinn*.[57]

Closely related to dietetic control of one's predisposition to cholera was the symptom of fear. Cholera-related fear was often associated with political anxieties that were still running high, especially in the aftermath of the July Revolution. In fact, Clarus's book was a good example of how political angst about the lower class was spreading among the elite. This was, however, neither the only nor the dominant articulation of fear in the context of cholera. The most elementary description of cholera-related fear came from the diagnosis of symptoms. Fear normally was listed as a common symptom of the early stages of cholera.[58] But because a symptom, according to traditional pathology, belonged to the essence of a disease, the doctors identified fear as a cause of the disease. Then, too, the strict cordoning, incarceration, and secretive methods of burying the victims or transporting them to hospitals caused fear among the population. Without protecting the population these measures did the opposite; they did not provide prophylaxis but, as the advocates of miasmism argued, caused fear and therefore cholera, or at least contributed to its spread.[59] Fear thus had two sources: the pathological state of the body and the misplaced measures of the autocratic state. It was articulated in popular uprisings, as in Königsberg, but also in different strategies of the educated middle class. These strategies tried to mediate between two social articulations of fear, fear of the unstable lower class and fear of governmental control of one's own body. Clearly, cholera provided a convenient relief for those who feared popular uprisings in the summer of 1831. Like an invisible hand, it seemed to punish the lower class most severely, giving it what it deserved for its immoral and disorderly lifestyle. Rahel Varnhagen von Ense expressed this common fear and hope in her letter to J.D. Assing:

> We are hopeful that the disease will not ravage here indiscriminately but, at best, remove some of those lives that properly enough have prepared themselves for that destiny through their psychic and moral nature. By doing this, they continue to offer themselves to the disease. These lives can hardly be saved, but orderly and careful people of the cultivated class are barely threatened [by the epidemic].[60]

This explanation of cholera as a moral punishment for lower-class uprisings was common indeed, as recent scholarship has shown.[61]

Closely associated with the moral explanation of cholera was the supplementary understanding of how the educated middle class could cope with fear of the state and its protective policies. Burdach, now a leading doctor and member of the cholera commission in Königsberg, provided the most elaborate articulation of this strategy. Authorized by the cholera commission, Burdach compiled a pamphlet in the early summer of 1831, *Belehrung für Nichtärzte über die Verhütung der Cholera*, addressing educated laity. They should be, so said Burdach, "in the position to correctly evaluate their situation regarding this epidemic and, consequently, to arrange their conduct appropriately."[62] To judge the situation correctly, a cultivated person needed to know how to prevent a predisposition to cholera.[63] He had to know the universal rules of dietetics to adjust his balance in everyday conduct. The most dangerous factors, according to Burdach, were exhaustion and overburdening of any kind, increased sensibility, and fear.[64] To control fear, one's social position and *Bildung* were important. This was so because the escalation of fear and, hence, cholera could be avoided only if the self-reflection of one's educational standing (*Bildungsstufe*) produced an example to emulate.[65] In short, Burdach reiterated the principles he had adopted in his early book on the dietetics of healthy persons and applied it to a situation in which middle-class conduct was challenged not only from below but also from above through the frightening terror of the state. As a matter of interest, Burdach and his colleagues were successful in protecting middle-class conduct of life. Soon after the disease broke out in Königsberg on June 22 and 23, 1831, severe control and restrictions were abandoned as ineffective. Yet the Prussian government delayed the release of the new liberal regulations, so the pathological and social tensions had time to erupt into violence by the end of July.[66]

The defense of bodily autonomy surfaced in Vienna in a striking way. Karoline Pichler recounts how cholera influenced her life. During the first epidemic in 1831, she and her husband tried to stay calm and fearless in the increasingly chaotic situation. The rapidly increasing number of victims, the nightly transportation of the diseased and the dead, and the medical personnel running around caused "fear, dismay, and misery."[67] In the second epidemic, the public reaction was quite different: "cordoning and disinfection, the measures of fearful [authorities], were not put into effect. One saw the disease for what it was, a painful fate, perhaps a punishment that God has sent to humankind."[68] Pichler was convinced that fearlessness was the best prophylaxis: the less one feared and panicked, the less one deviated from the customary way of life, the less likely one was to fall ill.[69] It had two benefits. It helped to protect one's health and it set the example for others to follow.[70] Personal prophylaxis, combined with new hygienic standards remained the most important protection against cholera until 1884, when Robert Koch identified its bacterial causes.

The implications of Burdach's position were clear. A cultivated person was capable of an orderly conduct of life because he could master the balance of his body and the environment. State regulation offered no benefits, only harm, for it could destroy this balance by creating unnecessary fear and angst and by imposing diets and measures that were not normal, average and moderate. It also deprived the educated middle class of its bodily autonomy and thus the means of cultural leadership. As a result, the liberal strategy of confronting the challenge of cholera had two different versions. The first was adopted during the fall of 1831 by Hamburg in its defense of commercial priorities. After 1832, it was introduced by Lübeck and, to a lesser extent, by most German principalities. The second one was based on the discourse of dietetics that Hufeland and Burdach had formulated at the beginning of the century as the cultivated autonomy of the body.

## Notes

1. Karl Rosenkranz, *Georg Wilhelm Friedrich Hegel's Leben*. Berlin: Duncker & Humblot, 1844, 419. Quoted in Günther Nicolin, *Hegel in Berichten seiner Zeitgenossen* (Hamburg: Meiner, 1970), 436.

2. Johann Wegener, a seaman, fell ill and died the following morning on his boat.

3. This is Arnold Ruge's version. See Arnold Ruge, *Aus früherer Zeit*, vol. 4 (Berlin,: Duncker & Humblot, 1867), 431, according to Nicolin, *Hegel*, 437–38.

4. According to Strauß, Hegel gave the "Eindruck des reinen Fürsichseins." He mentions both lectures; Jacoby only the one on the history of philosophy. For my depiction of Hegel's final lecture I have used D.F. Strauß's letter to Märklin, 11.15.1831, in Nicolin, *Hegel*, 466 and Johann Jacoby, *Bilder und Zustände aus Berlin*, vol. 1 (Altenberg, 1833), 268, according to Nicolin, *Hegel*, 438.

5. The most detailed account of Hegel's final days is Marie Hegel's letter to Christiane Hegel, November 11, 1831, which has been published in Nicolin, *Hegel*, 480–84. Her letter to Friedrich Immanuel Niethammer, December 2, 1831, published in Nicolin, *Hegel*, 496–500, also provides interesting insights into Hegel's agony. See also a detailed account by Barbara Markiewicz, "Hegels Tod," in *Die "Jahrbücher für wissenschaftliche Kritik." Hegels Berliner Gegenakademie*, ed. Christoph Jamme (Stuttgart-Bad Cannstatt: Fromman-Holzboog, 1994), 531–56. She duplicates the classic interpretation of Hegel's heroic death. Barbara Dettke provides a more sober and sensitive understanding of how cholera caused Hegel's death, *Die asiatische Hydra. Die Cholera von 1830/31 in Berlin und den preußischen Provinzen Posen, Preußen und Schlesien* (Berlin; New York: Walter de Gruyter, 1995), 185–88.

6. Marie Hegel to Christiane Hegel, November 11, 1831, in Nicolin, *Hegel*, 481.

7. *Ibid.*, 484.

8. Raimund Triml, "Die erste Cholera-Epidemie in Wien in den Jahren 1831 und 1832" (PhD diss., University of Vienna, 1992), 148, provides mortality figures as high as 178,780 for Hungary and 96,080 for Galicia; and for the whole Empire, 281,200 in 1831 and 105,300 in 1832. Compared with the total 4,158 dead when both epidemics struck metropolitan Vienna, the casualties were horrendous, Triml, *Cholera-Epidemie in Wien*, 138, 146–47. These figures are still in need of historical scrutiny, as is the course of cholera in Vienna. Triml's work provides only some preliminary outlines, though it is based on a fairly exhaustive inventory of archival materials. The connections between the medical profession, the city and state governments, and the general population need further study, after the manner in which Evans has conducted his seminal study on Hamburg. The emphasis of Evans' studies rest on the epidemics of the late nineteenth-century, though he traces its patterns of development to the 1830s. See Richard Evans, *Death in Hamburg. Society and Politics in the Cholera Years 1830–1910* (Oxford: Clarendon Press, 1987), on the early epidemics esp. 226–64.

9. Cholera in Munich has not been researched well enough, considering its wider ramifications for the history of hygiene in which Munich and Max von Pettenkofer played such a seminal role after the 1850s. Alida Christine Geßner's "Die Cholera-Epidemien in Bayern während des 19. Jahrhunderts unter besonderer Berücksichtigung der Statd Ingolstadt und ihrer Umgebung" (Munich: Diss., 1992) makes some general observations on Bavaria, esp. 20–40. More reliable and accurate is Johann Baier's *Armut, Not und Hoffnung am Rande einer Stadt. Haidhausen im Jahrhundert der Cholera-Epidemien. Ein Beitrag zur Sozialgeschichte Haidhausens* (Munich: Haidhausen-Verlag, 1988), esp. 31–39.

10. There is extensive literature on the political and social dimensions of cholera in European societies. On French history, see Catherine J. Kudlick, *Cholera in Post-Revolutionary Paris. A Cultural History* (London: University of California Press, 1996). She compares the two epidemics of 1832 and 1848. A more traditional class dichotomy between the conspiratorial upper class and the victimized lower class can be found in François Delaporte, *Le savoir de la maladie. Essai sur le choléra de 1832 à Paris* (Paris: Presses Universitaires de France, 1990). On cholera in the British Isles, see Michael Durey, *The Return of the Plague. British Society and the Cholera, 1831–32* (Dublin: Humanities Press, 1979), passim. The important case of Russia has been studied by Roderick E. McGrew, *Russia and the Cholera, 1823–1832* (Madison: University of Wisconsin Press, 1965). A scandinavian perspective is offered by Brita Zacke, *Koleraepidemien i Stockholm, 1834. En socialhistorisk studie* (Stockholm: Kommunalförvaltning, 1971). On Germany there is no modern overall presentation. The only work available is Walter Krehnke's *Der Gang der Cholera in Deutschland seit ihrem ersten Auftreten bis heute* (Berlin: Schoetz, 1937), although Richard Evans, *The Death in Hamburg*, 243–51, 470–78, and Barbara Dettke, *Die asiatische Hydra*, esp. 296–310, provide substantial materials through their local studies.

11. Carl Ignatius Lorinser, *Eine Selbstbiographie. Vollendet und herausgegeben von seinem Sohne Franz Lorinser*, vol. 1 (Regensburg: Georg Joseph Manz, 1864), 195.

12. Carl Ignatius Lorinser, *Eine Selbstbiographie. Vollendet und herausgegeben von seinem Sohne Franz Lorinser*, vol. 2 (Regensburg: Georg Joseph Manz, 1864), 13.

13. A detailed account of his travel can be found in Dettke, *Asiatische Hydra*, 66–73.

14. Dettke, *Asiatische Hydra*, 76–80, 152–68.

15. In November 1830, the Viennese government published a decree that regulated its protective measures, *Instruction fuer die Sanitaets-Behoerden, . . . die Graenzen der k.k. oesterr. Staaten vor dem Einbruche der im kaiserlichen russischen Reiche herrschenden epidemischen Brechruhr . . . zu sichern, und im möglichen Falle des Eindringens, ihre Verbreitung zu hemmen. Auf allerhöchsten Befehl verfasst* [Wien, 1830]. Reprinted (Hannover: Helwingsche Buch-Handlung, 1831). The existing *cordons sanitaires* on the eastern border—toward the Ottoman Empire—were strengthened, Triml, "Cholera-Epidemie in Wien," 67. Cf. Dettke, *Asiatische Hydra*, 77. Her observation of the early cordoning of the Austrian-Russian border needs a correction. According to Triml, hardly any quarantine institutions were used at the border, although the *Instruction* required their establishment. See Triml, "Cholera-Epidemie in Wien," 153.

16. Ernst Ludwig von Tippelskirch and Magnus Friedrich von Bassewitz, *Verordnung über das Verfahren bei der Annäherung und dem Ausbruche der Cholera in Berlin. Gesundheits-Commission für Berlin* (Berlin: Gesundheits-Commission für Berlin, 1831), 5.

17. Triml, "Cholera-Epidemie in Wien," 166–67. There is no indication that the model used in Vienna included participation by local lay members.

18. "Geeigneter Bewohner der Bezirke, welche die Stadtverordneten-Versammlung wählt," Tippelskirch and Bassewitz, *Verordnung über das Verfahren*, 6. Also in Baden, local lay participation was not only allowed but ordered. See Loetz, *Vom Kranken zum Patienten*, 263–64.

19. Tippelskirch and Bassewitz, *Verordnung über das Verfahren*, 10–13. Concerning Austrian regulations, see *Instruction für die Sanitäts-Behörden*, 11.

20. Tippelskirch and Bassewitz, *Verordnung über das Verfahren*, 28. Cf. *Instruction für die Sanitäts-Behörden*, 8.

21. Tippelskirch and Bassewitz, *Verordnung über das Verfahren*, 34.

22. Tippelskirch and Bassewitz, *Verordnung über das Verfahren*, 45.

23. *Instruction für die Sanitäts-Behörden*, 11.

24. Tippelskirch and Bassewitz, *Verordnung über das Verfahren. Beilage A*, 6–7.

25. Hufeland's interest in cholera appeared first in his article, "Athmosphärische Krankheiten und atmosphärische Ansteckung, Unterschied von Epidemie, Contagion und Infection. Ein Beitrag zu den Untersuchungen über die Contagiosität des gelben Fiebers," *Journal der practischen Heilkunde* 57.1 (1823): 3–41. In several articles published in the *Journal der practischen Heilkunde*, especially after 1829, Hufeland oscillated between contagionism and miasmism. His prophylactic recommendations shared this ambiguous approach, combining cordoning with personal diet, moderate and balanced nutrition, hygiene (washing with chloride etc.), fresh air, avoidance of alcohol, and a calm but cheerful mind (*guter Mut*) and "belief in one's own resistence against the disease." See Christoph Wilhelm Hufeland, "Ueber den Unterschied von epidemischer Constitution, Epidemie, und Contagion, und die Verschiedenheit mittelbarer und unmittelbarer, lebender und todter Contagiosität, mit Rücksicht auf die orientalische Cholera," *Journal der practischen Heilkunde* 72.4 (1831): 104–5. This interesting article presumably appeared in the summer of 1831 because Hufeland could justify his defense of *cordons sanitaires* by the Austrian experience. "Immediate separation of any diseased by cholera, namely the cordoning of the house . . . the cordoning of the district. By so doing one could abruptly stop the progress of the disease in Austria," Hufeland, "Unterschied von epidemischer," 106.

26. Erna Lesky, *Die Wiener medizinische Schule im 19. Jahrhundert* (Graz; Köln: Verlag Hermann Böhlaus Nachfolger, 1978), 45.

27. On Hildenbrand's contributions to the discussion and decisions, see J. Fischer, "Der erste Choleraausbruch in Österreich nach Akten der Wiener medizinischen Fakultät aus den Jahren 1831 und 1832," in *Historische Studien und Skizzen zu Natur- und Heilwissenschaft* (Berlin, 1930), 136–38. For Hildenbrand, even the thought of "morgenländische Brechruhr" (oriental cholera) was unacceptable because it implied the actuality of contagion.

28. This information is based on Krehnke, *Der Gang der Cholera in Deutschland*, 338–53.

29. Johann Peter Frank's work was classic in this field. The final supplemental volumes of his "System der medizinischen Polizei" were published as late as 1825 and 1827. But Frank was expelled from Vienna in 1805 and his disciples were carefully purged from academia. The public discussion was dominated after 1811 by the official journal, *Medicinische Jahrbücher des k.k. österreichischen Staates*. On the so-called reactionary Stifft-Era in Viennese medicine see, Lesky, *Wiener medizinische Schule*, esp. Chapter 2, 32–117.

30. *(Allgemeine Cholera-Zeitung.) Mittheilungen des Neuesten und Merkwürdigsten über die Asiatische Cholera*, ed. Justus Radius (Leipzig: Baumgärtners Buchhandlung, 1831–1832).

31. See Friedrich Schnurrer, *Die Cholera morbus, ihre Verbreitung, ihre Zufälle, die versuchte Heilmethode, ihre Eigenthümlichkeiten und die im Großen dagegen anzuwendenden Mittel. Mit der Charte ihres Verbreitungsbezirks*. Zweite vermehrte Auflage (Stuttgart und Tübingen: Cotta, 1834). Schnurrer's interest in cholera went back to 1828, when he published an extensive article on cholera in Ersch and Gruber's *Allgemeine Enzyklopädie*, vol. 17, 42–48. See Klaus Bauer, "Friedrich Schnurrer (1784–1833), ein Arzt aus Tübingen," in *Bausteine zur Tübinger Universitätsgeschichte*. Folge 7, ed. Volker Schäfer (Tübingen: Universitätsarchiv, 1995), 78. Gmelin responded to Schnurrer, whose explanation was extremely "atmospheric," i.e., environmental, by understanding cholera mainly as a contagious disease. Ferdinand Gmelin, "Comments," in John Mason Good, *Die ostindische Cholera*, aus dem Englischen des John Mason Good übersetzt und mit einigen Zusätzen versehen von Ferdinand Gottlieb Gmelin (Tübingen: Osiander, 1831), 58, 67.

32. See Evans, "Epidemics and Revolutions," 140. However, the protection of these *cordons sanitaires* is open to doubt because the government could afford only 280 men to guard the entire 270 km-long western border, see Loetz, *Vom Kranken zum Patienten*, 263.

33. "Die Vorschriften über die vorbereitenden Anstalten und sanitätspolizeilichen Anordnungen für den Fall des Ausbruchs der asiatischen Cholera im Innern des Landes," in Geßner, "Die Cholera-Epidemien," 132.

34. *Mannheimer Tageblätter* 115 (1832): 565–568. According to Martin Krauß, *Armenwesen und Gesundheitsfursorge in Mannheim vor der Industrialisierung, 1750-1850/-60* (Sigmaringen: Jan Thorbecke Verlag, 1993), 123.

35. Johann Christian August Clarus, *Ansichten eines Vereins praktischer Aerzte in Leipzig über die Verbreitung der asiatischen Cholera auf doppeltem Wege. Mit einer diätetischen Haustafel für die Cholerazeit* (Leipzig: Gerhard Fleischer, 1831), 14.

36. Johann Carl Georg Fricke, *Geschichtliche Darstellung des Ausbruchs der asiatischen Cholera in Hamburg. Nach Acten und amtlich angestellten Untersuchungen* (Hamburg: Perthes & Besser, 1831), 5. On the early *cordons sanitaires* See Richard J. Evans, *Tod in Hamburg. Stadt, Gesellschaft und Politik in den Cholera-Jahren 1830–1910*

(Reinbek bei Hamburg: Rowohlt, 1991), 316–17.

37. Fricke, *Geschichtliche Darstellung*, 7.

38. Lübeck, which had successfully erected *cordons sanitaires* and kept the city free of cholera, abruptly let almost all preventative measures lapse when the disease at last broke out in the city in July 1832. See Dietrich Helm, *Die Cholera in Lübeck. Epidemieprophylaxie und -bekämpfung im 19. Jahrhundert* (Neumünster: Karl Wachholtz Verlag, 1979), 22.

39. Triml, "Cholera-Epidemie in Wien," 173. Karoline Pichler saw the change in policy as quite dramatic; with the change in prophylactic measures from state intervention to divine intervention, cholera was seen as God's punishment to base humankind. See Karoline Pichler, *Denkwürdigkeiten aus meinem Leben*, vol. 2, ed. Emil Karl Blümmel (München: Georg Müller, 1914), 287.

40. Marie Hegel to Susanne von Tucher, 11.15.1831, in Nicolin, *Hegel*, 461.

41. *Allerhöchste Cabinetsordre vom 5ten Februar 1832, enthaltend die Bestätigung der Instruction über das, in Betreff der asiatischen Cholera in allen Provinzen des Preußischen Staats zu beobachtende Verfahren* (Berlin: Mittler, 1832), 3.

42. *Allerhöchste Cabinetsordre*, 6. As Evans correctly observes, Prussia remained, in general, committed to the assumption that cholera was contagious; this was also true after 1832, in the regulations of 1835 and 1850. Evans, "Epidemics and Revolutions," 141.

43. Clarus, *Ansichten*, 17.

44. A refreshing analysis of the "Leipzig unrest" in 1830 can be found in Robert Beachy's, *The Soul of Commerce. Credit, Property, and Politics in Leipzig, 1750–1840* (Leiden: Brill, 2005), 197–221.

45. Burdach, *Rückblick*, 391. Cf. Dettke, *Asiatische Hydra*, 134–37.

46. Concerning similar occasions in Paris during the 1832 epidemic, see Kudlick, *Cholera*, 186.

47. Marie Hegel to Susanne von Tucher, 11.15.1831, in Nicolin, *Hegel*, 460. Interestingly, right after mentioning this "disgusting word" (*gräßliches Wort*), Marie Hegel starts to depict Hegel's individual suffering as something exceptional, caused by a disease that destroyed his constitution but was not detectable on his body. "Such a cholera brings the most blessed death—such a disease is not rancorous," Marie Hegel to Susanne von Tucher, 11.15.1831, in Nicolin, *Hegel*, 461.

48. Evans identifies the request for psychological harmony, which the instructions emphasized, as an expression of social concern toward the lower class. Evans, *Death in Hamburg*, 247–48. Dettke also points out the strategies of the educated middle class in coping with cholera. Itwas not only fearful for its survival (just as the peasants were) but also concerned about social disturbances, social shame, and social equality brought about by cholera. In fact, to avoid public shame several upperclass persons asked their doctors not to use their names if they became ill or died of cholera. Dettke, *Asiatische Hydra*, 262–82. For the French and Parisian experience, Delaporte explains the prophylactic programs in Paris against cholera as an imposition of bourgeois morality over society, Delaporte, *Le savoir de la maladie*, 84–89.

49. Lorinser, *Selbstbiographie*. Vol. 2, 13.

50. Lorinser showed this difference in prophylaxis in his *Die Pest des Orients wie sie entsteht und verhütet wird. Drei Bücher* (Berlin: Enslin, 1837), 414, in dealing with the traditional plague: "The old plague order can be divided into two categories: those which emphasize miasma and those which stress contagium. In the first case, which is more

common, the main prophylaxis was in the protection of the individual through dietetic and medical measures. In the second case, the purpose was rather to prevent the progress of the disease by using methods of public policy."

51. Evans, *Death in Hamburg*, 233–34. On Paris, see Kudlick, *Cholera*, 178.

52. Christoph Wilhelm Hufeland, "Worüber streitet man. Was heisst Ansteckung. Was heisst Contagionist u. Nichtcontagionist bei der Cholera," *Journal der practischen Heilkunde* 74.1 (1832): 110–15.

53. "Die Cholera, eine neue, ausländische, aus Asien nach Europa verpflanzte, bedingt ansteckende, aber nicht sperrbare, Krankheit; Ihr Keim immer derselbe, ihre Ursache immer Uebertragung, aber nicht bloss persönliche," Christoph Wilhelm Hufeland, "Schlussresultat," *Journal der practischen Heilkunde* 74 (1832): 3-10.

54. Lorinser saw miasma as the cause of epidemic diseases, but because of the different mobility and resistance of different types of miasma, he also supported cordoning and public health policies as means of protection. Lorinser, *Pest des Orients*, 226, 434; Lorinser, *Selbstbiographie*, vol. 2, 13. Cf. Burdach, who defined the cause as an infectious matter in the air. See Karl Friedrich Burdach, Belehrung für Nichtärzte über die Verhütung der Cholera. Im Auftrage der Sanitätskommission zu Königsberg (Königsberg: Universitätsbuchhandlung, 1831), 8.

55. Tippelskirch and Bassewitz, *Verordnung über das Verfahren. Beilage A*, 5–6.

56. Clarus, *Ansichten*, 20–24.

57. Clarus, *Ansichten*, 18.

58. See the general instructions of Saxony, *Belehrung über die Asiatische Cholera für Nichtärzte. Auf allerhöchsten Befehl in dem Königsreich Sachsen bekannt gemacht* (Dresden: P.G. Hildersche Buchhandlung, 1831), 5. For Austria see *Instruction für die Sanitäts-Behörden*, 6. Cf. also Hufeland's explanation of cholera's influence on conception through fear in Christoph Wilhelm Hufeland, "Einfluss der Cholera auf die Conception," *Journal der practischen Heilkunde* 74.6 (1832): 137.

59. Burdach, *Rückblick*, 387. Cf. to Karoline Pichler's private experience about fearfulness and fearlessness in Vienna during the cholera epidemics of 1831 and 1832. See Pichler, *Denkwürdigkeiten*, 279, 287.

60. Rahel Varnhagen von Ense to J.D. Assing, 8.31.1831, according to Dettke, *Asiatische Hydra*, 262.

61. A critical but balanced overview of these interpretations can be found in Evans, "Epidemics and Revolutions," 128, 131–35.

62. Burdach, *Belehrung*, III.

63. Burdach, *Belehrung*, 21.

64. Burdach, *Belehrung*, 24–31.

65. Burdach, *Belehrung*, 31.

66. Burdach, *Rückblick*, 392.

67. Pichler, *Denkwürdigkeiten*, 280. For instance, the pan-German meeting of natural scientists in Vienna was postponed to 1832. "Several [of the visitors] stayed away, either because they feared cholera that ravaged Vienna by the beginning of September; or they stayed away because of the more reasonable fear for the quarantine (*Contumazanstalten*) that countries without cholera had established for traffic coming from the Austrian lands," "Das Fest der Naturforscher in Wien," *Zeitung für die elegante Welt* 205 (1832): 1634.

68. Pichler, *Denkwürdigkeiten*, 287.

69. Pichler, *Denkwürdigkeiten*, 282.

70. Pichler, *Denkwürdigkeiten*, 275–78. Through cholera, Pichler became interested in emulation and its influence on human behavior.

# Chapter Eight

# The *Überbürdung* Debate and *Gymnasium*

The delicate balance of bodily dietetics that state intervention threatened to destroy through its cholera prophylaxis seemed also to be threatened by another state institution, the school. The second important event of the 1830s was the seemingly innocent debate about overburdening at Prussian *Gymnasium*. It touched upon the rights of students to have their own time for leisure and recreation, and their own bodily autonomy and thus questioned the limits of the state and its ideology of education. But it also launched a reform that ultimately undermined the dietetic conception of the body and opened new avenues for the state to regulate the middle-class body.

Four years after cholera had invaded Prussia, Karl Ignaz Lorinser complained that "the essential energy of life has declined. The livelier the senses and the more desirous the instincts have become, the more the mind and body have lost their resistance."[1] As a leading cholera doctor, he accused, naturally, the increasing number of diseases that spread among the population; he also accused, as did many of his contemporaries, the detrimental consequences of children's premature sexual development and onanism.[2] But his main target was the school, especially the Prussian *Gymnasium*, which plagued students with "the plethora of subjects, lessons, and homework" so that it had become, according to Lorinser, a burdensome institution.[3] His article, which quickly made its author both a celebrity and a troublemaker, launched a debate that revealed an important facet of the political controversies revolving the bodily conduct of the German educated middle class.

The Lorinser-debate or the debate on *Überbürdung* (overburdening) has been discussed in two parallel fields of scholarship: the history of education and sports history. Friedrich Paulsen, the preeminent scholar of German education, characterized the overloaded curriculum as a master plot that loomed large in German secondary education, especially the *Gymnasium*, until the end of the nineteenth century.[4] But sports historians have adopted the Lorinser-debate as the second beginning of modern German gymnastics. These opposed interpretations indicate a problem in understanding Lorinser's article. Did he describe a genuine structural problem of German secondary education? Or was he writing the blueprint of modern German gymnastics? Rather than making one despair the lack of facts, these opposed interpretations mark the beginning of cleavage in German education. The article and ensuing debate can be seen as one of the last instances in the nineteenth century when German educators debated the relationship between the education of the mind and the body.

The discussion had started in eighteenth-century dietetics that emphasized moderation.[5] Krüger, Zückert, and especially Tissot were among those issuing the most vocal warnings against overloading the mind at the expense of the body. "The diseases of the scholars," maintained Tissot, "have two main sources: the busy occupation of the mind and the constant rest of the body."[6] The warning was reiterated in manuals for such dietetic practices as spa life and walking.[7] It is, however, difficult to determine whether these warnings were directed against specific activities and lifestyles or merely signified a rhetorical topos. In any case, ever since the mid-eighteenth century, their critical position was supported by Rousseau in his educational writings, the educational tracts of Johann Peter Miller, and the prescriptions of dietetic doctors who started to direct public attention to increased *Überbürdung* at secondary schools. Whereas Miller's call for an "education of pleasure" in the 1750s remained an isolated outcry against the current system of education, advocates of the *Philanthropismus* found broad support for their ideas of playful variation in learning.[8] Basedow was a vocal critic of the pedantic and sedentary lifestyle of scholars; he declared that at his institutions "no student will be coerced to study diligently."[9] The educational institutions of the *Philanthropismus* created a platform for those who saw traditional secondary schools as oppressive and burdensome. Yet the terms of discussion soon changed when, after 1800 and especially after the military defeats against Napoleonic troops at Auerstedt and Jena, Prussia and several other German principalities scrambled to compensate for the loss of political prestige with cultural and educational excellence. It was not the *Philanthropismus* but neohumanism, a modified version of the old school ideology, that set the parameters of the ensuing school reforms.

In fact, much of the spirit of German and especially Prussian and Bavarian educational reforms stemmed from the critique of the *Philanthropismus*. As a result, in 1808, Friedrich Immanuel Niethammer, the reformer of schools in Bavaria, found himself defending the neohumanistic school ideology against accusations of *Überbürdung*. Physical education had been one of the key ideas of the *Philanthropismus* to provide relief from academic burdens. But in his *Fight Between the Philanthropismus and Humanism,* Niethmammer declared defiantly that "one can say without reservation that more children are ruined by premature physical than by intellectual exertion."[10] This book, perhaps more than any other text or decision, contributed to the neohumanistic hegemony in German education and the subsequent decline of the overloaded curriculum as an educational problem.[11] The reformed curricula could hardly be accused of being too taxing, because they emphasized a small number of ancient languages and weeded out the auxiliary subjects that had congested every student's school day. At the same time, Jahn's gymnastics, which became increasingly acceptable and desirable, seemed to meet the requirement of the *Philanthropismus* for physical education that provided relief and variety from the hardships of intellectual exertion.

The Carlsbad Decrees changed the situation. Not only did it ban Jahn's gymnastics casting a shadow over physical education's place in the curriculum but it also undermined the influence of liberal reformers. The implementation of new school legislation, prepared by Süvern and other liberal administrators, was not feasible, and Prussian secondary education remained dependent on governmental decrees and temporary guidelines until the 1830s. In this political landscape, the neohumanists drifted away from the center of intellectual power. In 1818, Hegel assumed the professorship of philosophy at the University of Berlin. Johannes Schulze, the director of the department of education, found his way to Hegel's lectures, which he attended regularly between 1819 and 1821.[12] Subsequent discussions and, eventually, a close friendship made Hegel a trusted advisor to Schulze and allowed him to exercise considerable power over the department of education.[13] As a result of this relationship, a significant change took place in the ongoing debate over school reform. Under the pressure of Hegel's philosophy of realism, the philhellenic program of ancient learning was replaced by a program highlighted by the natural sciences, modern languages, philosophy, and a strong emphasis on Latin. But since the classical languages were retained, the additional requirements for natural sciences, mathematics, modern languages, and humanities were simply added to the 28–30 class-hours per week that all students attended.[14] This heavy and challenging curriculum was implemented in Prussian *Gymnasiums* during the 1820s.

In 1826, the critics raised their voices.[15] Friedrich von Raumer, professor of history at the University of Berlin, accused the new expanded curriculum of destroying students' joy in learning and, ultimately, their individuality.[16] He was seconded by the school reformer Friedrich Thiersch, a prominent philologist from Munich and an advocate of gymnastics, who responded to Schulze's acrimonious review of his *Über gelehrte Schulen mit besonderer Rücksicht auf Bayern* by angrily pointing out the exhaustion that the new Prussian curriculum would bring about. It would suppress, he said, the cheerful and free pursuit of knowledge that was the beginning of all genuine *Bildung*.[17] Thiersch and von Raumer were both traditional humanists. In the 1790s, Raumer had attended the *Gymnasium* of Joachimsthal in Berlin, known for its progressive spirit and its early adoption of gymnastics, while Thiersch was an alumni of Schulpforte, an elite grammar school that for centuries had practiced a strict humanistic program with a particularly light mandatory workload. Its curriculum contained one full day a week for the free pursuit of studies. Because of its exceptional results (Klopstock and Fichte were among its graduates) Schulpforte was named as an alternative to the emerging Prussian system.[18] Its classical, humanistic curriculum resonated well in Bavaria, Württemberg, and Saxony, which celebrated a strong and unchallenged tradition of grammar schools or *Lateinschule*.

From the perspective of educational history, Lorinser did not make a significant new contribution. As in the earlier curriculum debate in the 1820s, he built on the example of Saxonian elite schools;[19] and like the humanist critics of Hegelian reform, Lorinser challenged the competence of school authorities to shape a balanced curriculum for the *Gymnasium*. But in many ways his accusations merely skimmed the surface of the ongoing debate about the workload at the Prussian *Gymnasium*. It was the rhetorical form of his text, the way it articulated the symptoms of an educational crisis, that assured its political success.[20] The Prussian king, Frederick William III, strongly approved of Lorinser's analysis and ordered the secretary of education, von Altenstein, to respond to his accusations. Altenstein and the high officers of his department, especially Schulze, spent much energy and time countering Lorinser's allegations. They initiated an extensive and long-lasting investigation of all Prussian *Gymnasiums*. But as it was conducted by the local school authorities—the committees that were the very targets of Lorinser's attack—the results were predictable. The final report concluded that Lorinser's assertions lacked any empirical evidence and were invented in order to destroy the foundations of the Prussian school system and its raison d'etre, the classical *Bildung*. The "apology" of the administration was most successful: Rather than pushing the schools toward a more liberal curriculum, the Prussian administration used the criticism not for its specific suggestions but as an occasion to complete its own reform, which had remained temporary and incomplete in the 1820s. In the so-called Blue Book of 1837, a new curriculum was devised that left the old system basically the way it was.[21]

The same event that occasioned Paulsen's gloomy interpretation of an immutable and conservative Prussian school system appears in quite a different light if we look at sports history. After the Carlsbad Decrees had banned *Turnen*, the gymnastic tradition was preserved through secret meetings of student fraternities, *Burschenschaften*, and various projects of dietetic gymnastics, such as Werner's institutions in Dessau and Dresden. In Swabia and Hamburg, Jahn's gymnastics were never curtailed. After 1830, writers such as Koch, Kirchner, Maßmann, and Straß started to vindicate gymnastics and even to encourage the reintroduction of *Turnen*.[22] According to sports history, Lorinser, building on this revived enthusiasm for gymnastics, opened the discussion for crucial political decisions and institutional change.[23] The same investigation that doomed reductions in student workload launched, after 1838, a series of measures to reintroduce physical education and made it an optional subject in Prussian secondary education. After Frederick William IV, under the influence of national romanticism, assumed the throne and Minister von Altenstein died in 1840, the new policy received an additional boost. The ban on *Turnen* in Prussia was repealed in 1842. Saxony,

Baden, Bavaria, and Hesse legalized it in the following year, and Württemberg followed suit in 1845. There is, however, an important anomaly. Lorinser did not mention physical education or Jahn's gymnastics in his text nor did he suggest that physical exercise be introduced at the Prussian *Gymnasium*.[24] Ironically, Lorinser did not succeed in his intention—the reduction in student workload—but achieved the reintroduction of *Turnen*, which he had not intended at all.

To explain how this happened, it is advisable to return to the text itself. We find in Lorinser's article an argument that took its point of departure not from the theories of humanistic education or gymnastics but from Hufeland's dietetic analysis:

> In his outline on the history of health, C.W. Hufeland has attempted to describe the current physical character of humankind. Here he has discovered the refinement of the physiological constitution, particularly the neural system. Moreover, he has detected a decline in power and a corresponding increasing excitability, early development of intellectual activities and procreative desire, declining vision and elevated level of sickness (*Kräncklichkeit*). All these are conspicuous features of our time.[25]

Hufeland was one of several authors that Lorinser could have relied upon for his pamphlet. In *Medicinische Fastenpredigten*, Franz Anton May had made the detrimental lifestyle of scholars a powerful point of his argument. Like Tissot, he pointed out that by overloading their minds and avoiding physical exercise, scholars had become a serious pathological problem for the nation.[26] Yet by relying on Hufeland, Lorinser committed himself to a broad condemnation of the overrefined civilization, of which the secondary schools were concrete illustration.[27] They were unable to reach their stated purpose of genuine intellectual cultivation and harmony between physical and intellectual education, because, argued Lorinser, their practice "consists mainly in the development and cultivation of the intellectual faculties."[28] They had lost the balance between the mind and the body thanks to modernization, which had deprived humankind of its necessary harmony. The discovery of America, the "so-called" progress of the sciences, new raw materials, the compass, means of communication, industrial production, luxury, and, finally, the fever of revolution—all had conspired to produce a new type of soul and physical constitution, more mobile and unruly than ever before.[29] This accounted for increased irritability, sensibility, and capacity of mind. As a result, the body as the sensory medium of expanded intellectual operation grew ever more frail. The increased capacity of the mind and the hyperactivity of the sensory organs, Lorinser argued, fed themselves at the expense of the energy and tenacity of the body.

Instead of combating the morbid tendencies of civilization, Lorinser accused the Prussian *Gymnasium* of being an active accomplice in the process.[30] By increasing students' workload from 32 to 42 hours a week, the *Gymnasium* overburdened their intellectual capacity and contributed to the general pathology of modernization. With all the strain placed on the mind, there was not enough time in the day for recreation and recovery of the body, either at school or at home. "The old rules of a dietetics for the mind have virtually fallen into oblivion," and all kinds of ailments followed, from digestive problems to hemorrhoids.[31] Supported by Johann Christian Jahn, Lorinser suggested a radical reduction in the time spent sitting, enabled by a corresponding decrease in subjects and time for homework.[32] He had articulated a crucial problem and in a short time he had received more than seventy responses, mainly from Prussia but also from educators and administrations in other principalities. In 1838, the authorities in Württemberg encouraged medical doctors to discuss physiological problems that accompanied overburdened mind. Four years later, the problems were at the center of debates in the parliament, leading directly to the legalization of *Turnen* in Württemberg.[33] A. Schroeder, who reviewed the subsequent debate in the *Jenaische Allgemeine Literatur-Zeitung*, could not avoid a certain Hegelian pathos in describing Lorinser's historical contribution:

> In some periods in time and at some level of *Bildung*, ideas enter the universal feeling of rational humankind. By doing so, they elevate themselves from the dawn of incremental *Bildung* to the clarity of universal consciousness. In this process the encapsulated ideas need only a slight impulse in order to burst out to their full power. Dr. Lorinser has given such an impulse.[34]

In his millenarian rhetoric, Schroeder was right. Lorinser's text was historical in every sense of the word: It came at the right time, and it purported to restore the traditional and natural order of bodily and intellectual conduct. But even more historical was the subsequent discussion. Critics and defenders alike discussed the question of hours and their redistribution. While a vocal minority rejected Lorinser's findings and saw no excessive burden in classical languages and sciences, the educational mainstream accepted his statement.[35] And because the critical mass of Lorinser's readership endorsed the need for a physical corrective to intellectual exertion, *Turnen* and gymnastics were rehabilitated and reintroduced into the secondary educational system.

What kind of status and content this gymnastics should have was not clear. L.V. Jüngst had in mind diverse opportunities to enjoy fresh air and movement, swimming, mechanical work, games, and "hikes to collect objects of nature." Schroeder endorsed a similar program.[36] But such moderate exercises, which were little more than recreation, were not enough for most educators. Friedrich Kritz, a professor at the *Gymnasium* of Erfurt, advocated a moral hardening that could be improved through gymnastics,[37] while C.W.G. Marquard, a professor at a *Gymnasium* in Züllichau, spoke up for the return of Jahn's gymnastics: "The disappearance of the so-called *Turnkunst* (Jahn's gymnastics) from the grammar schools after 1819 has thrown the baby out with the bath water. By doing so we have made inestimable damage to . . . the well-being of the younger generation that has since then gone on to school and to state offices."[38]

Christa Kleindienst-Cachay has explained the striking medical and psychological language of the debates that led to the rehabilitation of *Turnen* in 1842 by a political situation that compelled reformers to find an apolitical vocabulary to promote their case.[39] We might call this a negative function of the dietetic language, but it had its merits as well. The Hegelian conception of *Bildung*, adapted to the existing system of secondary education, was hardly the instrument that could enable reforms that German societies of restoration needed and requested. The polemics of Lorinser's text show this clearly. Lorinser had wanted to create more space and time for the body's recreation and more autonomy for the individual. He received the endorsement of those who, much more than he, saw this space and time in a state of continuous erosion. Yet the debate indicated something more. It laid open a variety of options that Lorinser's critique suggested for the promotion of bodily *Bildung*. He did not exclude moderate exercise, dietetic "hardening" or Jahn's gymnastics. It was this multitude of physical education possibilities that gained momentum in the 1840s.

## The Revival of Gymnastics

In 1842, Frederick William IV issued a decree that permitted gymnastic exercise at educational institutions. Although the wording of the decree carefully avoided mentioning *Turnen*, the decree was generally perceived as the repeal of the 1819 ban.[40] As a further sign of political and ideological change, Friedrich Ludwig Jahn was rehabilitated.[41] The years immediately after the decree saw a surge in new gymnastic clubs and institutes in the Germanic Confederation, except in Austria.[42] In important ways, however, the revival of *Turnen* differed from its initial incarnation in 1811–19. No longer was *Turnen* a predominantly Prussian phenomenon. The new gymnastics movement was centered in Württemberg, Saxony, and Hesse (Frankfurt am Main and Hanau). In these principalities, we can find Wilhelm Klumpp from Stuttgart, Adolf Spieß from Gießen and Darmstadt, Moritz Kloss from Dresden, and other prominent figures of gymnastics at work. They were the new leaders, different from Jahn in personality as well as program and more influential than the *Turnvater* who remained passive and skeptical of the revival of his own invention.

Under Jahn, the gymnastics movement had emerged from a vision of a male tribal community. As a reaction against such politics, the scattered ventures of *Turnen* during the 1820s and 1830s had emphasized their educational or dietetic, hence normal, moderate, and harmless nature. The post-1842 revival of Jahn's gymnastics were different in at least three ways. First, we can distinguish a strong pull toward associational gymnastics. Second, equally strong, was the tendency to normalize gymnastics, to incorporate it into public education. Finally, a few efforts still promoted dietetic gymnastics.

The first gymnastic clubs for adult and adolescent males were founded in 1833 in Frankfurt am Main and Vogtland (Saxony).[43] If we include the club founded in Stuttgart by Klumpp in 1822, the map of semi-political gymnastics starts to take its shape. Württemberg, Saxony, and Hesse, with constitutions in place and dense populations, became the headquarters of the associational revival of *Turnen*. After 1842, the number of clubs accelerated significantly, so that by 1847 Düding has estimated between 80,000 and 90,000 gymnasts in the Germanic Confederation.[44] The gymnastics movement thus became with the choir movement and the German Catholic movement one of the first mass movements in Germany. Especially in Saxony, Württemberg, Baden, and Hesse, it provided a fertile environment for liberal, democratic, and even socialist mobilization. The fierce, though unsuccessful, efforts of Hanau gymnasts to start a local revolution in 1848 offers a good example of how closely bound up with politics were the revived gymnastics movement and how quickly political action took root in the clubs.[45] Although much of the historical interpretation of gymnastics concentrates on independent, associational gymnastics and its political aspirations and work, the febrile years 1811–19 and 1842–48 were only the highlights of active political involvement by German gymnastics. After 1850, the forces of restoration effectively suppressed political sentiment within the movement. The associational *Turnen*, acutely conscious of its independence and its tradition of self-determination, became institutionalized and politically harmless during the 1850s and the 1860s.

The main pressure on the institutionalization of *Turnen* came from state governments and their educational policies but, in fact, this pressure had been there from the very beginning. Jahn himself was unsure whether to pursue independent gymnastics or increase his influence by integrating gymnastics into public education.[46] Most of the gymnastic institutes that survived the ban or emerged after its implementation, were under strict governmental supervision. Hans Ferdinand Maßmann, who in 1828 became the director of the gymnastic institute in Munich, a facility under the patronage of Ludwig I, never quite reconciled himself to being removed from the sports field. Another disciple of Jahn, Eiselen, ran his gymnastics institute in Berlin as a private enterprise but under governmental supervision. By 1842, the question of educational gymnastics was not about its independence but about the specific conditions of its institutionalization. Maßmann realized this in a painful way when he was hired by the Prussian government in 1843 to organize gymnastic exercise in Berlin. After some successful gymnastic performances, familiar to those who had witnessed Jahn's gymnasts in Hasenhaide, public interest waned; moreover, conservative ministers became suspicious of Maßmann's motives. In 1845, Per Henrik Ling, a Swedish gymnastics leader who had developed gymnastics in a more rational and regimented direction, captured the official interest in gymnastics. From then on, Maßmann was a relict.[47]

The authorities, who had little interest in the kind of political activism that Jahn had promoted with *Turnen,* wanted gymnastics to prepare its initiates for military training and that is what they saw in Ling's gymnastics. It was Schulze who reinvented the military context to make *Turnen* acceptable, and it was his memorandum that defined the parameters of the decree of 1842.[48] Schulze saw in *Turnen* a perfect tool for uniting the population in defense of the Fatherland without undermining domestic calm. In addition to Ling, Friedrich Spieß was one of those who embraced the official interest in military exercise by developing his so-called free exercises or *Freiübungen*. In the wake of the July Revolution of 1830, when the authorities made a second crackdown on the public *Turnen*, Spieß became convinced that only the integration of gymnastics with public education could establish true physical education.[49] In the four-volume, *Die Lehre der Turnkunst* (1840–46), he crafted the conceptual and practical foundations for institutionalized *Turnen* as educational exercise. The work was widely read and influential in German schools and gymnastic clubs. The fourth volume in particular with its description of common exercise, *Gemeinübungen*, as semi-militaristic exercise in discipline, transformed *Turnen* from tribal community practice to drill. Spieß claimed that "school discipline and military discipline are essentially identical."[50] After years in Switzerland, Spieß returned to Darmstadt in 1850 and made it into one of the intellectual centers of the new gymnastics movement. From the perspective of 1818, when GutsMuths interpreted Jahn's gymnastics as military exercise, it seems that GutsMuths had won—posthumously.

Besides a political movement and a state institution, gymnastics developed another offshoot around 1830: dietetic gymnastics. It lacked the cohesion of the school gymnastics and the new gymnastics movement. Its proponents did not have systematic contacts and most of them were not even aware of each other. Yet their efforts show important structural similarities. Several were controversial figures in their lifetime: e.g., Roller, an outspoken dancing instructor at the Schulpforte, or Werner as the alter ego of the Saxonian gymnastics movement. Most were hardly noticed. But in their projects we find the continuation of dietetic tradition in German body culture.[51]

Throughout his tenure at the Schulpforte, Roller had tried to integrate dancing with *Turnen*. Although the liberal curriculum of a *Fürstenschule* allowed that, the neohumanistic ideas of its directors constantly impeded Roller's efforts. Yet the idea of combining gymnastics and dancing was gaining ground. In 1840, Spieß enthusiastically recommended gymnastic dancing for girls:

> The distinctive desire of girls to collectively express themselves in social settings can be animated and developed by gymnastics and connected to and satisfied in the realm of education. Dancing, according to its original meaning and nature, is so closely connected to Jahn's gymnastics. By using the free exercise it can be purified . . . and separated from its common superficiality and one-sidedness. By so doing it can be brought into a proper relation to life.[52]

Koch was more skeptical. Like Roller, who only reluctantly accepted the disappearance of the minuet, Koch suggested that the merging of dancing and *Turnen* was possible if dances were transformed, "gymnasticized."[53] Given the limits of gymnastic dancing as a way of changing the prevalent physical exercise, the return to dietetics seemed to provide another and, one could argue, better option because, as Koch observed, medicine and gymnastics had common roots.[54] This mission animated Schreber, who not only lectured on dietetics and published a medical treatise on *Turnen* but also was involved in the gymnastics movement in Leipzig for several years. But in a most interesting way it was reflected in the career of Johann Adolph Ludwig Werner, who started as a gymnastic and fencing teacher and finished his career as the head of an orthopedic institute in Dessau.[55]

Several years younger than Jahn, Werner participated in the same war as the gymnastics leader Jahn, but his experience was completely different, far away from romantic guerrilla camps and fierce ambushes. As a 19-year-old student, he was recruited into the cavalry of the Saxonian militia. After 1815, as a member of the occupation army in Northern France, Werner was exposed to exercises popular among French troops and civilians: swimming, single-stick, archery, gymnastic games, and, above all, fencing.[56] Within a few months, he had developed an obsession for fencing and became an instructor for his detachment. In 1820, we find Werner, who in the meanwhile had persuaded himself of the one-sided and politically harmful nature of Jahn's gymnastics, as fencing and vaulting instructor at the University of Leipzig.[57] But unlike Eiselen, who at the same time was working on a Germanized version of rapier, the classical form of French and Italian fencing, Werner concentrated on saber, the classical German fencing that had become enormously popular for student dueling in the fraternities. Werner attempted to create an art of saber, to civilize it along the lines of rapier.[58]

After a few years, Werner became interested in the educational application of gymnastics. He acquired students from local *Gymnasiums* and instructed them in physical exercise. According to the auditing report, Werner superbly trained his disciples in military gymnastics. When they marched in, "it was most delightful to see how dexterous and skillful they were in doing their exercise with rifle. . . . How precisely they, young as well as older ones, followed the commands."[59] In addition to marching, Werner had instructed them in etiquette and in agreeable and charming behavior. By this time he also discovered the dietetic and therapeutic benefits of gymnastics.[60] Military drill, aesthetic education, and dietetics now constituted the basis of his gymnastics, in diametric opposition to Jahn's ideas but still appropriating and embracing the same subjects. Werner wanted to divorce political agitation from physical exercise, creating what his biographer Rasmus called scientific gymnastics.[61]

And he succeeded. Between 1824 and 1849, Werner published more than ten extensive manuals on such topics as fencing, girls' physical education, educational gymnastics, military gymnastics, and medical gymnastics. His work on physical education and orthopedics in Leipzig and, after 1830, in Dresden was well recognized. In 1839, the prince of Dessau invited Werner to be director of the recently founded gymnastic academy, where he remained until his death in 1866.[62] Along with his work in Dessau, Werner became instrumental in introducing physical exercise at Saxonian grammar schools and threatened to overshadow Jahn and his followers.[63] By doing so he gained a permanent seat in the folklore of the gymnastics movement as the black sheep of physical educators. In 1846, Moritz Kloss, a Saxonian gymnastics leader, remembered Werner bitterly as the one whose appearance made clear the division between genuine *Turnen* and its superficial imitation, *Gymnastik*.[64] Jahn, never shy in voicing his antagonism for the aristocratic French and effeminate physical exercise, called Werner the *Manschettenturner* (the gymnast with cuffs). Werner, an admirer of military exercise, used systematic drilling in his training. For Jahn and Maßmann, this revived the debates of 1818, when GutsMuths had "misinterpreted" Jahn's ideas and tried to redefine gymnastics as military training. In their eyes, Werner was now the one who tried to smuggle in this old and dangerous idea.[65] But Werner, his institutes, and his literary work provide an important testimony to the increased diversity of gymnastic projects at the local level after 1830.[66]

What men such as Koch, Schreber, and Werner were looking for, and what the dietetic gymnastics aimed at, was not so much the therapeutic effects of gymnastics or the development of specific physical skills but the understanding of gymnastics as a form of bodily autonomy. In the 1830s, dietetics was challenged at several levels. In academic medicine, it was obviously losing ground: new findings and conceptualizations in natural science quickly made it an outdated form of therapy. Yet cholera overwhelmed standard medical therapy with such force that within a few months dietetics was a more respected remedy than ever. It was back not only in the gray zone of public health but, above all, in the strategies of the educated middle class to defend its bodily autonomy against state intervention and the social and political threats of the lower class. The debate on *Überbürdung* further confirmed the dietetic championship of bodily autonomy but also helped *Turnen* regain its legitimacy which indirectly challenged the dietetic tradition. In the 1840s, the revival of Jahn's gymnastics movement set the agenda of bodily *Bildung*. Instead of discussing whether dancing and walking or other moderate exercises should be preferred to Jahn's gymnastics, the public debated whether or how its exercise could or should be integrated with Jahn's program and in what institutional setting. This shows the curious trajectory of dietetics in nineteenth-century Germany. It was first revived by romantic doctors by the turn of the century, then again revived by cholera in 1831, then recaptured by the educational movement against the overburdened lives of cultivated young men, and continued by several individual projects of dietetic gymnastics well into the second half of the century.

## Notes

1. Karl Ignaz Lorinser, "Zum Schutze der Gesundheit in den Schulen," in *Führer in der Zeit der Turnsperre. Maßmann, v. Klumpp, Lorinser, Straß, Diesterweg, E.F. Koch, Kirchner, Nachtegall, Ling, Eiselen*, ed. Franz Paul Wiedemann (Dresden: Wilhelm Limpert-Verlag, 1933), 113.

2. "Die wesentliche Energie des Lebens ist gesunken, und in dem Maaße, wie die Sinne beweglicher und die Triebe begierlicher geworden, haben Geist und Körper an Festigkeit und Widerstand verloren," Lorinser, "Schutze der Gesundheit," 113–14.

3. "Vielheit der Unterrichtsgegenstände, in der Vielheit der Unterrichtsstunden und in der Vielheit der häuslichen Aufgaben," Lorinser, "Schutze der Gesundheit," 114.

4. Paulsen, *Geschichte des gelehrten Unterrichts*, 335. After Paulsen, overburdening was no longer considered an issue worthy of scholarly reflection. Only recently has it reemerged as a topic in the history of education. In the recent re-edition of his *Das preußische Gymnasium in Staat und Gesellschaft*, vol. 2, *Höhere Bildung zwischen Reform und Reaktion, 1817–1859* (Stuttgart: Klett-Cotta, 1996), 233–56, Karl-Ernst Jeismann reinvigorates Paulsen's narrative by paying renewed attention to the Lorinser debate. Uwe Keiler's dissertation, "Die Lorinserschrift und die dazu erstellten Gutachten unter besonderer Berücksichtigung der Leibeserziehung" (PhD diss., University of Mainz, 1978), is a thorough inventory of the archival and literary materials related to the Lorinser controversy. More recently, in the third volume of the *Handbuch der Bildungsgeschichte* (1987), Georg Jäger and Heinz-Elmar Tenorth mention playfulness and *Überbürdung* as correlated topics. See Georg Jäger and Heinz-Elmar Tenorth, "Pädagogisches Denken," in *Handbuch der deutschen Bildungsgegschichte*, vol. 3. *1800–1870. Von der Neuordnung Deutschlands bis zur Gründung des Deutschen Reiches*, ed. Karl-Ernst Jeismann and Peter Lundgreen (München: Beck, 1987), 94. See also Jeismann's detailed analysis in *Das preußische Gymnasium*, vol. 2, 233–56. He emphasizes the importance of internal divisions within the Prussian school administration; several schools were more than reluctant to adopt the new, heavily loaded neohumanistic program.

5. Paulsen starts his analysis with the so-called complaint of overburdening (*Überbürdungsklage*) of the late 1820s.

6. "Die Krankheiten der Gelehrten haben zwo Hauptquellen; die emsige Beschäftigungen des Geistes, und die stete Ruhe des Leibes," Tissot, *Gesundheit der Gelehrten*, 11.

7. Marcard, *Pyrmont*, vol. 2, 298. According to Schelle, promenading was suppose to entertain the spirit and "Jede anstrengende Geistesbeschäftigung würde diesen doppelten Zweck vereiteln." Schelle, *Spatziergänge*, 41.

8. Johann Peter Miller, "Die Schule des Vergnügens," *Acta Scholastica, Worinnen Nebst einem gründlichen Auszuge derer auserlesensten Programmatum, Der gegenwärtige Zustand Derer Berühmtesten Schulen und der dahin gehörigen Gelehrsamkeit entdecket wird* 2 (1753): 206. Miller's idea of pleasure was not hedonistic but Christian, influenced by Moravian notions of positive, transcendental love. See Miller, "Die Schule," 209–20.

9. "Zum Fleiße in Studien wird also kein Pensionist gezwungen," Johann Bernhard Basedow, "Das in Dessau errichtete Philanthropinum, eine Schule der Menschenfreundschaft," in *Ausgewählte pädagogische Schriften* (Paderborn: Ferdinand Schöningh, 1965), 217.

10. Friedrich Immanuel Niethammer, *Der Streit des Philanthropinismus und Humanismus in der Theorie des Erziehungsunterrichts unserer Zeit* (Jena: Frommann, 1808), 241.

11. On Niethammer's influence on the educational system of the early nineteenth century, see Peter Euler, *Pädagogik und Universalienstreit. Zur Bedeutung von F.I. Niethammers pädagogischer "Streitschrift"* (Weinheim: Deutscher Studien Verlag, 1989), esp. 52–53. Cf. Michael Schwarzmaier, *Friedrich Immanuel Niethammer, ein bayerischer Schulreformator*, vol. 1, *Niethammers Leben und Wirken bis zum Jahre 1807*. (1937)

(Aalen: Scientia, 1974), 68–72.

12. On Hegel's influence on Schulze see Jeismann, *Das preußische Gymnasium*, vol. 2, 225–26. Cf. Paulsen, *Geschichte des Gelehrten Unterrichts*, 347–48. The most important decrees and laws were the decree concerning the teachers' exam (*Lehrerprüfung*), 4.20.1831; law of the maturity exam (*Abiturientenprüfung*), 6.4.1834; and the curriculum for the *Gymnasium* (*Lehrordnung mit Stundenplan*), 10.24.1837.

13. Conrad Varrentrapp, *Johannes Schulze und das höhere preußische Unterrichtswesen in seiner Zeit* (Leipzig: Teubner, 1889), 452–53, according to Nicolin, *Hegel*, 209–10. Cf. Paulsen, *Geschichte des Gelehrten Unterrichts*, 320–30. Barbara Schneider, *Johannes Schulze und das preußische Gymnasium* (Frankfurt am Main: Peter Lang, 1989), 222–26, 282–84.

14. On the curriculum of the Prussian *Gymnasium* see Paulsen, *Geschichte des Gelehrten Unterrichts*, 291–92, 327, 354.

15. I follow the presentation of Keiler, *Die Lorinserschrift*, 34–36 and Paulsen, *Geschichte des Gelehrten Unterrichts*, 335–43.

16. Jeismann, *Das preußische Gymnasium*. Vol. 2, 222.

17. See Hans-Martin Kirchner, *Friedrich Thiersch. Ein liberaler Kulturpolitiker und Philhellene in Bayern* (Munich: Hieronymus, 1996), 72–74. Richter, *Hans Ferdinand Maßmann*, 181. Thiersch was also the most important contact person for Hans Ferdinand Maßmann in Munich, Kirchner, *Friedrich Thiersch*, 204. Paulsen, *Geschichte des Gelehrten Unterrichts*, 335–36.

18. On the Saxonian school system, see Paulsen, *Geschichte des Gelehrten Unterrichts*, 410–20. On the curriculum and influence of Schulpforte, see Gerhard Arnhardt, *Schulpforte. Eine Schule im Zeichen der humanistischen Bildungstradition* (Berlin: Volk und Wissen, 1988), esp. 113–63. In 1815, Schulpforte came under Prussian control, which increased pressure upon it to adapt its special program to the neohumanistic ideology of Prussian school administration. On the controversy between Thiersch and Schulze over the reform of Schulpforte, see Arnhardt, *Schulpforte*, 97.

19. Lorinser, "Schutze der Gesundheit," 127, pointed out the light curriculum of a 25–26 hour weekly workload at Saxonian public schools (*Fürstenschule*).

20. See Keiler, "Die Lorinserschrift," 17–36 and Paulsen, *Geschichte des Gelehrten Unterrichts*, 335–43.

21. Jeismann, *Das preußische Gymnasium*. Vol. 2, 246–48.

22. Koch, *Gymnastik*, 281–82, already supported in 1830 the revival of Jahn's gymnastics but wanted to reorder it as military exercise. Also Friedrich Straß, "Über die Nothwendigkeit geordneter Leibesübungen für die Gelehrtenschulen," in *Führer in der Zeit der Turnsperre*. Maßmann, v. Klumpp, Lorinser, Straß, Diesterweg, E.F. Koch, Kirchner, Nachtegall, Ling, Eiselen, ed. Franz Paul Wiedemann (Dresden: Limpert Verlag, 1933), 150, saw it necessary to subordinate Turnen to moral control. See also Hans Ferdinand Maßmann's *Leibes-Uebungen. Erstes Werk. Zur Militair-Gymnastik in's Besondere* (Landshut: Thomann, 1830), which contained long passages on gymnastics in general. C. Kirchner, "Oratio de gymnastices in gymnasiis restituendae necessitate. Rede von der Nothwendigkeit der Wiedereinführung der Leibesübungen auf den Gymnasien," in, *Führer in der Zeit der Turnsperre*. Maßmann, v. Klumpp, Lorinser, Straß, Diesterweg, E.F. Koch, Kirchner, Nachtegall, Ling, Eiselen, ed. Franz Paul Wiedemann (Dresden: Limpert Verlag, 1933), 246, saw gymnastics as a form of recreation, but one that required public support and organization.

23. Michael Krüger, *Einführung in die Geschichte der Leibeserziehung und des Sports*, vol. 2, *Leibeserziehung im 19. Jahrhundert. Turnen fürs Vaterland* (Schorndorf: Verlag Karl Hofmann, 1993), 64–76. On Württemberg in German context, see Kleindienst-Cachay, *Die Verschulung*, 112–21.

24. This discrepancy also was noticed by some critics. G.....r, *Ueber die Nothwendigkeit der Trennung von Gymnasien und Realschulen und einer Reform des Gymnasialiunterrichts. Eine Abhandling veranlaßt durch Lorinser's Aufsatz "Zum Schutz der Gesundheit auf Schulen"* (Berlin: Ludwig Hold, 1836), 8–9.

25. Lorinser, "Schutze der Gesundheit," 107–8.

26. May, *Fastenpredigten*, vol. 1, 260. Hufeland had elaborated on the overloading of mental powers and neglect of physical exercise in his *Makrobiotik*, 122–23.

27. Lorinser, "Schutze der Gesundheit," 108, referred to Christoph Wilhelm Hufeland's short essay, *Geschichte der Gesundheit nebst einer physischen Karakteristik der jetzigen Zeitalters* (Berlin: Realschulbuchhandlung, 1812).

28. Lorinser, "Schutze der Gesundheit," 109.

29. Lorinser, "Schutze der Gesundheit," 112. Cf. Krüger, *Einführung*, 66–69.

30. Lorinser, "Schutze der Gesundheit," 114.

31. Lorinser, "Schutze der Gesundheit," 108.

32. Lorinser, "Schutze der Gesundheit," 125–27.

33. Lorinser, *Selbstbiographie*, vol. 2, 40–41. Friedrich August Gotthold listed 41 public contributions to the debate in his *Abfertigung eines zweiten Lorinser. Nebst eilf Beilagen pädagogisches, bibliographisches und polemisches Inhaltes* (Königsberg: Gräfe und Unser, 1836), 4–45. Some comments were sent to Lorinser personally. In regard to Württemberg, see Kleindienst-Cachay, *Die Verschulung*, 112, 119–21.

34. A. Schroeder, "Pädagogik. Rezension von Überbürdungsschriften," *Jenaische Allgemeine Literatur-Zeitung* 157–60 (1836): 290.

35. S.G. Reiche, *Lorinser und die Gymnasien oder des Versuchs, die Frage: Können höhere Bürgerschulen gedeihen, ohne dass die bestehenden Gymnasien, jedoch unbeschadet ihrer Grundverfassung, eine Veränderung erfahren? Zu beantworten und einige verwandte Gegenstände zu beleuchten, zweytes Fragment* (Breslau: Grass, Barth & Comp., 1837), 10, even endorsed Lorinser's critique of civilization. More moderate yet positive statements on Lorinser's ideas can be found in N. Bach, "Review. Lorinser's Zum Schutz der Gesundheit," in *Neue Jahrbücher für Philologie und Paedagogik oder kritische Bibliothek für das Unterrichtswesen.* 16 (1836): 449, in C.W.G. Marquard, *Mens sana in Corpore sano! Ein freimüthiges Wort über die Schriftdes M.R. Dr. Lorinser: Zum Schutz der Gesundheit* (Züllichau: F.A. Lange, 1836), 8, in L.V. Jüngst, *Freimüthige Gedanken über eine zweckmäßige Umgestaltung der Gymnasien* (Bielefeld: Velhagen & Klasing, 1836), 7, whereas G.....r, *Trennung von Gymnasien*, 8–9, and Friedrich Kritz, *Zur Beleuchtung der Schrift des Herrn Medicinalraths Dr. Lorinser: "Zum Schutz der Gesundheit in den Schulen* (Erfurt; Gotha: Hennings und Hopf, 1836), 39, were skeptical about Lorinser's analysis yet saw the importance of physical exercise as part of a well-rounded education.

36. Jüngst, *Freimüthige Gedanken*, 66–67; Schroeder, "Pädagogik," 309. On the great variation of responses even in Prussia, see Jeismann, *Das preußische Gymnasium*, vol. 2, 245.

37. Kritz, *Zur Beleuchtung*, 40. Kritz referred to a text by Straß, a colleague at the *Gymnasium* in Erfurt. Straß saw the effect of physical exercise on moral education, in hardening and controlling the body and mind, Straß, "Über die Nothwendigkeit," 152.

38. Marquard, *Mens sana*, 19. Georg Köpke put forward the same straightforward proposal in his *Zu öffentlichen Prüfung der Zöglinge des Berlinischen Gymnasiums zum grauen Kloster*... (Berlin, 1836), according to Schroeder, "Pädagogik," 294. Froriep even suggested Jahn's gymnastics during regular school hours. See Robert Froriep, *Bemerkungen über den Einfluss der Schulen auf die Gesundheit* (Berlin, 1836), according to Schroeder, "Pädagogik," 299. In Köngisberg, a dispute on the reintroduction of *Turnen* continued awhile, as Friedrich August Gotthold, a leading figure of dogmatic neohumanism, reports in his critique of Lorinser, Gotthold, *Abfertigung*, 57. On Gotthold see Jeismann, *Das preußische Gymnasium*, vol. 2, 236–37.

39. Kleindienst-Cachay, *Die Verschulung*, 111. See also Neuendorff, *Neuere Deutsche Leibesübung*, vol. 3, 27–32.

40. For a detailed discussion on the rise of this decree, see Düding, *Organisierter*, 217–18.

41. As Neumann shows, this estrangement was mutual: Jahn, as a constitutional monarchist, did not accept the increasingly democratic and republican tendencies in the gymnastics movement. Those who had high hopes for Jahn as a democratic leader and symbol were disappointed by their idol's conservative opinions at the diet of Frankfurt, Neumann, *Die deutsche Turnbewegung*, 37–41.

42. In addition to the restrictive policies of the Metternich regime, Berlin also was one of the few cities without any gymnastic clubs (*Turnverein*), Düding, *Organisierter*, 231.

43. Düding sees essential differences between "nationalistic vs. non-nationalistic," "adult vs. student," and "institutionalized vs. associational" gymnastic clubs. See Düding, *Organisierter*, 204–12, 219–22. In reality, they often intertwined, as Düding's own depiction shows. For instance, Heuber's "real" gymnastic club in Vogtland gave rise to several gymnastic institutes or *Turnanstalte*, Düding, *Organisierter*, 209. For a more specific analysis of the political aspects of gymnastic clubs see Hannes Neumann, *Die deutsche Turnbewegung in der Revolution 1848/49 und in der amerikanischen Emigration* (Schorndorf bei Stuttgart: Hofmann, 1968). For a cultural analysis of the gymnastic movement in the 1840s, see McMillan, "Germany Incarnate," esp. 357–405. See also the introductory chapters in Krüger, *Körperkultur und Nationsbildung*, 25–39.

44. Düding, *Organisierter*, 233.

45. For a detailed analysis of the German gymnasts in the Revolution of 1848, and especially the events in Hanau, see Neumann, *Die deutsche Turnbewegung*, 26–34.

46. Although Jahn understood gymnastics to be a part of universal education (*Gesamtausbildung*), he was not sure of its institutional nature. *Die Deutsche Turnkunst* mentioned the sports field as an organizational unit. Despite his constant wishes for state protection of the sports field, Jahn was still skeptical of efforts to integrate *Turnen* into the system of public education. See "Jahn to Altenstein, Berlin, March 15, 1819," in *Unbekannte Briefe von Ludwig Friedrich Jahn*, 79. Without completely excluding this option, he saw it as happening only in the distant future and only after authorities reopened the sports fields that they had recently closed.

47. Richter, *Hans Ferdinand Maßmann*, 318–26.

48. On the rise of military interest in *Turnen* see Heinz Denk, "Schulturnen. Leibesübungen im Dienste autoritärer Erziehung," in *Geschichte der Leibesübungen*, vol. 3/1, ed. Horst Ueberhorst (Berlin: Verlag Bartels & Wernitz KG, 1980), 328–37. Denk argues that Schulze's memorandum anticipated and predestined the trajectory of educational gymnastics before 1918, Denk, "Schulturnen," 332.

49. Geiss, *Adolf Spieß*, 103.

50. Adolf Spieß, *Die Lehre der Turnkunst*, vol. 4. Die Gemeinübungen (Basel: Schweighauser, 1846), IX. According to Spieß, the *Ordnungsübungen* contributed to the instruction of dancing, hiking, and all kinds of gymnastic exercise. In Hugo Rothstein's *Die Gymnastik nach dem Systeme des schwedischen Gymnasiarchen P.H. Ling* (Berlin: Schroeder, 1848) drill was introduced in shaping *Turnen* for the purposes of state.

51. This almost forgotten tradition of German gymnastics has been noticed by Neuendorff, *Neuere Deutsche Leibesübung*, vol. 3, 19–27.

52. Adolf Spieß, *Die Lehre der Turnkunst*, vol. 1 Die Freiübungen (Basel: Schweighäuser, 1840), 6.

53. Roller, "Unser jetziger Tanz," 69; Roller, *Systematisches Lehrbuch*, 19; Koch, *Gymnastik*, 281–82.

54. Koch, *Gymnastik*, V.

55. Johann Adolf Ludwig Werner, *Medicinische Gymnastik oder die Kunst, verunstaltete und von ihren natürlichen Form- und Lagerverhältnissen abweichende Theile des meschlichen Körpers nach anatomischen und physiologischen Grundsätzen in die ursprünglichen Richtungen zurückzuführen und darin zu kräftigen* (Dresden; Leipzig: Arnold, 1838), IV, referred to the ancient roots of gymnastics: "Bei den Griechen trieben nur Aerzte Gymnastik, weil man wohl wußte, daß nur diese dazu geeignet wären, sie zum Wohle der Menschheit in Anwendung zu bringen." Cf. also Neuendorff, *Neuere Deutsche Leibesübung*, vol. 3, 92. See also Euler, *Geschichte des Turnunterrichts*, 189.

56. G. Rasmus, *Dr. Adolf Werner in seinem Wirken auf dem Felde der Gymnastik* (Dessau, 1848), 3. Rasmus called these exercises on sticks *Bâton- und Fléuretschlagen*.

57. Rasmus, *Adolf Werner*, 9.

58. Rasmus, *Adolf Werner*, 13.

59. Quoted by Rasmus, *Adolf Werner*, 21.

60. In 1838, still in Dresden as teacher of a gymnastic-pediatric institute, Werner published his *Medicinische Gymnastik oder die Kunst, verunstaltete und von ihren natürlichen Form- und Lagerverhältnissen abweichende Theile des meschlichen Körpers nach anatomischen und physiologischen Grundsätzen in die ursprünglichen Richtungen zurückzuführen und darin zu kräftigen* (Dresden; Leipzig: Arnold, 1838).

61. Rasmus, *Adolf Werner*, 22.

62. On Werner's activities in Saxony and Anhalt-Dessau, see Euler, *Geschichte des Turnunterrichts*, 188–97; Neuendorff, *Neuere deutsche Leibesübung*, vol. 3, 90–95.

63. See Jahn to W. Lübeck, December 19, 1837, in Jahn, *Briefe* (1930), 347–48, and Jahn to Priest Lippold, January 19, 1839, in Jahn, *Briefe* (1930), 362.

64. Moritz Kloss, *Pädagogische Turnlehre oder Anweisung, den Turnunterricht als einen wesentlichen Theil des allgemeinen Erziehungs- und Unterrichtswesens zu behandeln* (Zeitz: Schieferdecker, 1846), 8–9.

65. See Jahn to W. Lübeck, December 19, 1837, in Jahn, *Briefe* (1930), 347–48, and Jahn to Priest Lippold, January 19, 1839, in Jahn, *Briefe* (1930), 362. See also Maßmann's warnings against the militarization of gymnastics, Maßmann, *Die öffentliche Turnanstalt*, VII.

66. Clearly, Jahn did not gain much influence in Leipzig before the 1840s; see Kneschke, *Leipzig*, 427. Leipzig witnessed an early effort to establish a gymnastic club among the students. This was, however, weak, consisting mainly of secret meetings at the outskirts of the city, in Gohlis and Leutzsch, during the 1820s. Werner's contributions were publically recognized and thus more important.

# Chapter Nine

# Conclusion

In the preceding pages, I have tried to draw the historical outlines of change in middle-class perceptions and practices of the body in the first half of the nineteenth century. While a specific year does not mark a definite closure to the history of German physical culture, there is evidence of a logical stopping place in the middle of the century. During the latter part of the nineteenth century, German body culture moved in directions that anticipated the industrialized twentieth century. Through three parallel but loosely connected developments—the careers of Johann Strauss Sr. and Daniel Gottlob Moritz Schreber, and the construction of the *Ringstrasse* of Vienna—I want to illustrate these changes and point out possible continuities.

## The Dawn of the New

German ballroom dancing, especially as practiced in dancing clubs, was characterized by a delicate balance between diversion and moral education. By the mid-nineteenth century, this balance started to show signs of breakage. One can be traced to the Museums-Gesellschaft of Tübingen. Professor Serth, a leading member of the Museums-Gesellschaft, was concerned by the decline in the society's membership and suggested, in a letter dated October 8, 1851, to his friend Professor Helferich, a remedy.

> I had made it known last winter in the finance committee of the Museum that, instead of delegating the balls to a club within the club, one should have the committee itself in charge of the balls in order to invigorate the club's activities. The fact that our club has to do something to keep its members and recruit new ones has been repeated by the committee several times during the past two years. As soon as possible, I intend to propose in the meeting of the committee
> 1. that the Museum itself regularly organize balls for its members and for that purpose request a single payment or . . . an entrance fee;
> 2. that the committee commission two or three of its members to organize this matter.
> I believe I can no longer postpone this message to you, my dear colleague, because I have heard that other agents—I don't know which ones—have already collected signatures to establish a dancing club (*Casino*) in the Museum. Perhaps you could ask the manager (*Diener*) to encourage the dancers to be patient until the coming resolution of the committee.[1]

An increased interest in dancing, to attract new members and to bring in revenues was successful in the following years. In 1854, for instance, a series of four carnival balls was organized, aggressively advertised through letters and public announcements in the Tübinger Intelligenzblatt.[2] No less striking was the same commercial drive in a carnival society of Tunnel in Leipzig. By 1864, it had increased the ball activities to such an extent that Lange, the chronicler of the society, saw it as a mere dancing club.[3] This scattered evidence of the increasing commodification of social clubs is supported by observations of the waltz industry and its Viennese purveyor, the Strauss family.[4]

Johann Strauss Sr., son of an impoverished pub-owner, became the golden boy of Viennese ballrooms in the 1820s.[5] Starting in 1819, he was employed in Joseph Lanner's dance orchestra as a violinist. Lanner had made his name as a conductor skilled in combining popular music with his own operetta themes and waltzes. Strauss, three years younger than Lanner, followed his employer's practice, trying his skill at composing waltzes and, finally, as a conductor, when Lanner was compelled to divide the orchestra to meet the increasing popularity of his music. The two went their separate ways in 1825. Lanner held on to his reputation as Vienna's foremost ballroom musician, while Strauss not only challenged his former master's position as conductor and composer but took the whole craft to a new level of production. In 1829, he signed a contract for six years with the leading ballroom of Vienna, the Sperl. Access to fame automatically guaranteed access to revenues. The audience was always in the thousands, and Strauss's share of the entrance fees guaranteed him a handsome income; by then the custom was that the orchestra collected its honorary by circulating a silver plate in the audience. Especially at carnival time, Strauss was busy directing an ensemble of more than 200 musicians divided into smaller orchestras that played simultaneously in different ballrooms. He also produced a stream of dancing music, mainly waltzes, by using a team of second-string composers—he prepared the themes and the leading melodies himself—and secretaries who finished the details of orchestration and polished the text. Sometimes a waltz was finished only an hour before performance. By the beginning of the 1830s, Strauss and Lanner, who learned quickly from his former disciple, had become local industrialists in ballroom music.

What made Strauss's contribution so extraordinary was neither his intuitive grasp of local commerce nor the skills to attract a mass audience but his systematic and successful effort to open European markets for his music. Encouraged by his first great success in Pest, Hungary in 1833, Strauss took his orchestra the following year on a long and exhausting tour of Berlin, Leipzig, Dresden, and Prague. In 1835, he toured Southern Germany, and a year after that we find him in Prague, Leipzig, Hannover, and Hamburg. Strauss opened Paris and London, the capitals of the nineteenth century, to his products in 1837 and 1838, also paying visits to French and English provinces, Belgium, and Holland. The ecstatic reception of his music in Western European capitals is part of the Strauss mythology.[6] What is not so well known—and in need of a thorough analysis—are the impacts of his marketing strategies on the local dancing culture. Leipzig was a case in point. After his initial visit in 1834, Strauss had again made the commercial center of Saxony a stop on his tour in the fall of 1845. His main concert was scheduled on Monday, Novemeber 17. An *Extra-Tunnel* with a concert and dancing program was organized to accommodate the famous conductor from Vienna.[7] Shortly before his arrival, hectic maneuvering took place to arrange additional concerts for him. Several restaurant owners approached the presidium of the Tunnel, offering either their attractive ballrooms or simply requesting to "borrow" Strauss for an evening. An important question was the size of the ballroom, which one offer set at 800 seated guests.[8] These mass concerts would change the nature of the ball from an intimate regulated arena of social recognition to an anonymous entertainment hall. Ballroom dancing in clubs followed the course set by commercial masquerades and started its long journey to commodification.[9]

At the beginning of the nineteenth century, Johann Gottlob Schelle had envisioned walking as an aesthetic activity whose social character was formed by one's interest in being disinterested in others and the environment. For Schelle, walking was an end in itself. But even as he preached his gospel, there were processes at work that seriously undermined his ideas. We have seen how gymnastics and the new culture of trekking changed the whole concept of meaningful walking by making it an exercise. In addition to this "internal" challenge, there appear a host of structural arrangements in city planning that played against the ideals of walking as well. As early as the sixteenth century, in commercial German cities with small and crowded city centers, space was made available for merchants by connecting major central buildings with passages (*Durchhäuser*) that normally reached several stories. These covered and protected areas soon became popular gathering places; in addition to facilitating commerce, they were sites of social bonding and strolling for the patrician class. One of the most famous was the Auerbach Hof in Leipzig, built in 1530 by Dr. Heinrich Stromer von Auerbach. During the eighteenth century, it became one of the most renowned gathering points for the social elite of Leipzig.[10] Similar covered walking areas can be found in Vienna's Seitzer Hof.[11] These early shopping malls combined walking with commercial transaction.

Unlike some later passages and arcades, these covered pedestrian areas did not separate the customer/walker from goods. Several shops were no more than stands on which the owners displayed their products, encouraging potential customers to touch, smell, and taste. Through the invention of pressed glass (*Gußglas*), an aesthetically more gratifying arrangement became possible. By the middle of the eighteenth century, shop windows had become common in England and France. By 1781, this invention was brought into the arcades when the Duc d'Orleans opened the famous Palais-Royal. Its galleries, which hosted numerous luxury stores, were carefully designed to keep the strolling area and the shopping area apart, separated by the shop window, which now displayed all the commodities in their most seductive beauty to the passing promenaders. The seduced promenader of the Palais-Royal became the *flâneur* that Walter Benjamin has described in his book on nineteenth-century Paris.[12]

Germany was slow in adopting the shopping arcades. The first was built in Hamburg after the Great Fire of 1842, when a local businessman W. Sillem opened a passage called Sillem's Bazar. The fire occasioned a further architectural overhaul of Hamburg, creating space for the so-called Alster arcades on the famous river of Hamburg, Alster.[13] But the arcades remained the exception in German cities before 1850; according to Geist, the next full-fledged arcade in Germany did not open until 1863 in Cologne.[14] This late adoption of shopping passages in Germany seems to support the thesis that undisturbed strolling, made possible by walking paths and new boulevards, remained unchallenged. Yet a closer look proves otherwise. Although the shopping passage was superior in casting its material spell over the innocent stroller, several similar arrangements had nearly the same impact. When German spas started to enhance their facilities after the Seven Years War, they paid attention to commerce, which traditionally played an important role in improving the comfort of guests. For instance, in Pyrmont the selling stands that had already appeared by the end of the seventeenth century became boutiques selling mainly luxury items. Not accidentally, they were placed along the main strolling boulevard, the Hauptallee.[15] In Wiesbaden, another exclusive spa, the wooden shops, erected in 1805, were replaced in 1810 by luxury boutiques sheltered by the colonnades located to the left and right of the new main building.[16] The goods and the strollers were now connected to the same space, and this connection moved to the cities once the shopping passages and, later, sidewalks emerged to allow safe and protected walking.

In 1857, the Emperor Francis Joseph launched a project to support safe and protected walking in a modern setting: the *Ringstrasse* of Vienna. This street, which connected the inner city to the suburbs and became the site of an architectural *Gesamtkunstwerk* comparable only to Hausmann's accomplishments in Paris, was the cultural hub and landmark of *fin-de-siècle* Vienna and Europe. Yet its impact on the city structure reveals another story as well. The *Ringstrasse* was the result of two socio-political interests: to solve the constant traffic problems caused by the huge defenses and glacis between the inner city and the suburbs of Vienna and to create a monumental cultural center worthy of the imperial capital.[17] When the contours of this gigantic enterprise started to take shape in the 1860s, local critics could feel more than justified about the concerns they had voiced throughout the planning process. In particular, the glacis had provided an excellent recreational area for city dwellers as well as residents living in adjacent suburbs. The *Ringstrasse*, residents argued, would bring about an irrevocable loss of the city's green.[18]

Table 9.1. The Use of Land on the Glacis in 1857[19]

| *Use of Land* | *% of the Whole Area* |
|---|---|
| Built | 3.7 |
| Parks and free land | 64.8 |
| Traffic areas | 26.7 |
| *Wienfluß* | 4.8 |
| Total | 100.0 |

Table 9.2. The Use of Land in Vienna According to the Plan of 1859[20]

| *Use of Land* | *% of the Whole Area* |
|---|---|
| Buildings | 21.2 |
| Traffic | 50.5 |
| Parks and green areas | 18.7 |
| Waterways | 9.6 |
| Total | 100.0 |

This free and unregulated military area, covered with lawns after 1781, had been an ideal space for promenades, picnics, and children's play. As the statistics show (Tables 9.1. to 9.3.), the so-called *Grundplan* of 1859, envisioned a reduction of green areas on the glacis and the walls, from 64.8% of the area to 18.7% and of this only 28.1% was supposed to become public parkland. By the time the *Ringstrasse* was finished in 1917, the public parks had shrunk to 20%.[21]

Table 9.3. Division of Parks in Vienna According to the Original Plan of 1859[22]

| *Use of Area* | *% of All Park Areas* |
|---|---|
| Public parks | 28.1 |
| Private parks | 6.6 |
| Parade ground | 25.8 |
| Other green areas | 39.5 |
| Total | 100.0 |

The loss of free green space was not the only outcome of the *Ringstrasse* project. The parks and green areas that state authorities and architects envisioned, planned, and created on the former glacis were dramatically different from those created in other German cities at the beginning of the century. Their tree-lined and shaded promenades were diametrically opposed to the artistic principles of *Ringstrasse* architects. Instead of major landscape gardens, they suggested small decorative parks with few trees because the trees would obscure the view of their architectural creations.[23] This left little space for traditional walking in public parks. The major area of pedestrian activity was created along the *Ringstrasse* itself. It was lined with sidewalks and a broad promenade with rows of trees on both sides. Carriages, riders, and, later, streetcars, which before the new construction had enormous problems both entering and circumventing the inner city, now could use four broad driveways, more than 65% of the street capacity.[24] In short, the *Ringstrasse* became primarily a transportation venue, rather than a public space for social interaction. It was dominated by majestic and overwhelming architectural structures and broad driveways that dictated the terms of environmental design. Pedestrian Vienna had lost much of its space to transportation Vienna.

## The Persistence of the Old

The signs were clear that dietetics was going through a similar demise to that undergone by walking and dancing. After the 1850s, the science of the six non-naturals rapidly disappeared from the teaching of medicine.[25] When Jacob Moleschott published the *Handbuch der Diätetik* (1850), his focus was on the physiology of nutrition. But while old dietetics was losing ground in academic medicine, its influence remained strong. It was still widely used by spa doctors, and, as the career of Moritz Schreber shows, became a staple of medical gymnastics. Two years before his premature death Schreber declared that one of the greatest triumphs of his time was the attempt to "harmonize the endogenous forces of the body among themselves and in relation to the environment, by using them reasonably" and avoiding medicine whenever possible.[26] The guiding principle of dietetics was to "live moderately, actively, and happily."[27] What else could a Hufeland or a Burdach have said about a good life?

Soon after their author's death, Schreber's ideas took on a life of their own. In 1864, a group of educational enthusiasts in Leipzig, under the leadership of Ernst Hausschild and inspired by Schreber's proposal of a children's playground, founded an association whose main function was to organize and maintain a playground for their children. A part of the playground was a small garden plot. Originally for children to cultivate, it soon was taken over by their parents. This was the first Schreber Garden (*Schrebergarten*) and starting point of the Schreber Association (*Schreber-Verein*). It took a decade until the second Schreber Garden was founded; but once the idea gained momentum around the turn of the century, associations were founded in Leipzig and other German cities. Soon the Schreber Movement became international. But it resembled nothing that Schreber or Hausschild had imagined. By the turn of the century, the allotment movement was one of dozens of social organizations that fostered a natural lifestyle in Germany. Vegetarianism, macrobiotics, nudism, and various proponent groups of natural healing were part of a wholesale effort to reform a lifestyle corrupted by capitalism and industrialization.[28] As we know, these societies and movements not only carried a significant influence in the Weimar Republic but became a staple of German culture in the later twentieth century.

Michael Hau has traced the ideological model and beginning of the lifestyle reform movement to Hufeland and his dietetics.[29] As we have seen, Hufeland was only one of the several dietetic reformers that shaped German life in the first half of the nineteenth century. It was no single individual but the culture itself that persisted in its respect for the dietetic tradition. Hufeland was one of those who articulated its benefits and rationalized its methods. Why did he defend a body of knowledge that was not scientific and, as Kant argued, a personal narrative incapable of becoming a science? Or, to take his own words, why did he insist on the existence of an animating force that, by definition, escaped scientific scrutiny? We can, of course, see the influence of Romanticism on his thinking, with its yearning for individuality, wholeness, and hidden qualities. We can also understand the overwhelming impact of the cholera epidemics that seemed invincible to medical science, severely undermined public trust in medicine, and made a dietetic lifestyle the only viable option, in the view of many, for avoiding contamination.

But why did the arguments and institutions of dietetics hold such sway after the first shock of cholera had passed and even after a cure was found in the 1890s? Because dietetics included a view of political and social status that reached far beyond medicine and therapeutic practices. As Burdach so clearly argued, dietetics was a profoundly middle class strategy to regulate one's own body. In fact, despite the efforts of Hufeland and Burdach to create a scientific vocabulary for dietetics, the art of the six non-naturals always remained accessible to the educated layman. And this everyman's knowledge implied a utopian vision of control over one's body, of autonomy from state control, and of protection from the physical and social threats of the lower class to the middle class. Dietetics included a vision of wholeness: a body in harmony with its environment, in which an autonomous individual could regulate his well-being by finding for himself the rules of moderation. It was this utopia of self-regulation and bodily autonomy that contributed to the tremendous appeal of promenades, dancing clubs, and spas to the educated German middle class. In a curious way, an old science, dietetics, supported a political strategy that was strikingly modern: the strategy of individual autonomy. This is an important legacy of nineteenth-century Germany. But why did this legacy turn into that flagrantly autocratic culture of the body that characterized Nazi Germany? Quite often the answers have included the statement on the lack of modernization and modernity in German culture and society. The answer, however, is much more difficult once we realize that pre-modern arguments were fully capable of producing modern political strategies. Rather than the use it might have been the careful hiding of the modern characteristics of German pre-modern body culture that made the Nazi revolution of German society so successful.

## Notes

1. *Universitätsarchiv Tübingen*. 406/202: "Organisation von Bällen der Museumsgesellschaft," Fol.. 31. Professor Serth to Professor Helferich, October 8, 1851. On the declining activities at the Museumsgesellschaft see Schmucker and Kolb, *Die Museumsgesellschaft*, 73–4.

2. *Universitätsarchiv Tübingen*. 406/202: "Organisation von Bällen der Museumsgesellschaft," Fol. 32. List of Museumsbälle in Winter 1853–54, 20. November 1853.

3. Lange, *Der Tunnel*, 66.

4. On the theoretical discussion of commodification see Wolfgang Fritz Haug, *Kritik der Wahrenästhetik* (Frankfurt am Main: Suhrkamp, 1971). Some of Haug's central statements can be traced back to the Frankfurt School, especially to Walter Benjamin's *Charles Baudelaire. A Lyric Poet in the Era of High Capitalism* (London: Verso, 1983) and his analysis of the *flâneur*, the arcades, the soul of the commodity (Haug, *Kritik*, 26), and

Siegfried Kracauer's reflections on the "agreeable exterior" (*angenehmes Äußeren*) in commercial interaction, Haug, *Kritik*, 79–80. A good theoretical introduction to the current historical debate can be found in Ann Bermingham's "Introduction" to Ann Bermingham and John Brewer, *The Consumption of Culture 1600–1800. Image, Object, Text* (London: Routledge, 1995), 1–20, esp. 6–14, where she derives the classical separation of production vs. consumption from Hegel's *Phenomenology*.

5. On popular music in Vienna see Alice Hanson, *Musical Life in Biedermeier Vienna* (Cambridge: Cambridge University Press, 1989), esp. 150–76. On Strauss see Peter Kemp's *Die Familie Strauß. Geschichte einer Musikerdynastie* (Stuttgart: Verlags-Anstalt, 1987), esp. 11–85 and Otto Schneidert, *Johann Strauss und die Stadt an der schönen Donau* (Berlin: VEB Lied der Zeit/Musikverlag, 1982), 7–90. As Gramit, *Cultivating Music*, 131–32, observes, Strauss "knew his place" as a waltz-composer, a man of lower, popular music.

6. See, for instance, Kemp, *Die Familie Strauß*, 35–42, and Schneidert, *Johann Strauss*, 42–47.

7. *Statdtarchiv Leipzig*. Kap. 35, Gesellschaft Tunnel, Nr. 1. "Acta: die Angelegenheiten des Tunnels betreffend. 23. Juni 1845–1846." Fol. 48: Extra Tunnel für Strauß and Einladungskarten.

8. *Stadtarchiv Leipzig*. Kap. 35, Gesellschaft Tunnel, Nr. 1. "Acta: die Angelegenheiten des Tunnels betreffend. 23. Juni 1845–1846." Fol. 41.

9. As Andreas Ballstaedt and Tobias Widmaier show in their *Salonmusik. Zur Geschichte und Funktion einer bürgerlichen Musikpraxis* (Stuttgart: Franz Steiner Verlag, 1989), 306, in the second half of the nineteenth century, one-third of the highly commercialized and even industrialized production of salon music was dance music, especially the compositions of Strauß and Lanner.

10. Johann Friedrich Geist, *Passagen. Ein Bautyp des 19. Jahrhunderts* (Munich: Prestel-Verlag, 1969), 49.

11. Geist, *Passagen*, 50.

12. Benjamin, *Charles Baudelaire*, 55.

13. Geist, *Passagen*, 183–88. On the Alster arcades see Jung-Köhler's instructive, *Verlust und Chance*, 128–32.

14. Geist, *Passagen*, 191–93.

15. Schäfer-Schmidt, "Die Entwicklung," 430–31. An arcade was created in Pyrmont fairly late, in 1843, Schäfer-Schmidt, "Die Entwicklung," 443. On colonnades and arcades in spas see Bothe, ed., *Kurstädte*, 17–25, and the view of the arcades in Wiesbaden, 25. In Driburg, a competitor of Pyrmont, the arcades were built in 1822. According to Bothe, "Bad Driburg," 307–0, it also contained boutiques and became a paragon of spa arcades in the first half of the nineteenth century.

16. Fuhs, *Mondäne Orte*, 209. Because no detailed descriptions of these boutiques are available, we do not know about the arrangement of space and the use of shop windows.

17. Kurt Mollik, Hermann Reining, Rudolf Wurzer, *Planung und Verwirklichung der Wiener Ringstrassenzone*. Renate Wagner-Rieger, ed., *Die Wiener Ringstrasse. Bild einer Epoche*, vol. 3 (Wiesbaden: Franz Steiner Verlag, 1980), 125–26.

18. Mollik, *Planung*, 80–81.

19. Mollik, *Planung*, 65.

20. Mollik, *Planung*, 158.

21. Mollik, *Planung*, 172.

22. Mollik, *Planung*, 159.

23. Mollik, *Planung*, 287.

24. In 1905, the final profile of the *Ringstrasse* was from left to right: a sidewalk (5.55 m), local access road (*Zufahrtweg*, 6.25 m), riding road (*Reit-Allee*, 8.95 m), tramway (*Strassenbahn*, 1.10 m), driveway (14.90 m), promenade (*Geh-Allee*, 9.00 m), access road (6.25 m), sidewalk (5.55 m). See Mollik, *Planung*, 238.

25. Eulner, "Die Lehre von der Ernährung," 95–97. On the rise of modern dietetics, see Nikolaus Mani's "Die wissenschaftliche Ernährungslehre," in *Ernährung und Ernährungslehre im 19. Jahrhundert*, ed. Edith Heischkel-Artelt (Göttingen: Vandenhoeck & Ruprecht, 1976), esp. 22–36.

26. "Das Streben nach Harmonisirung der dem Organismus inwohnenden Kräfte, unter sich und in ihrer Beziehung zur Aussenwelt, durch wohlberechte Benutzung ihrer selbst," Schreber, *Zimmer-Gymnastik*, III.

27. Schreber, *Zimmer-Gymnastik*, 21.

28. On the natural health movement see Claudia Huerkam''s "Medizinische Lebensreform im späten 19. Jahrhundert. Die Naturheilbewegung in Deutschland als Protest gegen die naturwissenschaftliche Universitätsmedizin," *Vierteljahrsschrift für Sozial- und Witschaftsgeschichte* 73 (1986): 179–82.

29. Michael Grover Hau, *The Cult of Health and Beauty in Germany. A Social History, 1890–1930* (Chicago: The University of Chicago Press, 2003), 110. Hau shows how "Hufeland propagated a rational and natural lifestyle, one that aimed for a stronger life force due to moderation in all things." As we have seen, the question is exactly what do we mean by "rational and natural lifestyle."

# Bibliography

*Archival Sources*


*Landeshauptarchiv Sachsen-Anhalt (Außenstelle Oranienbaum)*

"Acta, enth. einzelne Sachen über das Philanthropin zu Dessau, dessen Lehrer, dessen Einrichtungen und sonst Anhängendes. 1771–1780."

*Staatsarchiv Hamburg*

Bibliothek A 507/54/1. "Verfassung und Gesetze der Harmonie. Revidirt im November 1815. Hamburg: Hermann Restler, 1815."

*Museum für die Geschichte der Stadt Leipzig*

Blauer Kasten E 2/51–128. "Gesellschaft Erholung."

Blauer Kasten E 2/14–24. "Verein Erheiterung, Gesetze, Programme, Tafellieder, 1836–1872,"

Sig.: I M 319. *Geschichtliche Rückblicke auf das Glockenleben 1837–1937. Zur Erinnerung an das 100jährige Jubelfest zusammengestellt als Festgabe* (S.l., s.a.)

*Stadtarchiv Leipzig*

Kap. 35, Tanzgesellschaft im Gewandhaus.

Kap. 35, Gesellschaft Tunnel.

*Bayerisches Hauptstaatsarchiv*

Staatsarchiv München, RA 21208: "Die Gesellschaft des Museums in München betr. De anno 1819–1846."

*Bayerische Staatsbibliothek*

Handschriften, CGM 6054: "Harmonie, Museum, Landwirtschaftlicher Verein."

*Stadtarchiv München*

Vereine 336, Fol. 15/a.

Vereine 338, Fols. 8/a, 10/a, 14/a, 24/b.

*Staatsbad Pyrmont Archiv*
Einzelabhandlungen
*Staatsarchiv Marburg*
Best. 121
*Stadtarchiv Tübingen*
A 70/3330: "Verschönerung des Wöhrds."
*Universitätsarchiv Tübingen*
406/3. "Vorschlag zur Vereinigung der hier bestehenden einzelnen Lesegesellschaften und zur Errichtung eines allen Klassen hiesiger Gebildeten gemeinsamen Verbands für Umgang und Zeitlektüre."
406/202: "Organisation von Bällen der Museumsgesellschaft,"
*Universitätsbibliotek Tübingen*
16 A 9129. "Statuten des Tanz-Sängerkränzchens der Sängerkranz-Mitglieder."
*Wiener Stadt- und Landesarchiv*
Bibliothek B 1372 1–3. Pemmer, Hans, *Alt-Wiener Gast- und Vergnügunsstätten*. Manuscript, 1969.

*Primary Sources: Journals, Encyclopedias, Dictionaries*

Adelung, Johann Christoph. *Grammatisch-Kritisches Wörterbuch der hochdeut schen Mundart*. 4 vols. Leipzig: Breitkopf und Härtel, 1793–1801.

*Allgemeine Literatur-Zeitung Halle*. Halle: Schwetschke; Leipzig: Churfürstl. Sächsische Zeitungsexpedition, 1785-1849.

*Allgemeine deutsche Real-Encyclopädie für die gebildeten Stände. Conversations-Lexikon*. Vol. 2. Leipzig: Brockhaus, 1851.

Biedermann, Johann Gottlieb, ed. *Altes und Neues von Schulsachen*. 8 vols. Halle, 1752–1755.

Campe, Joachim Heinrich. *Wörterbuch der Deutschen Sprache*. 4 vols. Braunschweig: Schulbuchhandlung, 1807–1809.

———, ed. *Allgemeine Revision des gesammten Schul- und Erziehungswesens von einer Gesellschaft praktischer Erzieher*. 16 vols. Hamburg: Bohn; Wolfenbüttel: Schulbuchhandlung; Vienna; Gräffer, 1785–1792.

Ersch, J.S. and J. G. Gruber, eds. *Allgemeine Encyclopädie der Wissenschaften und Künste in alphabetischer Folge*. Leipzig: Gleditsch, 1818.

*Göttingisches Magazin der Wissenschaft und Literatur*. Göttingen: Dieterich, 1780-85.

*Hamburg und Altona. Eine Zeitschrift zur Geschichte der Zeit, der Sitten und des Geschmacks*. Hamburg: Reftler, 1801–6.

*Intelligenz-Blatt für die Oberamts-Bezirke Tübingen, Rottenburg, Horb und Herrenberg*. Tübingen: Schramm, 1827–54.

*Jenaische allgemeine Literatur-Zeitung*. Jena: Literaturzeitung; Leipzig: Kurfürstl.-Sächs. Zeitungsexpedition, 1804-41.

*Journal des Luxus und der Moden*. Weimar: Landes-Ind.-Compt., 1788–1827.

*Journal der practischen Arzneykunde und Wundarzneykunst.* Berlin: Wittich, 1795-1836.

Krug, Wilhelm Traugott, *Allgemeines Handwörterbuch der philosophischen Wissenschaften nebst ihrer Literatur und Geschichte.* Vol. 2. Leipzig: Brockhaus, 1833.

Mannheimer Tageblätter 115. 1832.

Nachrichten aus Schnepfenthal. Für die Eltern und Freunde der dasigen Zöglinge, Schnepfenthal, 1794.

*Neues Conversations-Lexicon oder encyclopädisches Handwörterbuch für gebildete Stände. Herausgegeben von einer Gesellschaft rheinländischer Gelehrten*. Köln: Comptoir für Kunst und Literatur, 1824.

*Pädagogische Unterhandlungen*. Dessau: Institut, 1777–84.

*Toilettengeschenk. Ein Jahrbuch für Damen.* IV vols. Leipzig: Georg Voss, 1805–8.

Zedler, Johann Heinrich, ed. *Grosses vollständiges Universal-Lexikon aller Wissenschafften und Künste*. Halle and Leipzig: Johann Heinrich Zedler, 1732–54.

*Zeitung für die elegante Welt*. Leipzig: Voß, 1801–59.

## *Primary Literature*

A.H. "Kurze Uebersicht von neuen und interessanten Kompositionen für die musikalischen Leserinnen dieses Toilettengeschenks," *Viertes Toilettengeschenk. Ein Jahrbuch für Damen*. Leipzig: Georg Voss, 1808), 61–63.

*Allerhöchste Cabinetsordre vom 5ten Februar 1832, enthaltend die Bestätigung der Instruction über das, in Betreff der asiatischen Cholera in allen Provinzen des Preußischen Staats zu beobachtende Verfahren*. Berlin: Mittler, 1832.

Ammon, Friedrich August von. *Brunnendiätetik. Anweisungen zum zweckmässigen Gebrauche der Gesundbrunnen und Mineralbäder Deutschlands*. Leipzig: Weidmann'sche Buchhandlung, 1841.

Apinus, Sigmund Jakob, *Vernünftiges Studenten Leben, welches zeiget, Was sowol ein Candidatus Academiae, als auch ein würcklicher Studiosus, bey dem Anfang, Fortgang und Ende seiner Academischen Fahrt zu thun und zu lassen hat*. Jena: Johann Matthäus Kaltenbrunner, 1726.

"Aus den Taunusbädern, Ende Julius." *Zeitung für die elegante Welt* 166 (1827): 1327.

"Aus Karlsbad. Ende Julius." *Zeitung für die elegante Welt* 165 (1833): 659–60.

"Aus Karlsbad. Ende Julius." *Zeitung für die elegante Welt* 164 (1833): 655–56.

B. & H., "Landeck." *Journal des Luxus und der Moden* (Januar 1798): 18–25.

"Bade- und Reise-Epoque. Wanderung durch die Bäder von Driburg, Pirmont und Geismar 1807." *Journal des Luxus und der Moden* (September 1807): 584–88.

Bahrdt, Carl Friedrich. *Philanthropinischer Erziehungsplan oder vollständige Nachricht von dem ersten wirklichen Philanthropin zu Marschlins*. Frankfurt am Main: Eisenberg, 1776.

Balling, Franz Anton. *Die Heilquellen und Bäder zu Kissingen. Für Kurgäste*. Frankfurt am Main und Kissingen: Carl Jügel, 1855.

Bartholomay, Paul Bruno. *Die Tanzkunst in Beziehung auf die Lehre und Bildung des wahren Anstandes und des gefälligen Aeußern*. Giessen: Selbstverlag, 1838.

Basedow, Johann Bernhard. "Das in Dessau errichtete Philanthropinum, eine Schule der Menschenfreundschaft." In *Ausgewählte pädagogische Schriften*. Paderborn: Ferdinand Schöningh, 1965), 215–23.

Bechstein, Ludwig and O. Kleinknecht. *Leipzig*. Schweinfurt: Kleinknecht und Schäfer's Kunstverlag, 1844.

*Belehrung über die Asiatische Cholera für Nichtärzte*. Dresden: P.G. Hildersche Buchhandlung, 1831.

Beneke, Otto. *Hamburgische Turnanstalt von 1816. Erinnerungen aus der Zeit ihres Entstehens und Aufblühens*. Hamburg: Johann August Meißner's Verlags-Buchhandlung, 1866.

"Blasibad." *Intelligenz-Blatt für die Oberamts-Bezirke Tübingen, Rottenburg, Horb und Herrenberg* 82. 10.13.1828.

Blumenbach, Johann Friedrich. "Über den Bildungstrieb (Nisus formativus) und seinen Einfluß auf die Generation und Reproduction." *Göttingisches Magazin der Wissenschaft und Literatur* 1, no. 5 (1780): 247–66.

———. *Über den Bildungstrieb und das Zeugunsgeschäfte*. Göttingen: Dieterich, 1781.

Boerhaave, Hermann. *Institutiones Medicæ, in usus annuæ exercitationis domesticos digestæ. Cum præfatione nova de studio medico difficili, sed jucundo, Johannis Philippi Burggravii*. Francofurti ad Moenum: Georgii Heinrici Oehrlingii, 1710.

Bruchstück einer Reise von Frankfurt nach Wisbaden, Langenschwalbach, Schlangenbad und Brückenau, nebst Nachrichten von diesen Bädern im Monat August 1808." *Journal des Luxus und der Moden* (September 1808): 622–38.

Bruckbräu, Friedrich Wilhelm. *Neuestes Taschenbuch der Haupt- und Residenzstadt München*. Munich: Lindauer, 1828.

Buek, Friedrich Georg. *Wegweiser durch Hamburg und die umliegende Gegend*. Hamburg: Pethes & Besser, 1836.

Bühren, Adolph. *Vier Wochen in Pyrmont, oder Wer's Glück hat, führt die Braut heim. Erzählung in Briefen*. Braunschweig: G.C.E. Meyer, 1824.

Burdach, Karl Friedrich. *Belehrung für Nichtärzte über die Verhütung der Cholera*. Königsberg: Universitätsbuchhandlung, 1831.

———. *Die Diätetik für Gesunde*. Vol. 1. Leipzig: Wichmann, 1805.

———. *Rückblick auf mein Leben. Selbstbiographie*. Leipzig: Leopold Voß, 1848.

"Carlsbad und Töplitz." *Journal des Luxus und der Moden* (November 1798): 626–32.

Casorti, Louis. *Der instructive Tanzmeister für Herren und Damen, oder die Kunst, sich in kurzer Zeit durch bloßen Selbstunterricht*. Iimenau: Bernh. Fr. Voigt, 1826.

Charles, Jean [pseud. of Karl Johann Braun von Braunthal]. *Wien und die Wiener. Ihr öffentliches und häusliches, geistiges und materielles Leben. Ein Wegweiser für Einheimische und Fremde*. Stuttgart: Metzler, 1840.

Clarus, Johann Christian August. *Ansichten eines Vereins praktischer Aerzte in Leipzig über die Verbreitung der asiatischen Cholera auf doppeltem Wege. Mit einer diätetischen Haustafel für die Cholerazeit*. Leipzig: Gerhard Fleischer, 1831.

Clias, Phokion Heinrich. *Kalisthenie. Oder Uebungen zur Schönheit und Kraft für Mädchen*. Bern: Jenni, 1829.

Conrath, Niklas Benedikt. "Heilquellen zu K. Franzensbad bei Eger. Mit einer Nachschrift von Osann und Hufeland." *Journal der practischen Arzneykunde und Wundarzneykunst* 78, no. 3 (1834): 120.

"Correspondenz aus Ems." *Zeitung für die elegante Welt* 219 (1841): 875–76.

"Correspondenz aus Teplitz." *Zeitung für die elegante Welt* 133 (1842): 531–32.

"Das Augustusbad bei Radeberg." *Journal des Luxus und der Moden* (October 1805): 677–84.

"Das Fest der Naturforscher in Wien." *Zeitung für die elegante Welt* 205 (1832): 1633–37.

"Das Ronneburger Bad im Herzogthum Altenburg." *Journal des Luxus und der Moden* (October 1812): 669–76.

"Die Würtembergischen Bäder und Gesundbrunnen." *Journal des Luxus und der Moden* (September 1814): 580–87.

Domingo, Santo [Eduard Lehmann]. *Hamburg, wie es ist*. Leipzig: Reclam, 1838.

Dürre, Christian Eduard Leopold. *Aufzeichnungen, Tagebücher und Briefe aus einem deutschen Turner- und Lehrerleben*, edited by Ernst Friedrich Dürre. Leipzig: Strauch, 1881.

"Eger." *Journal des Luxus und der Moden* (November 1799): 555–63.

"Einige der allgemeinen Pflichten." In *Philanthropisches Lesebuch*. Vol. 2, 120–27.

Eiselen, Ernst. *Abriß des Deutschen Stoßfechtens, nach Kreuslers Grundsätzen dargestellt*. Berlin: Dümmler, 1826.

Eisenmann, Gottfried. *Die Heilquellen des Kissinger Saalthales. Physisch, chemisch und therapeutisch*. Erlangen: Palm und Enke, 1837.

"Erinnerungen an Karlsbad, Eger und Töplitz." *Journal des Luxus und der Moden* (October 1804): 493–95.

Faust, Bernhard Christian. *Gesundheits-Katechismus zum Gebrauche in den Schulen und dem häuslichen Unterrichte*. Bückeburg: Althaus, 1794.

Feiler, Johann Nepomuk. *Handbuch der Diätetik*. Landshut: Krull, 1821.

Fichte, Johann Gottlieb. "Einige Vorlesungen über die Bestimmung des Gelehrten (1794)." In *J.G. Fichte-Gesamtausgabe der Bayerischen Akademie der Wissenschaften*. Vol. 1, 3. Stuttgart: Friedrich Frommann Verlag, 1966.

———. "Grundriss des Eigenthümlichen der Wissenschaftlehre in Rücksicht auf das theoretische Vermögen als Handschrift für seine Zuhörer. (1795)." In *J.G. Fichte-Gesamtausgabe der Bayerischen Akademie der Wissenschaften*. Vol. 1, 3. Stuttgart: Friedrich Frommann Verlag, 1966.

———. *Reden an die deutsche Nation*. Hamburg: Felix Meiner, 1955.

Fleckles, Leopold. *Die Krankheiten der Reichen. Diätetische Grundlinien für das höhere und conversationelle Leben*. Wien: Carl Gerold, 1834.

Florencourt, Wilhelm Ferdinand Chaßot von. *Sittliche Schilderungen entworfen auf einer Reise von Braunschweig, über Pyrmont, Rinteln etc. nach Cassel in Briefen an einen Freund*. Berlin: Felischische Buchhandlung, 1801.

Francke, August Hermann. "Was von dem weltüblichen Tanzen zu halten sei, Vorrede, 1697." In *Werke in Auswahl*, edited by Erhard Peschke. Berlin: Luther-Verlag, 1969.

Fricke, Johann Carl Georg. *Geschichtliche Darstellung des Ausbruchs der asiatischen Cholera in Hamburg. Nach Acten und amtlich angestellten Untersuchungen*. Hamburg: Perthes & Besser, 1831.

G.....r, *Ueber die Nothwendigkeit der Trennung von Gymnasien und Realschulen und einer Reform des Gymnasialiunterrichts. Eine Abhandling veranlaßt durch Lorinser's Aufsatz 'Zum Schutz der Gesundheit auf Schulen.'* Berlin: Ludwig Hold, 1836.

*Ganz Leipzig für Acht Groβchen. Neuer und vollständiger Wegweiser für Fremde und Einheimische. Mit Plan von Leipzig und Karte des Laufes der Leipzig-Dresdner Eisenbahn*. Leipzig: Weber, 1838.

Geisler, Christian Friedrich. *Turnfreund. Eine Sammlung hochachtbarer, aus alter und neuer Zeit, für den Werth und die Nothwendigkeit absichtlicher, wohlgeordneter Leibesübungen der Jugend*. Berlin: G.C. Nauck's Buchhandlung, 1819.

*Gesetze der Gesellschaft Harmonie 1845. Berathen und genehmigt in einer am 15. März 1845 gehaltenen Generalversammlung*. Leipzig: Wilhelm Vogel, 1845.

*Gesetze für die Turnergemeinde zu Tübingen*. Tübingen: Richter und Eberhardt, 1819.

*Geseze des Museums zu Tübingen*. Tübingen: Schramm, 1822.

"Gesundbrunnen in Liebenstein." *Journal des Luxus und der Moden* (October 1799): 496–508.

Gmelin, Ferdinand, "Comments." In John Mason Good, *Die ostindische Cholera, aus dem Englischen des John Mason Good übersetzt und mit einigen Zusätzen versehen von Ferdinand Gottlieb Gmelin*. Tübingen: Osiander, 1831.

Goethe, Johann Wolfgang von, *Briefe an Goethe*. Vol. 1. Hamburg: Christian Wegener Verlag, 1965.

Goethe, Johann Wolfgang von. *Briefe an Goethe. Gesamtausgabe in Regestform*. Vol. 1. Weimar: Hermann Böhlau, 1980.

———. "Faust." In *Sämtliche Werke*. Vol. 7/1. Frankfurt am Main: Deutscher Klassiker Verlag, 1994.

———. *Goethes Briefe*. Vol. 2. Hamburg: Christian Wegener Verlag, 1964.

———. *Sämtliche Werke nach Epochen des Schaffens. Münchner Ausgabe.* Vol. 14. *Autobiographische Schriften*, edited by Reiner Wild. Munich: Carl Hanser Verlag, 1986.

———. *Scientific Studies*. New York: Suhrkamp, 1988.

———. *Werke*. Vol. 9. Munich: Deutscher Taschenbuch Verlag, 1974.

———. *Wilhelm Meisters Wanderjahre*. Stuttgart: Reclam, 1982.

Gotthold, Friedrich August. *Abfertigung eines zweiten Lorinser. Nebst eilf Beilagen pädagogisches, bibliographisches und polemisches Inhaltes*. Köngisberg: Gräfe und Unser, 1836.

Gourdoux-Daux, J. H. *Die Tanzkunst als Bildungsmittel der Jugend oder Methodik, Grundsätze und Elementar-Kenntnisse dieser Kunst, mit Hinsicht auf die Art sich in guter Gesellschaft zu zeigen un zu benehmen.* 3rd ed. Wien: Verlage der C. Haas'schen Buchhandlung, 1830.

Groß, Gustav W. *Diätetisches Handbuch für Gesunde und Kranke mit vorzüglicher Berücksichtigung der homöopathischen Heilkunst*. Leipzig: Reclam, 1824.

GutsMuths, Johann Christoph Friedrich. "An den Herrn geheimen Kanzley-Sekretär Brandes in Hannover. Gegen dessen Behauptung die Revolution in der Erziehung sey am verminderten Sinne des Vergnügens Schuld" *Braunschweigischer Journal* (June 1791): 219–45.

———. *Gymnastik für die Jugend. Enthaltend eine praktische Anweisung zu Leibesübungen. Ein Beytrag zur nöthigsten Verbesserung der körperlichen Erziehung*. Schnepfenthal: Buchhandlung der Erziehungsanstalt, 1793.

———. *Gymnastik für die Jugend enthaltend eine praktische Anweisung zu Leibesübungen. Ein Beytrag zur nöthigsten Verbesserung der körperlichen Erziehung* (1804). Frankfurt am Main: Limpert, 1970.

———. *Spiele zur Uebung und Erholung des Körpers und Geistes für die Jugend, ihre Erzieher und alle Freunde unschuldiger Jugendfreuden*. Schnepfenthal: Verlag der Buchhandlung der Erziehungsanstalt, 1796.

———. *Turnbuch für die Söhne des Vaterlandes. Beigebunden: Katechismus der Turnkunst*. Wiesbaden: Sändig, 1973.

———. "Was müssen Aeltern, erzieher und Lehrer als Freunde des deutschen Vaterlandes bey der Erziehung der Ihrigen von jetzt an thun, und das Schicksal unseres Vaterlandes und die freie Selbständigkeit unseres Volks auch für unsere Nachkommen zu sichern?" *Neue Bibliothek für Pädagogik, Schulwesen und die gesammte pädagogische Literatur* (January 1814 and 1815): 7–27, 97–127, 193–220.

Hamburgisches Wörterbuch. Vol. 1. Neumünster: Karl Wachholtz Verlag, 1985.

Harnisch, Wilhelm. *Das Turnen in seinen allseitigen Verhältnissen*. Breslau: Lenz, 1819.

Hebenstreit, Wilhelm. *Der Fremde in Wien und der Wiener in der Heimath*. Wien: Leop. Grund, 1840.

Hecker, August Friedrich. *Therapia Generalis oder Handbuch der allgemeinen Heilkunde*. Berlin: Christian Friedrich Himburg, 1789.

Hegel, Georg Wilhelm Friedrich. *Phänomenologie des Geistes*. Frankfurt am Main: Suhrkamp, 1973.

———. "Rechts-, Pflichten- und Religionslehre für die Unterklasse (1810)." In *Werke in zwanzig Bänden*. Vol. 4. Frankfurt am Main: Suhrkamp, 1969.

Helmke, Eduard David. *Almanach der neuesten Modetänze auf das Jahr 1833. Für Freunde und Freundinnen der höheren Tanzkunst*. Merseburg: Fr. Weidemann, 1835.

———. *Die Kunst, sich durch Selbstunterricht in kurzer Zeit zum feinen Weltmann und sehr geschickten Tänzer zu bilden*. Merseburg: Sonntagsche Buchhandlung, 1831.

———. *Neue Tanz- und Bildungsschule. Ein gründlicher Leitfaden für Eltern und Lehrer bei der Erziehung der Kinder und für die Erwachsene Jugend, um sich einen hohen Grad der feinen Bildung zu verschaffen und sich zu kunstfertigen und ausgezeichneten Tänzern zu bilden*. Leipzig: Christian Ernst Rollmann, 1829.

Hentschke, Theodor. *Allgemeine Tanzkunst. Theorie und Geschichte, antike und moderne (gesellschaftliche und theatralische) Tanzkunst und Schilderung der meisten National- und Charaktertänze*. Stralsund: Hausschildt, 1836.

Herbart, Johann Friedrich. "Allgemeine Pädagogik aus dem Zweck der Erziehung abgeleitet. 1806." In *Pädagogische Schriften*. Vol. 1, edited by Fr. Bartholomäi. Langensalza: Beyer, 1896.

Herder, Johann Gottfried. *Ideen zur Philosophie der Geschichte der Menschheit*. Vol. 1. Leipzig: Hartknoch, 1821.

Hlawaczek, Eduard. *Karlsbad in medicinischer, pitoresker und geselliger Beziehung. Für Kurgäste*. Prag: Kronbergers Wittwe und Weber, 1838.

Hoffmann, Friedrich. *Kurzgefaßte Diätetic oder hinlänglicher Unterricht*. Jena: Goller, 1744.

Hoser, Joseph Carl Eduard. *Beschreibung von Karlsbad*. Prag: Calve, 1797.

Huber, Alois. *München im Jahre 1819*. Vol. 1. *Mit einer Ansicht, einem Grundrisse der Stadt, und Anhange*. Munich: Zängl, 1819.

Hufeland, Christoph Wilhelm. "Athmosphärische Krankheiten und atmosphärische Ansteckung, Unterschied von Epidemie, Contagion und Infection. Ein Beitrag zu den Untersuchungen über die Contagiosität des gelben Fiebers." *Journal der practischen Heilkunde* 57.1 (1823): 3–41.

———. "Einfluss der Cholera auf die Conception." *Journal der practischen Heilkunde* 74.6 (1832): 136–37.

———. *Enchiridion medicum oder Anleitung zur medizinischen Praxis. Vermächtniss einer fünfzigjährigen Erfahrung* 5th ed. Berlin: Jonas Verlagsbuchhandlung, 1839.

———. *Hufeland. Leibarzt und Volkserzieher. Selbstbiographie von Christoph Wilhelm Hufeland*. Stuttgart: Verlag Robert Lutz, 1937.

———. *Makrobiotik oder die Kunst, das menschliche Leben zu verlängern*. Baden-Baden: Insel Taschenbuch, 1984.

———. *Praktische Uebersicht des vorzüglichsten Heilquellen Deutschlands nach eignen Erfarungen*. Berlin: Reimer, 1820.

———. "Schlussresultat." *Journal der practischen Heilkunde* 74 (1832): 3-10.

———. *System der practischen Heilkunde. Ein Handbuch für academische Vorlesungen und für den practischen Gebrauch.* Vol. 1. *Allgemeine Therapeutic.* Jena und Leipzig: Friedrich Frommann, 1800.

———. "Worüber streitet man. Was heisst Ansteckung. Was heisst Contagionist u. Nichtcontagionist bei der Cholera." *Journal der practischen Heilkunde* 74.1 (1832): 109–16.

———. "Ueber den Unterschied von epidemischer Constitution, Epidemie, und Contagion, und die Verschiedenheit mittelbarer und unmittelbarer, lebender und todter Contagiosität, mit Rücksicht auf die orientalische Cholera." *Journal der practischen Heilkunde* 72.4 (1831): 91–106.

Hufeland, Christoph Wilhelm and Friedrich Justin Bertuch. "Nöthige Erinnerung an die Bäder und ihre Wiedereinführung in Teutschland; nebst einer Einweisung zu ihrem Gebrauch und bequemer Einrichtung derselben in den Wohnhäusern." *Journal des Luxus und der Moden* (May 1801): 237–50.

Humboldt, Wilhelm von. "Bericht der Sektion des Kultus und Unterrichts an den König—Dezember 1809." In *Schulreform in Preußen 1809–1819. Entwürfe und Gutachten*, edited by Lothar Schwiem. Weinheim: Beltz, 1966.

———. "Die Sprache als Ausdruck eigentümlicher Geistesform." In *Schriften zur Anthropologie und Bildungslehre*, edited by Andreas Flitner. Frankfurt am Main: Ullstein, 1984.

———. *Gesammelte Schriften*. Vol. 15. *Tagebücher I.* Berlin: B. Behr's Verlag, 1918.

———. "Über den Geist der Menschheit." In *Gesammelte Schriften*. Vol. 2. Berlin: B. Behr's Verlag, 1904.

———. "Über die Liegnitzer Ritterakademie. 7. September 1809." In *Gesammelte Schriften* Vol. 10. Berlin: B. Behr's Verlag, 1903.

———. *Wilhelm und Caroline von Humboldt in ihren Briefen.* Vol. 3. *Weltbürgertum und preußischer Staatsdienst* 1808–10. Berlin, Ernst Siegfried Mittler und Sohn, 1909.

———. *Wilhelm von Humboldt. Sein Leben und Wirken, dargestellt in Briefen, Tagebüchern und Dokumenten seiner Zeit*, edited by Rudolf Freese. Berlin: Verlag der Nation, 1955.

Ideler, Carl Wilhelm. *Die allgemeine Diätetik für Gebildete*. Halle: C.A. Schwetschke und Sohn, 1846.

*Instruction für die Sanitäts-Behörden, und für das bei den Contumaz-Anstalten verwendete Personale, zum Behufe die Gränzen der k.k. österreichischen Staaten vor dem Einbruche der im skaiserlich-russischen Reiche herrschenden epidemischen Brechruhr (Cholera morbus) zu sichern, und im möglichen Falle des Eindringens, ihre Verbreitung zu hemmen*. Hannover: Helwingsche Buch-Handlung, 1831.

Ivensen, Dietrich Alexander Valentin. *Terpsichore, ein Taschenbuch für Freunde und Freundinnen des Tanzes in Liv-, Kur- und Estland.* Riga: Steffenhagen und Sohn, 1806.

Jahn, Christian. *Norma Diaetetica oder regelmäßige Abhandlung wie ein Mensch . . . sein Leben und Gesundheit nebst wenigen Arzeneyen lange erhalten.* Dresden: Johann Nicol. Gerlach, 1757.

———. *Bereicherung des hochdeutschen Sprachschatzes versucht im Gebiethe des Sinnverwandtschaft, ein Nachtrag zu Adelung's und eine Nachlese zu Eberhard's Wörterbuch.* Leipzig: Adam Friedrich Böhme, 1806.

———. *Deutsches Volksthum.* Leipzig: Philipp Reclam, 1813.

———. *Die Briefe F.L. Jahns*, edited by Wolfgang Meyer. Dresden: Wilhelm Limpert-Verlag, 1930.

———. *Die Briefe Friedrich Ludwig Jahns gesammelt und im Auftrage des Ausschusses der Deutschen Gymnastschaft*, edited by Wolfgang Meyer. Leipzig: Paul Eberhardt, 1913.

———. "Runenblätter (s.l., 1814)." In *Werke*, edited by Carl Euler. Vol. 1. Hof: Verlag von Rud. Lion, 1884.

———. "Werke zum deutschen Volkstum (1833)." In *Werke*, edited by Carl Euler. Vol. 2,2. Hof: Verlag von Rud. Lion, 1887.

Jahn, Friedrich Ludwig and Ernst Eiselen. *Die deutsche Turnkunst zur Einrichtung der Turnplätze.* Berlin: Auf Kosten der Herausgeber, 1816.

———. *Die deutsche Turnkunst*, edited by Max Schwarze. Dresden: Wilhelm Limpert-Verlag, 1928.

———. *Die deutsche Turnkunst.* Berlin: Sportverlag, 1960.

Jahn, Johann Christian. "Die in dem voranstehenden Aufsatze besprochene Anklageschrift des Herrn Med.-Raths Lorinser." *Neue Jahrbücher für Philologie und Paedagogik oder kritische Bibliothek für das Unterrichtswesen* 16 (1836): 456–83.

Jean Paul, *Werke.* Section 1. Vol. 1, edited by Norbert Miller. Munich: Hanser Verlag, 1969.

Jörg, Johann Christian Gottfried. *Zehn Gebote zur Diätetik.* Leipzig: Brockhaus, 1847.

Juncker, Johann. *Conspectus Therapiae Generalis, cum Notis in Materiam Medicam Tabulis XX. Methodo Stahliana Conscriptus.* 2nd ed. Halle: Impensis Orphanotrophei, 1736.

Jüngst, L.V. *Freimüthige Gedanken über eine zweckmäßige Umgestaltung der Gymnasien.* Bielefeld: Velhagen & Klasing, 1836.

Kahn, Anton Friedrich *Anfangsgründe der Fechtkunst.* Göttingen: L. Schultze, 1739.

Kant, Immanuel. *Critique of Judgment*, translated by Werner S. Pluhar. Indianapolis: Hackett, 1987.

———. "Über Pädagogik," edited by Friedrich Theodor Rink. 1803. In Immanuel Kant, *Gesammelte Schriften. Akademieausgabe.* Vol. 9. Berlin: de Gruyter, 1923.

———. *Werke*. Vol. 7. Berlin: Cassirer, 1912.

Käppel, Gottfried. *Pyrmont's Merkwürdigkeiten. Eine Skizze für Reisende und Kurgäste*. Pyrmont: Helwingsche Buchhandlung, 1810.

"Karlsbad, im August 1804." *Journal des Luxus und der Moden* (September 1804): 438–42.

Kirchner, C. "Oratio de gymnastices in gymnasiis restituendae necessitate. Rede von der Nothwendigkeit der Wiedereinführung der Leibesübungen auf den Gymnasien." In *Führer in der Zeit der Turnsperre. Maßmann, v. Klumpp, Lorinser, Straß, Diesterweg, E.F. Koch, Kirchner, Nachtegall, Ling, Eiselen*, edited by Franz Paul Wiedemann. Dresden: Limpert Verlag, 1933.

Kirchner, Carl. *Kurze Nachricht von der Königlichen Landesschulen Pforta*. Leipzig: Vogel, 1839.

*Kissingen Spa: the International Health-resort, in its Medical and Social Aspects*. Munich: Kurverein Bad Kissingen, 1900.

Kloss, Moritz. *Pädagogische Turnlehre oder Anweisung, den Turnunterricht als einen wesentlichen Theil des allgemeinen Erziehungs- und Unterrichtswesens zu behandeln*. Zeitz: Schieferdecker, 1846.

Klumpp, Friedrich Wilhelm. *Eine Selbstbiographie*. Essen: Bädeker, 1838.

Koch, Friedrich. *Der wohlunterrichtete Fremdenführer in der kaiserl. königl. Haupt- und Residenzstadt Wien und ihren nahen Umgebungen*. Wien: Singer et Goering, 1844.

Koch, Karl Friedrich. *Die Gymnastik aus dem Gesichtspuncte der Diätetik und Psychologie, nebst einer Nachricht von der gymnastischen Anstalt zu Magdeburg*. Magdeburg: Creuß'sche Buchhandlung, 1830.

Koenig, Heinrich. *Eine Pyrmonter Nachcur. Roman*. Leipzig: Brockhaus, 1869.

Köhnke, Markus Christian. *Erinnerungen aus meinem Leben nebst Bemerkungen über mancherlei Gegenstände*. Ottensen: Perthes-Besser & Mauke, 1839.

Körner, Theodor. "Lützow's wilde Jagd." In *Sämmtliche Werke*. Vol. 1. Berlin: Grote, 1892.

Krimer, Wenzel. *Erinnerungen eines alten Lützower Jägers 1795–1819*. Vol. 1. Stuttgart: Lutz, 1913.

*Kritik über den Apollosaal nebst einigen rezensirenden Bemerkungen über die bereits erschienenen Schilderungen desselben*. Wien, 1808.

Kritz, Friedrich. *Zur Beleuchtung der Schrift des Herrn Medicinalraths Dr. Lorinser: 'Zum Schutz der Gesundheit in den Schulen.'* Erfurt; Gotha: Hennings und Hopf, 1836.

Krüger, Johann Gottlob. *Gedancken von der Erziehung der Kinder*. Vol. 2. *Von der Bildung der Seele*. Halle: Hemmerde, 1752.

———. *Diät oder Lebensordnung*. Halle: Hemmerde, 1751.

Kühne, Ferdinand Gustav. "Bade-Leiden und Freuden. Ein Capriccio." *Zeitung für die elegante Welt* 251 (1835): 1001–5.

———. "Bade-Leiden und Freuden. Ein Capriccio." *Zeitung für die elegante Welt* 252 (1835): 1006–7.

Kurländer, Franz August von. "Briefe an eine Dame über den diesjährigen Fasching in Wien." *Zeitung für die elegante Welt* 85 (1832): 673–76, 708–10, 761–64.

Kümmerle, L.F. *Praktische Anleitung zu Leibesübungen für Mädchen. Nebst einem Anhang über die Haltung des Körpers und über die Anfangsgründe der Tanzkunst.* Stuttgart: Metzler, 1832.

L. "Oeffentliche Spaziergänge." *Hamburg und Altona* I (1801): 14–16.

Länger, Christian. *Terpsichore. Ein Taschenbuch der neuesten gesellschaftlichen Tänze, worin zugleich Anweisung gegeben wird, wie man 40 Touren und 76 Tänze ohne orchesigraphische Zeichnungen und ohne Lehrer erlernen kann. Zum Nutzen und Vergnügen für Freude der Tanzkunst.* Würzburg: Etlingersche Buch- und Kunsthandlung, 1824.

Lahire, P. *Das non plus ultra der Tanzkunst. Eine gründliche Anweisung, nach welcher Jeder in sehr kurzer Zeit ohne Tanzlehrer der geschickteste Tänzer werden kann.* 2nd ed. Nordhausen: Ernst Friedrich Fürst, 1842.

"Lauchstädt." *Journal des Luxus und der Moden* (Januar 1798): 25–30.

"Leben in München. Februar 1817." *Journal des Luxus und der Moden* (März 1817): 200–3.

"Leipzig. Verzeichniss der Vorlesungen auf der Universität daselbst im Winterhalbjahre 1837." *Intelligenzblatt der Allgemeinen Literatur-Zeitung* (October 1837): 521–26.

"Leipzig. Verzeichniss der Vorlesungen auf der Universität daselbst im Winterhalbjahre 1839/40." *Intelligenzblatt der Allgemeinen Literatur-Zeitung* (October 1839): 500.

"Leipzig. Verzeichniss der Vorlesungen auf der Universität daselbst im Sommerhalbjahre 1840." *Intelligenzblatt der Allgemeinen Literatur-Zeitung* (Mai 1840): 201–8.

"Leipzig. Verzeichniss der Vorlesungen auf der Universität daselbst im Winterhalbjahre 1840/41." *Intelligenzblatt der Allgemeinen Literatur-Zeitung* (October 1840): 397.

"Leipzig. Verzeichniss der Vorlesungen auf der Universität daselbst im Sommerhalbjahr 1845." *Intelligenzblatt zur Allgemeinen Literatur-Zeitung* (April 1845): 205.

Leupoldt, Johann Michael. *Eubiotik. Oder Grundzüge der Kunst als richtig, tüchtig, wohl und lang zu leben.* Berlin; Leipzig: Reimer, 1828.

Lewald, August. *Panorama von München.* Vol 1. Stuttgart: Hallberg'sche Verlagsbuchhandlung, 1835.

"Liebenstein und Brückenau." *Journal des Luxus und der Moden* (August 1805): 550–54.

Lippold, Adolf. *Erinnerungen eines alten Leipzigers. Humoristische Chronika aus Leipzigs jüngerer Vergangenheit.* Vol. 1. Leipzig: Lenz, 1893–95.

Lorinser, Karl Ignaz. *Die Pest des Orients wie sie entsteht und verhütet wird.* Berlin: Enslin, 1837.

———. *Eine Selbstbiographie.* 2 vols. Regensburg: Georg Joseph Manz, 1864.

———. "Zum Schutze der Gesundheit in den Schulen." In *Führer in der Zeit der Turnsperre. Maßmann, v. Klumpp, Lorinser, Straß, Diesterweg, E.F. Koch, Kirchner, Nachtegall, Ling, Eiselen*, edited by Franz Paul Wiedemann. Dresden: Wilhelm Limpert-Verlag, 1933.

Ludwig, Christian Gottlieb. *Institutiones Therapiae generalis praelectionibus academicis accommodatae*. Lipsiae: Gleditschiana, 1754.

Mädel, Ernst Christian. *Anfangsgründe der Tanzkunst oder genaueste Angabe zur Erlernung und Wiederholung aller jezzo üblichen Tänze, ohne Beihülfe eines Tanzmeisters*. Erfurt: Ernst Christian Mädel, 1801.

Marcard, Henrich Matthias. *Beschreibung von Pyrmont*. 2 vols. Leipzig: Weidmanns Erben und Reich, 1784–85.

———. *Kleines Pyrmonter Brunnenbuch für Curgäste zu Hause und an der Quelle*. Pyrmont: Helwingsche Buchhandlung, 1805.

Marquard, C.W.G. *Mens sana in Corpore sano! Ein freimüthiges Wort über die Schriftdes M.R. Dr. Lorinser: Zum Schutz der Gesundheit*. Züllichau: F.A. Lange, 1836.

Maßmann, Hans Ferdinand. *Die öffentliche Turnanstalt zu München. Nebst Anlagen über Einrichtung von Turnanstalten und Beyträgen zur Geschichte älterer deutscher Leibesübungen*. Munich: Lindauer'sche Buchhandlung, 1838.

———. *Leibes-Uebungen. Erstes Werk. Zur Militair-Gymnastik in's Besondere*. Landshut: Thomann, 1830.

May, Franz Anton. *Die Kunst die blühende Gesundheit zu erhalten und die verlorne durch zweckmäßige Krankenpflege wieder herzustellen. Eine Einleitung zu Vorlesungen über die Gesundheit-Erhaltungs-Lehre und vernünftige Krankenpflege*. Vol. 1. 3rd ed. Mannheim: Tobias Löffler, 1820.

———. *Medicinische Fastenpredigten oder Vorlesungen über Körper und Seelen-Diätetik, zur Verbesserung der Gesundheit und Sitten*. Vol. 1. Mannheim: Schwan und Götz, 1793.

———. "Von den Krankheiten der Schauspieler, und der Schwierigkeit, dieselbe zu behandeln." In *Vermischte Schriften*. Mannheim: Neue Hof- und akademische Buchhandlung, 1786.

Menke, Karl Theodor. *Pyrmont und seine Umgebungen mit besonderer Hinsicht auf seine Mineralquellen; historisch, geographisch, physikalisch und medicinisch dargestellt*. Pyrmont: Georg Uslar, 1840.

Merkel, Garlieb. *Briefe über Hamburg und Lübeck*. Leipzig: Hartknoch, 1801.

Meyer, Anton Johann Heinrich, *Hamburg und Altona nebst Umgegend. topographisch-statistisch-historisches Handbuch für Einheimische und Fremde*. Hamburg: Schuberth & Niemeyer, 1836.

Meyer, Friedrich Johann Lorenz. *Skizzen zu einem Gemälde von Hamburg*. 2 vols. Hamburg: Friedrich Hermann Nestler, 1801–2.

Miller, Johann Peter. "Die Schule des Vergnügens." *Altes und Neues von Schulsachen* 2 (1753): 201–20.

Minding, Julius. "Geschichtliche Bemerkungen über die Struveschen Nachbildungen, nebst Nachrichten über das Leben des Erfinders." *Annalen der Struveschen Brunnenanstalten.* Vol. 1 (Berlin: August Hirschwald, 1841), 1–45.

"Miscellen aus München." *Journal des Luxus und der Moden* (März 1808): 202–22.

Mohl, Robert von. *Lebenserinnerungen (1799–1875).* Vol. 1. Stuttgart; Leipzig: Deutsche Verlags-Anstalt, 1902.

Most, Georg Friedrich. *Gesundheit und Krankheit. Ein diätetisch-medicinisches Handbuch für alle Stände.* 2nd ed. Hannover: Hahn, 1827.

*Nachrichten aus Schnepfenthal für Eltern und Erzieher.* Leipzig: Siegfried Lebrecht Crusius, 1788.

Nadler, Franz Xaver. *Kallischematik, oder Anleitung zu einem edlen Anstande und zur schönen, gefälligen Haltung des Körpers.* Munich: George Jaquet, 1834.

"Neue Beschreibung von Eger und Schwalbach." *Journal des Luxus und der Moden* (Februar 1800): 74.

"Neue Anlagen in Karlsbad." *Journal des Luxus und der Moden* (January 1801): 10–13.

*Neue vollständige Tanzschule für die elegante Welt oder faßliche und umfassende Anleitung zum gesellschaftlichen und theatralischen Tanz: Zum Selbstunterricht sowohl wie auch zum Handbuch für den Tanzlehrer bestimmt.* Ilmenau: Bernhard Fr., 1830.

*Neuer Tanz- und Ball-Kalender für 1801.* Berlin: Johann Friedrich Unger, 1800.

Nicolin, Günther. *Hegel in Berichten seiner Zeitgenossen.* Hamburg: Meiner, 1970.

Niemeyer, A. H. "Anstand." In *Allgemeine Encyclopädie der Wissenschaften und Künste in alphabetischer Folge.* Vol. 3, edited by. J.S. Ersch and J.G. Gruber. Leipzig: Gleditsch, 1818.

Niethammer, Friedrich Immanuel. *Der Streit des Philanthropinismus und Humanismus in der Theorie des Erziehungsunterrichts unserer Zeit.* Jena: Frommann, 1808.

Nietzsche, Friedrich. "Über die Zukunft der Bildungs-Anstalten." In *Werke in drei Bänden.* Vol. 3, edited by Karl Schlechta. Gütersloh: Harenberg Kommunikation, 1982.

Osann, Emil. *Physikalisch-medicinische Darstellung der bekannten Heilquellen der vorzüglichsten Länder Europa's.* Berlin: Dümmler, 1829.

Paracelsus. *Vom Licht der Natur und des Geistes.* Stuttgart: Reclam, 1984.

Pasch, Johann. *Beschreibung wahrer Tanz-Kunst, Nebst einigen Anmerckungen über Herrn J.C.L.P.P. zu G. Bedencken gegen das Tanzen (1707).* Munich: Reimer Verlag, 1978.

Pestalozzi, Johann Heinrich. "Über Körperbildung als Einleitung auf den Versuch einer Elementargymnastik, in einer Reihenfolge körperlicher Übungen." In *Sämtliche Werke* Vol. 20. Zürich: Orell Füssli Verlag, 1963.

Pichler, Karoline. *Denkwürdigkeiten aus meinem Leben.* Vol. 2, edited by Emil Karl Blümmel. Munich: Georg Müller, 1914.

"Pyrmont im Jahr 1797. Mein Vermächtniß für das Moden-Journal." *Journal des Luxus und der Moden* (September 1798): 497–511.

"Pyrmont im Sommer 1812." *Journal des Luxus und der Moden* (September 1812): 624–28.

"Pyrmont im Sommer 1806 (Aus dem Brief einer Dame)." *Journal des Luxus und der Moden* (October 1806): 645–47.

"Pyrmont." *Journal des Luxus und der Moden* (September 1801): 493

"Pyrmont." *Journal des Luxus und der Moden* (September 1801): 492–93.

Rambach, Johann Jakob. *Versuch einer physisch-medizinischen Beschreibung von Hamburg*. Hamburg: Carl Ernst Bohm, 1801.

Reiche, S.G. *Lorinser und die Gymnasien oder des Versuchs, die Frage: Können höhere Bürgerschulen gedeihen, ohne dass die bestehenden Gymnasien, jedoch unbeschadet ihrer Grundverfassung, eine Veränderung erfahren? Zu beantworten und einige verwandte Gegenstände zu beleuchten, zweytes Fragment*. Breslau: Grass, Barth & Comp., 1837.

Review of Kant's *"Macht des Gemüthes* (1798)" *Allgemeine Literatur-Zeitung* 184 (1799): 645–48.

Reyscher, August.Ludwig. *Erinnerungen aus alter und neuer Zeit (1802 bis 1880)*. Freiburg im Breisgau und Tübingen: Mohr, 1884.

Richter, Josef. *Der wiederaufgelebte Eipeldauer. Mit Noten von einem Wiener*. Heft 3 (1809). Wien: Rehm, 1799–1821.

———. *Der wiederaufgelebte Eipeldauer. Mit Noten von einem Wiener*. Heft 36. Wien: Rehm, 1799–1821.

Roller, Franz Anton. "Die Allemande." *Viertes Toilettengeschenk. Ein Jahrbuch für Damen*. Leipzig: Georg Voss, 1808, 54–58.

———. "Körperliche Bildung oder Erziehung der Jugend." *Drittes Toilettengeschenk. Ein Jahrbuch für Damen*. Leipzig: Georg Voss, 1807, 103–6.

———. "Leibchen für Damen, zu Beförderung einer schöneren Haltung des Körpers." *Erstes Toilettengeschenk. Ein Jahrbuch für Damen*. Leipzig: Georg Voss, 1805, 77–78.

———. *Systematisches Lehrbuch der bildenden Tanzkunst und körperlichen Ausbildung* (1843). Leipzig: Zentralantiquariat der DDR, 1989.

———. "Ueber die Bildung des Körpers zum Tanzen." *Erstes Toilettengeschenk. Ein Jahrbuch für Damen*. Leipzig: Georg Voss, 1805, 57–64.

———. "Unser jetziger Tanz." *Erstes Toilettengeschenk. Ein Jahrbuch für Damen*. Leipzig: Georg Voss, 1805, 64–71.

———. "Versuch einer Theorie der Tanzkunst." *Zweites Toilettengeschenk. Ein Jahrbuch für Damen*. Leipzig: Georg Voss, 1806, 116–23.

———. "Wahrscheinliche Ursache des Verfalls der Tanzkunst als Privatvergnügen." *Toilettengeschenk. Ein Jahrbuch für Damen*. Leipzig: Georg Voss, 1807, 106–9.

Rosenhain, August von. *Bemerkungen über das Tanzen; nebst einer gründlichen Anleitung zu den jetzt beliebtesten Tänzen. Besonders für seine Scholaren bearbeitet*. Schleswig: Königliches Staubstummen-Institut, 1821.

Roux, Johann Adolph Karl. *Die Deutsche Fechtkunst, enthaltend eine theoretisch-praktische Anweisung zum Stoßfechten.* 2nd ed. Leipzig: Johann Ambrosius Barth, 1817.

———. *Gründliche und vollständige Anweisung in der deutschen Fecht-Kunst auf Stoss und Hieb.* Jena: Wolfgang Stahls Buchhandlung, 1798.

S., Fr.W. "Ueber Sichersreut in Franken." *Journal des Luxus und der Moden* (December 1798): 673–82.

"Scene aus dem Carlsbad im Jahr 1802, in einem Briefe." *Journal des Luxus und der Moden* (November 1802): 620–28.

Schaarschmidt, Samuel. *Therapia Generalis oder Abhandlung von denen üblichen Artzneien, nach ihren wahren Eigenschaften und Würckungen, nebst der Anweisung zu deren gehörigen Gebrauch, auf Verlangen seiner Zuhörer*, edited by J.C.W. Moehsen. Berlin: Verlag Joh. Jacob Schützens, 1749.

Scheerer, Wilhelm. *Turn-Fehde, oder: Wer hat Recht?* Berlin: Krause, 1818.

Schelle, Karl Gottlob. *Die Spatziergänge oder die Kunst spatzierenzugehen.* Leipzig, 1802. Reprint. Hildesheim; Zürich; New York: Olms-Weidemann, 1990.

Schilderung der Sächsischen und Böhmischen Bäder Radeberg, Schandau, Sieshübel und Töplitz im Sommer 1804." *Journal des Luxus und der Moden* (August 1804): 401–8.

Schiller, Friedrich. "Der Spaziergang." In *Schillers Werke. Nationalausgabe.* Vol. 2/1. Weimar: Hermann Böhlaus nachfolger, 1983.

Schleiermacher, Friedrich Daniel Ernst. "Versuch einer Theorie des geselligen Betragens." (Berlinisches Archiv der Zeit und ihres Geschmacks 5, Teilband 1, Berlin 1799). In *Kritische Gesamtausgabe. Erste Abteilung. Schriften und Entwürfe.* Vol. 2. Berlin; New York: Walter de Gruyter, 1984.

Schmidl, Adolf. *Wien, wie es ist. Ein Gemälde der Kaiserstadt und ihrer nächsten Umgebungen in Beziehung auf Topographie, Statistik und geselliges Leben, mit besonderer Berücksichtigung wissenschaftlicher Anstalten und Sammlungen.* Wien: Carl Gerold, 1833.

Schmidt. "Das Buschbad, bey Meißen." *Journal des Luxus und der Moden* (February 1799): 76–81.

Schmidt-Lisber, H. *Die Reise nach Pyrmont. Wahrheit und Dichtung.* Braunschweig: Waisenhaus, 1828.

Schneider, " Statistische Übersicht von Gymnasten und Turnplätzen in Preußen." In *Unbekannte Briefe von Friedrich Ludwig Jahn und Hugo Rothenstein als Quellen zur Frühgeschichte des Turnens*, edited by Hans Langenfeld and Josef Ulfkotte. Oberwerries: WTB, 1990.

Schönwald, Andreas. *Grundregeln der Tanzkunst.* Freyburg: Herdersche Buchhandlung, 1812.

Schreber, Daniel Gottlob Moritz. *Aertzliche Zimmer-Gymnastik oder Darstellung und Anwendung der unmittelbaren—d.h. ohne Geräth und Beistand, mithin stets und überall ausführbaren—heilgymnastischen Bewegungen für beide Geschlechter, jedes Alter und die verschiedenen speciellen Gebrauchszwecke*

*als ein einfach natürliches System entworfen*. 6th ed. Leipzig: Friedrich Fleischer, 1859.
———. *Kallipädie oder Erziehung zur Schönheit durch naturgetreue und gleichmäßige Förderung normaler Körperbildung, lebenstüchtiger Gesundheit und geistiger Veredelung. Für Aeltern, Erzieher und Lehrer*. Leipzig: Fleischer, 1858.
Schroeder, A. "Pädagogik. Rezension von Überbürdungsschriften." *Jenaische Allgemeine Literatur-Zeitung* 157–60 (1836): 290–318.
Senff, Adam Andreas. *Gesundheitskatechismus für das Landvolk und den gemeinen Mann*. Berlin und Stettin: Friedrich Nicolai, 1781.
Senff, Barthoff. *Buntes Leipzig. Skizzen und Genrebilder*. Vol. 2. Leipzig: Louis Rocca, 1842.
"Skizzen zum neuesten Gemälde von München." *Journal des Luxus und der Moden* (März 1811): 158–62.
"Skizzen zum neuesten Gemälde von München." *Journal des Luxus und der Moden* (Julius 1811) 462–69.
Spieß, Adolf. *Die Lehre der Turnkunst*. Vol. 1. *Die Freiübungen*. Basel: Schweighäuser, 1840.
———. *Die Lehre der Turnkunst*. Vol. 4. *Die Gemeinübungen*. Basel: Schweighauser, 1846.
Stahl, Georg Ernst. *Theoretische und practische Abhandlung von der Diaet*. Leipzig: Grießbach, 1739.
"Statistische Tabelle von der Stadt Leipzig (1788)." In *Leipziger Stadtpläne. Verzeichnis der in Leipziger Institutionen verfügbarer Karten und Pläne*, edited by Heike Boden, Alice Hecht, and Thomas Nabert. Leipzig: Klingenberg, 1994.
Steffens, Henrich. *Caricaturen des Heiligsten*. Vol. 1. Leipzig: Brockhaus, 1819.
Steinmetz, Friedrich. *Pyrmont und seine Mineralquellen. Anleitung zu Trink- und Badecuren, in Bezug auf die neueste Analyse*. Pyrmont: G. Uslar, 1825.
Straß, Friedrich. "Über die Nothwendigkeit geordneter Leibesübungen für die Gelehrtenschulen." In *Führer in der Zeit der Turnsperre. Maßmann, v. Klumpp, Lorinser, Straß, Diesterweg, E.F. Koch, Kirchner, Nachtegall, Ling, Eiselen*, edited by Franz Paul Wiedemann. Dresden: Limpert Verlag, 1933.
Straß, Karl Friedrich Heinrich. *Pyrmont und dessen Umgebungen. Ein Taschenbuch für Curgäste und Reisende. Aus Dankbarkeit gegen die kräftigenden Quellen des herrlichen Bades*. Pyrmont: Georg Uslar, 1850.
Struve, Friedrich Adolf August. "Bemerkungen über einige gegen seine künstlichen Mineralwässer gemachten Einwendungen." *Journal der practischen Arzneykunde und Wundarzneykunst* 68, no. 4 (1829): 82–101.
Süvern, Johann Wilhelm. "Entwurf eines allgemeinen Gesetzes über die Verfassung des Schulwesens im preußischen Staate." In *Schulreform in Preußen 1809–1819. Entwürfe und Gutachten*, edited by Lothar Schwiem. Weinheim: Beltz, 1966.

———. "Unterrichts-Verfassung der Gymnasien und Stadtschulen. Vom 12. Jan. 1816." In *Schulreform in Preußen 1809–1819. Entwürfe und Gutachten*, edited by Lothar Schwiem. Weinheim: Beltz, 1966.

Taubert, Gottfried. *Rechtschaffener Tanzmeister, oder gründliche Erklärung der Frantzösischen Tanz-Kunst.* 3 vols. Leipzig: Friedrich Lanckischens Erben, 1717.

Teubern, E.A.L. von. "Das Bad zu Liebenstein im Sachsen-Meiningischen im Sommer 1804." *Journal des Luxus und der Moden* (September 1804): 442–56.

Thomasius, Christian. "Additamenta ad notas praecedentes." In *Christian Thomasius. Leben und Lebenswerk*, edited by Max Fleischmann. Halle: Max Niemeyer Verlag, 1931.

———[propable author]. *Bericht von Einrichtung des Paedagogii zu Glaucha an Halle. Nebst der von einem gelehrten Manne verlangten Erinnerung über solche Einrichtung*. Franckfurt; Leipzig, 1699.

———. "Der Studierenden Jugend zu Leipzig in einem Discours, Von denen Mängeln der Aristotelischen Ethic, und von andern das Jus Publicum betreffenden Sachen. Zwey Collegia Über die Christliche Sitten-lehre und über das Jus Publicum." In *Allerhand bißher publicirte Kleine Deutsche Schriften. Mit Fleiß colligiret und zusammen getragen. Nebst etlichen Beylagen und einer Vorrede*. Halle: Christoph Salfeld, 1701.

———. *Kurtzer Entwurff der politischen Klugheit, sich selbst und andern in allen menschlichen Gesellschaften wohl zu rathen und zu einer gescheiden Conduite zu gelangen*. Franckfurth; Leipzig: Gross, 1713.

———. *Von der Kunst, vernünfftig und tugendhaft zu lieben. Als dem eintzigen Mittel zu einen glückseligen, galanten und vergnügten Leben zu gelangen. Oder Einleitung zur Sitten-Lehre*. Halle: Christoph Salfeld, 1692.

Tippelskirch, Ernst Ludwig von and Magnus Friedrich von Bassewitz. *Verordnung über das Verfahren bei der Annäherung und dem Ausbruche der Cholera in Berlin*. Berlin: Gesundheits-Commission für Berlin, 1831.

Tissot, Samuel André. *Anleitung für das Landvolk in Absicht auf seine Gesundheit*. Translated by H.C. Hirzel. Zürich: Fueßlin, 1768.

———. *Von der Gesundheit der Gelehrten*. Zürich: Fueßlin, 1770.

Trapp, Ernst Christian. "Ueber das Hallische Erzihungsinstitut." *Pädagogische Unterhandlungen 5* (1783): 32–70.

Tschütter, Gotthelf. *Terpsichore. Ein Taschenbuch der neueren Tanzkunst für Anfänger und solche, die bereits einige Kenntnisse erlangt haben und sich darin vervollkommnen wollen*. Dresden; Leipzig: Arnold'sche Buchhandlung, 1828.

"Ueber das Seebad zu Doberan am heiligen Damme an der Ostsee." *Journal des Luxus und der Moden* (März 1799): 134–46.

"Ueber die Hazard-Spiele im Bade zu Flinsberg in Schlesien." *Journal des Luxus und der Moden* (May 1798): 289–94

"Ueber Pyrmont. Mlle Kirchgeßner. Feten in Pyrmont." *Journal des Luxus und der Moden* (November 1803): 610–12.

"Ueber Pyrmont 1798." *Journal des Luxus und der Moden* (Februar 1799): 72–75.
"Ueber Warmbrunn." *Journal des Luxus und der Moden* (October 1803): 540–47.
Valentiner, Theodor. "Allgemeine Balneotherapie." In *Handbuch der allgemeinen und speciellen Balneotherapie*, edited by Theodor Valentiner. Berlin: G. Reimer, 1873, 1–74.
———. *Pyrmont für Kurgäste und Fremde*. Kiel: Carl Schröder & Comp., 1859.
Valentiner, Theodor. "Vorwort." In *Handbuch der allgemeinen und speciellen Balneotherapie*, edited by Theodor Valentiner. Berlin: G. Reimer, 1873.
Verschönerungen der Städte unsers Zeitalters." *Journal des Luxus und der Moden* (July 1810): 404–7.
Vetter, August. "Beantwortung der gegen den Ersatz natürlicher durch künstliche Mineralwasser von Hrn Prof. A. Pleischl in Wien erhobenen Einwände." *Annalen der Struveschen Brunnenanstalten*. Vol. 3. Berlin: August Hirschwald, 1843, 137–58.
———. "Die Saison von 1840 in der Berliner Brunnenanstalt." *Annalen der Struveschen Brunnenanstalten*. Vol. 1. Berlin: August Hirschwald, 1841, 170–83.
———. "Vorrede." *Annalen der Struveschen Brunnenanstalten*. Vol. 1. Berlin: August Hirschwald, 1841, III–X.
Vieth, Gerhard Ulrich Anton. *Versuch einer Encyklopädie der Leibesübungen*. Vol. 2. *System der Leibesübungen*. Berlin: Carl Ludwig Hartmann, 1795.
Villaume, Peter. "Ob und in wie fern bei der Erziehung die Vollkommenheit des einzelnen Menschen seiner Brauchbarkeit aufzuopfern sey?" In *Allgemeine Revision des gesammten Schul- und Erziehungswesens*. Vol. 3, edited by Joachim Heinrich Campe. Hamburg: Carl Ernst Bohn, 1785.
———. "Von der Bildung des Körpers in Rücksicht auf die Vollkommenheit und Glückseligkeit der Menschen, oder über die physische Erziehung insonderheit." In *Allgemeine Revision des gesammten Schul- und Erziehungswesens von einer Gesellschaft praktischer Erzieher*. Vol. 8, edited by Joachim Heinrich Campe. Wolfenbüttel: Gräffer, 1787.
———. *Von der Bildung des Körpers in Rücksicht auf die Vollkommenheit und Glückseligkeit der Menschen oder über die physische Erziehung insonderheit* (1787). Dresden: Wilhelm Limpert Verlag, 1929.
Vischer, Friedrich Theodor. *Briefwechsel zwischen Strauß und Vischer*. Vol. 1. Stuttgart: Klett Verlag, 1952.
———. "Das akademische Leben und die Gymnastik. Ein frommer Wunsch." In *Kritische Gänge*. Vol. 3. Berlin: Meyer & Jessen, 1920.
"Von den täglichen Aufsicht im Philanthropin und von den Sitten unserer Zöglinge." In *Philanthropisches Archiv*. Vol. 3, 115–17.
*Vorschläge zu einigen provisorischen Einrichtungen in der Gesellschaft der Harmonie*. Leipzig, 1829.
Wedel[ius], Georg Wolfgang. [Johannes Rottenberger] *Diæta Literatorum*. Editio Quarta cum Additamenta Paradoxis. Erfurt: Müller, 1704.
Welsch, Hermann. *The Springs and Baths of Kissingen*. Kissingen: Author, 1888.

Wendt, Johann. *Die Heilquellen zu Kissingen im Königreiche Baiern*. Breslau: Gosohorsky, 1837.

———. *Ueber den Tanz als Vergnügen und Schädlichkeit. Ein Beytrag zur Diätetik*. 2nd ed. Breslau: August Schall, 1804.

Werner, Johann Adolf Ludwig. *Medicinische Gymnastik oder die Kunst, verunstaltete und von ihren natürlichen Form- und Lagerverhältnissen abweichende Theile des meschlichen Körpers nach anatomischen und physiologischen Grundsätzen in die ursprünglichen Richtungen zurückzuführen und darin zu kräftigen*. Dresden; Leipzig: Arnold, 1838.

Wolf, Georg Jacob, ed. *Ein Jahrhundert München 1800–1900. Zeitgenössische Bilder und Dokumente*. Munich: Hanfstaengl, 1919.

Z. "Erster Spazziergang in und um Altona." *Hamburg und Altona* 1 (1801): 273–82.

Z. "Zweiter Spazziergang in und um Altona." *Hamburg und Altona* 1 (1801): 311–18.

Z. "Der Tanz, wie er ist, und seyn könnte." *Journal des Luxus und der Moden* (Januar 1802): 5–7.

Zangen, Carl Georg von. *Etwas über das Walzen, nebst einigen Gedichten und Anhang einiger Oden*. Wetzlar: Philipp Jacob Winkler, 1782.

Zeller, Eduard. *Erinnerungen eines Neunzigjährigen*. Stuttgart: Uhland'sche Buchdruckerei, 1908.

Zückert, Johann Friedrich. *Von der diätetischen Erziehung der entwöhnten und erwachsenen Kinder bis in ihr mannbares Alter*. Berlin: August Mylius, 1765.

*Secondary Literature*

*90 Jahre Casino-Gesellschaft Mannheim e.V.* Als Festgabe unseren Mitgliedern und Freunden zum 90jährigen Jubiläum gewidmet. Mannheim, 1925.

Ackerknecht, Erwin H. "The End of Greek Diet." *Bulletin of the History of Medicine* 45 (1971): 242–49.

Adamson, Melitta Weiss. *Medieval Dietetics. Food and Drink in Regimen Sanitatis Literature from 800 to 1400*. Frankfurt am Main: Lang, 1995.

Albrecht, Wolfgang and Hans-Joachim Kertscher, *Wanderzwang—Wanderlust. Formen der Raum- und Sozialerfahrung zwischen der Afklärung und Frühindustrialisierung*. Tübingen: Max Niemeyer Verlag, 1999.

Arnhardt, Gerhard. *Schulpforte. Eine Schule im Zeichen der humanistischen Bildungstradition*. Berlin: Volk und Wissen, 1988.

Arz, Maike. *Literatur und Lebenskraft. Vitalistische Naturforschung um 1800*. Stuttgart: M&P, 1996.

Assmann, Aleida. *Arbeit am nationalen Gedächtnis. Eine kurze Geschichte der deutschen Bildungsidee*. Frankfurt am Main: Campus Verlag, 1993.

Bähr, Marion. "Erziehung zur Lebenstüchtigkeit durch harmonische Miteinander von Körper und Geist. Zum 125. Jahrestag der Gründung des ersten deutschen

Schrebervereins." In *Leipzig. Aus Vergangenheit und Gegenwart.* Beiträge zur Stadtgeschichte 7. Leipzig: VEB Fachbuchverlag, 1990.

Baier, Johann. *Armut, Not und Hoffnunf am Rande einer Stadt. Haidhausen im Jahrhundert der Cholera-Epidemien. Ein Beitrag zur Sozialgeschichte Haidhausens.* Munich: Haidhausen-Verlag, 1988.

Ballstaedt, Andreas and Tobias Widmaier. *Salonmusik. Zur Geschichte und Funktion einer bürgerlichen Musikpraxis.* Stuttgart: Franz Steiner Verlag, 1989.

Barnard, Frederick M.. "Rightful Decorum and Rational Accountability. A Forgotten Theory of Civil Life." In *Christian Thomasius 1655–1728. Interpretationen zu Werk und Wirkung. Mit einer Bibliographie der neueren Thomasius-Literatur. Studien zum achtzehnten Jahrhundert.* Vol. 11, Werner Schneiders. Hamburg: Meiner, 1989.

Barthel, Christian. *Medizinische Polizey und medizinische Aufklärung. Aspekte des öffentlichen Gesundheitsdiskurses im 18. Jahrhundert.* Frankfurt am Main: Campus Verl., 1989.

Bauer, Klaus. "Friedrich Schnurrer (1784–1833), ein Arzt aus Tübingen." In *Bausteine zur Tübinger Universitätsgeschichte.* Folge 7, edited by Volker Schäfer. Tübingen: Universitätsarchiv, 1995.

Bauer, Reinhard and Ernst Piper *München. Die Geschichte einer Stadt.* Munich/Zürich: Pier, 1993.

Beachy, Robert, *The Soul of Commerce. Credit, Property, and Politics in Leipzig, 1750–1840.* Leiden: Brill, 2005.

Beetz, Manfred. "Ein neuentdeckter Lehrer der Conduite. Thomasius in der Geschichte der Gesellschaftsethik." In *Christian Thomasius 1655–1728. Interpretationen zu Werk und Wirkung. Mit einer Bibliographie der neueren Thomasius-Literatur. Studien zum achtzehnten Jahrhundert.* Vol. 11, edited by Werner Schneiders. Hamburg: Meiner, 1989.

Benjamin, Walter. *Charles Baudelaire. A Lyric Poet in the Era of High Capitalism.* London: Verso, 1983.

Benzenhöfer, Udo. *Psychiatrie und Anthropologie in der ersten Hälfte des 19. Jahrhunderts.* Hürtgenwald: Guido Pressler Verlag, 1993.

Berg, Fredrik. "Hygienens omfattning i äldre tider. Sex res non naturales." *Lychnos* (1962): 91–127.

Bermingham, Ann. "Introduction." In Bermingham, Ann and John Brewer, *The Consumption of Culture 1600–1800. Image, Object, Text.* London: Routledge, 1995.

Bernett, Hajo. *Die pädagogische Neugestaltung der bürgerlichen Leibesübungen durch die Philanthropen.* Stuttgart: Karl Hofman, 1960.

Björnsson, Páll. "Making the New Man. Liberal Politics and Associational Life in Leipzig, 1845-1871." PhD diss., University of Rochester, 1999.

Bleeck, Klaus. *Adelserziehung auf deutschen Ritterakademien. Die Lüneburger Adelsschulen 1655–1850.* Vol. 1. Frankfurt am Main: Peter Lang, 1977.

Bocklitz, Klaus. "Hamburgische Festungsanlagen." In Clasen, Armin and Klaus Bocklitz, *Studien zur Topographie Hamburgs. Beiträge zur Geschichte Hamburgs.* Vol. 14. Hamburg: Hans Christians Verlag, 1979.

Böhme, Hartmut and Gernot Böhme. *Das Andere der Vernunft. Zur Entwicklung von Rationalitätsstrukturen am Beispiel Kants.* Frankfurt am Main: Suhrkamp, 1985.

Bollenbeck, Georg. *Bildung und Kultur. Glanz und Elend eines deutschen Deutungsmusters.* Frankfurt am Main: Insel Verlag, 1994.

Bothe, Rolf. "Bad Driburg." In *Kurstädte in Deutschland. Zur Geschichte einer Baugattung*, edited by Rolf Bothe. Berlin: Frölich & Kaufmann, 1984.

———, ed. *Kurstädte in Deutschland. Zur Geschichte einer Baugattung.* Berlin: Frölich & Kaufmann, 1984.

Brandt, Peter. "Einstellungen, Motive und Ziele von Kriegsfreiwilligen 1813/14: Das Freikorps Lützow." In *Kriegsbereitschaft und Friedensordnung in Deutschland 1800–1814*, edited by Jost Düffler. Jahrbuch für historische Friedensforschung. Vol. 3. (1994).

Braun, Rudolf and David Gugerli, *Macht des Tanzes—Tanz der Mächtigen. Hoffeste und Herrschaftszeremoniell 1550–1914.* Munich: Beck, 1993.

Brecht, Martin. *Geschichte des Pietismus* Vol. 1. *Der Pietismus vom siebzenhten bis zum frühen achtzehnten Jahrhundert.* Göttingen: Vandenhoeck & Ruprecht, 1993.

Brednow, Walter. *Christoph Wilhelm Hufeland, Arzt und Erzieher im Lichte der Aufklärung.* Berlin: Akademie-Verlag, 1964.

Broman, Thomas S. *The Transformation of German Academic Medicine 1750–1820.* New York: Cambridge University Press, 1996.

Brückner, Jutta. *Staatswissenschaften, Kameralismus und Naturrecht. Ein Beitrag zur Geschichte der Politischen Wissenschaft im Deutschland des späten 17. und frühen 18. Jahrhunderts.* Munich: Beck, 1977.

Bruford, Walter. *The German Tradition of Self-Cultivation. 'Bildung' from Humboldt to Thomas Mann.* Cambridge: Cambridge University Press, 1975.

Buchmann, Bertrand Michael. *Der Prater. Die Geschichte des unteren Werd.* Wien; Hamburg: Zsolnay, 1979.

Busse, Gerhard. *Schreber, Freud und die Suche nach dem Vater. Über die realitätsschaffende Kraft einer wissenschaftlichen Hypothese.* Berlin: Peter Lang, 1991.

Conze, Werner and Jürgen Kocka, eds. *Bildungsbürgertum im 19. Jahrhundert.* Vol. 1. *Bildungssystem und Professionalisierung im internationalen Vergleich.* Stuttgart: Klett-Cotta, 1985.

Craig, Gordon. *The Politics of the Prussian Army 1640–1945.* London: Oxford University Press, 1964.

Czeike, Felix. *Geschichte der Stadt Wien.* Vienna: Molden, 1981.

*Das Preußische Heer der Befreiungskriege.* Vol. 2. *Das Preußische Heer im Jahre 1813. Der Große Generalstab. Kriegsgeschichtliche Abteilung II.* Berlin: Ernst Siegfried Mittler und Sohn, 1914.

Delaporte, François. *Le savoir de la maladie. Essai sur le choléra de 1832 à Paris.* Paris: Presses Universitaires de France, 1990.

Denk, Heinz. "Schulturnen. Leibesübungen im Dienste autoritärer Erziehung." In *Geschichte der Leibesübungen.* Vol. 3.1, edited by Horst Ueberhorst. Berlin: Verlag Bartels & Wernitz KG, 1980.

Dettke, Barbara. *Die asiatische Hydra. Die Cholera von 1830/31 in Berlin und den preußischen Provinzen Posen, Preußen und Schlesien.* Berlin: Walter de Gruyter, 1995.

Diamant, Adolf. *Chronik der Juden in Leipzig.* Chemnitz: Verlag Heimatland Sachsen, 1993.

Dinges, Martin. "Die Ehre als Thema der Stadtgeschichte." Zeitschrift für Historische Forschung 16 (1989): 409–40.

Dohmen, Günther. *Bildung und Schule. Die Entstehung des deutschen Bildungsbegriffs und die Entwicklung seines Verhältnisses zur Schule* Vol. 1. Weinheim: Beltz, 1964–65.

Dombart, Theodor. *Der Englische Garten zu München. Geschichte seiner Entstehung und seines Ausbaues zur großstädtischen Parkanlage.* Munich: Hornung Verlag, 1972.

Düding, Dieter. *Organisierter gesellschaftlicher Nationalismus in Deutschland (1808–1847). Bedeutung und Funktion der Turner- und Sängervereine für die deutsche Nationalbewegung.* Munich: R. Oldenbourg Verlag, 1984.

Dülmen, Richard van. *Die Kultur und Alltag in der Frühen Neuzeit.* Vol. 2. *Dorf und Staat 16.–18. Jahrhundert.* Munich: Beck, 1992.

Dumont, Louis. *German Ideology. From France to Germany and Back.* Chicago: University of Chicago Press, 1993.

Duquette, David. "The Political Significance of Hegel's Concept of Recognition." In *Hegel's Phenomenology of Spirit: A Reappraisal*, edited by Gary K. Browning. Dordrecht: Kluwer, 1997.

Durey, Michael. *The Return of the Plague. British Society and the Cholera, 1831–32.* Bristol: Gill and Macmillan, 1979.

Eichberg, Henning. *Leistung, Spannung, Geschiwindigkeit. Sport und Tanz im gesellschaftlichen Wandel des 18./19. Jahrhunderts.* Stuttgart: Klett-Cotta, 1978.

———. "Sport im 19. Jahrhundert—Genese einer industriellen Verhaltensform." In *Geschichte der Leibesübungen.* Vol. 3.1, edited by Horst Ueberhorst. Berlin: Bartels & Wernitz, 1980.

Eichel, Wolfgang, ed. *Geschichte der Körperkultur in Deutschland.* Vol. 2. *Die Körperkultur in Deutschland von 1789 bis 1917.* Berlin: Sportverlag, 1969.

Eifert, Max. *Geschichte und Beschreibung der Stadt Tübingen.* Tübingen: Ludwig Friedrich Fues, 1849.

Eisenberg, Christiane. "Charismatic National Leader. Turnvater Jahn." *the International Journal of the History of Sport* 13 no. 1 (1996): 14–23.

———. *"English Sports" und deutsche Bürger. Eine Gesellschaftsgeschichte 1800–1939.* Paderborn: Ferdinand Schöningh, 1999.

Emch-Dériaz, Antoinette. "The Non-Naturals Made Easy." In *The Popularization of Medicine, 1650–1850*, edited by Roy Porter. London: Routledge, 1992.

Engelhardt, Ulrich. *"Bildungsbürgertum." Begriffs- und Dogmengeschichte eines Etiketts*. Stuttgart: Klett & Cotta, 1986.

Euler, Carl. *Friedrich Ludwig Jahn. Sein Leben und Wirken*. Stuttgart: Verlag von Karl Krabbe, 1881.

———. *Geschichte des Turnunterrichts*. Gotha: Thienemann, 1891.

Euler, Peter. *Pädagogik und Universalienstreit. Zur Bedeutung von F.I. Niethammers pädagogischer "Streitschrift."* Weinheim: Deutscher Studien Verlag, 1989.

Eulner, Hans-Heinz. "Die Lehre von der Ernährung im Universitätsunterricht." In *Ernährung und Ernährungslehre im 19. Jahrhundert.* Vorträge des Symposiums am 5. und 6. Januar 1973 in Frankfurt am Main, edited by Edith Heischkel-Artelt. Göttingen: Vandenhoeck & Ruprecht, 1976.

Evans, Richard. *Death in Hamburg. Society and Politics in the Cholera Years 1830–1910.* Oxford: Clarendon Press, 1987.

———. "Epidemics and Revolutions. Cholera in Nineteenth-Century Europe." *Past and Present* 120 (1988): 123–46.

Fambach, Oscar, ed. *Das Repertorium des Stadttheaters zu Leipzig 1817–1828.* Bonn: Bouvier Verlag Herbert Grundmann, 1980.

Fauser, Markus. "Promenade als Kunstwerk. Karl Gottlob Schelles Theorie des Spaziergangs." In Karl Gottlob Schelle, *Die Spatziergänge oder die Kunst spatzierenzugehen* (Leipzig, 1802). Hildesheim: Olms, 1990.

Fehrenbach, Elisabeth. "Einführung." In *Adel und Bürgertum in Deutschland 1770–1848*, edited by Elisabeth Fehrenbach. Munich: R. Oldenbourg Verlag, 1994.

———, ed. *Adel und Bürgertum in Deutschland 1770–1848*. Munich: R. Oldenbourg Verlag, 1994.

Feilchenfeldt, Konrad. "Karl August Varnhagen von Ense und Hegel. Anhang: Anzeige in der J.G. Cotta'schen Buchhandlung erscheinen im künftigen Jahre fortgesetzt und beginnen ihren dritten Jahrgang die Jahrbücher für wissenschaftliche Kritik." In *Die "Jahrbücher für wissenschaftliche Kritik." Hegels Berliner Gegenakademie*, edited by Christoph Jamme. Stuttgart-Bad Cannstatt: Fromman-Holzboog, 1994.

Fink, Monika. *Der Ball. Eine Kulturgeschichte des Gesellschaftstanzes im 18. und 19. Jahrhundert*. Innsbruck: Studien Verlag, 1996.

Fischer, J. "Der erste Choleraausbruch in Österreich nach Akten der Wiener medizinischen Fakultät aus den Jahren 1831 und 1832." In *Historische Studien und Skizzen zu Natur- und Heilwissenschaft*. Berlin, 1930.

Foucault, Michel. "Preface to *The History of Sexuality*, Vol. 2." In *The Foucault Reader. An Introduction to Foucault's Thought, with Major New Unpublished Material*, edited by Paul Rabinow. London: Peregrine Books, 1984.

———. "Nietzsche, Genealogy, History." In *The Foucault Reader. An Introduction to Foucault's Thought, with Major New Unpublished Material*, edited by Paul Rabinow. London: Peregrine Books, 1984.

Franke, Annelore. *Leipzig um die Wende vom 18. zum 19. Jahrhundert*. Leipzig: Offprint, s.a.

Freudenthal, Herbert. *Vereine in Hamburg. Ein Beitrag zur Geschichte und Volkskunde der Geselligkeit*. Hamburg: Museum für Hamburgische Geschichte, 1968.

Frevert, Ute. *Ehrenmänner. Das Duell in der bürgerlichen Gesellschaft*. Munich: Beck, 1991.

———. "Das jakobinische Modell: Allgemeine Wehrpflicht und Nationsbildung in Preußen-Deutschland." In *Militär und Gesellschaft im 19. und 20. Jahrhundert*, edited by Ute Frevert. Stuttgart: Klett-Cotta, 1997, 17–47.

———. *Krankheit als politisches Problem 1770–1880. Soziale Unterschichten in Preußen zwischen meidizinischer Polizei und staatlicher Sozialversicherung*. Göttingen: Vandenhoeck & Ruprecht, 1984.

———. "*Mann und Weib, und Weib und Mann.*" Geschlechter-Differenzen in der Moderne. Munich: Beck, 1995.

———. "Soldaten, Staatsbürger. Überlegungen zur historischen Konstruktion von Männlichkeit." In *Männergeschichte—Geschlechtergeschichte. Männlichkeit im Wandel der Moderne*, edited by Thomas Kühne. Frankfurt: Campus Verlag, 1996.

Frey, Manuel. *Der reinliche Bürger. Entstehung und Verbreitung bürgerlicher Tugenden in Deutschland, 1760–1860*. Göttingen: Vandenhoeck & Ruprecht, 1997.

Friedmann, Helmut. *Alt-Mannheim im Wandel seiner Physiognomie, Struktur und Funktionen (1606–1965)*. Mannheim: Bundesforschungsanstalt für Landeskunde und Raumordnung, 1968.

Fritsche, Herbert. *Pyrmont. Aus der Gnadengeschichte einer Stätte*. Bad Pyrmont: Verlag Leonhard Friedrich, 1946.

Fuhs, Burkhard. *Mondäne Orte einer vornehmen Gesellschaft. Kultur und Geschichte der Kurstädte 1700–1900*. Hildesheim: Georg Olms Verlag, 1992.

Gall, Lothar. "Liberalismus und 'bürgerliche Gesellschaft.' Zu Charakter und Entwicklung der liberalen Bewegung in Deutschland." *Historische Zeitschrift* 220 (1975): 324–56.

———. "Vom alten zum neuen Bürgertum. Die mitteleuropäische Stadt im Umbruch 1780–1820." In *Vom alten zum neuen Bürgertum. Die mitteleuropäische Stadt im Umbruch 1780–1820. Historische Zeitschrift. Beihefte (Neue Folge)* 14, edited by Lothar Gall. Munich: Oldenbourg, 1991.

———. "Die Bassermanns. Eine Mannheimer Bürgerfamilie zwischen Ancien Régime und moderner Welt." In *Bildungsbürgertum im 19. Jahrhundert*. Vol. 3. *Lebensführung und ständische Vergesellschaftung*, edited by M. Rainer Lepsius. Stuttgart: Klett-Cotta, 1992.

Gallagher, Catherine and Thomas Laqueur. *The Making of the Modern Body. Sexuality and Society in the Nineteenth Century*. Berkeley/Los Angeles/London: University of California Press, 1987.

Gasch, Rudolf. *Festschrift zur fünfzigjährigen Jubelfeier des Allgemeinen Turnvereins zu Leipzig*. Leipzig: Allgemeiner Turnverein, 1895.

Gaulhofer, Karl. *Die Fußhaltung. Ein Beitrag zur Stilgeschichte der menschlichen Bewegung*. Vol. 1. Kassel: Rudolph'sche Verlagsanstalt, 1930.

Geiss, Philipp H. *Das Leben des Turnpädagogen Adolf Spieß (1810–1858. Ein Beitag zur Geschichte des deutschen und des schweizer Schulturnens*. Idstein: Schulz-Kirchner, 1991.

Geist, Johann Friedrich. *Passagen. Ein Bautyp des 19. Jahrhunderts*. Munich: Prestel-Verlag, 1969.

Geßner, Alida Christine. "Die Cholera-Epidemien in Bayern während des 19. Jahrhunderts unter besonderer Berücksichtigung der Stadt Ingolstadt und ihrer Umgebung." PhD diss., University of München, 1992.

Göckenjan, Gerd. *Kurieren und Staat machen. Gesundheit und Medizin in der bürgerlichen Welt*. Frankfurt am Main: Suhrkamp, 1985.

Goldmann, Stefan. *Christoph Wilhelm Hufeland im Goethekreis. Eine psychoanalytische Studie zur Autobiographie und ihrer Topik*. Stuttgart: M & P, 1993.

Golterman, Svenja. *Körper der Nation. Habitusformierung und die Politik des Turnens 1860-1890*. Göttingen: Vandenhoeck & Ruprecht, 1998.

Grobe, Peter. *Die Entfestigung Münchens*. Munich: Oppermann, 1970.

Gramit, David, *Cultivating Music. The Aspirations, Interests, and Limits of German Musical Culture, 1770–1848*. Berkeley: University of California Press, 2002.

Groll, Hans. *Die Systematiker der Leibesübungen. Vergleichende Systemkunde der pädagogischen Leibesübungen*. Vienna: Österreichischer Bundesverlag für Unterricht, Wissenschaft und Kunst, 1959.

Haas, Erwin. *Die Sieben Württembergischen Landesfestungen*. Reutlingen: Verlag Harwalik, 1996.

Habermas, Jürgen. *Strukturwandel der Öffentlichkeit. Untersuchungen zu einer Kategorie der bürgerlichen Gesellschaft*. Neuwied: Luchterhand,1965.

Habermas, Rebekka. *Frauen und Männer des Bürgertums. Eine Familiengeschichte (1750–1850)*. Göttingen: Vandenhoeck & Ruprecht, 2000.

Hagemann, Karen. "Heldenmütter, Kriegerbräute und Amazonen. Entwürfe 'patriotischer' Weiblichkeit zur Zeit der Freiheitskriege" In *Militär und Gesellschaft im 19. und 20. Jahrhundert*, edited by Ute Frevert. Stuttgart: Klett-Cotta, 1997.

———. "Heran, heran, zu Sieg oder Tod! Entwürfe patriotisch-wehrhafter Männlichkeit in der Zeit der Befreiungskriege." In *Männergeschichte— Geschlechtergeschichte. Männlichkeit im Wandel der Moderne*, edited by Thomas Kühne. Frankfurt: Campus Verlag, 1996.

Hahlweg, Werner. *Guerrilla. Krieg ohne Fronten*. Stuttgart: W. Kohlhammer Verlag, 1968.

Hanson, Alice. *Musical Life in Biedermeier Vienna*. Cambridge: Cambridge University Press, 1989.

Hardtwig, Wolfgang. "Auf dem Weg zum Bildungsbürgertum. Die Lebensführungsart der jugendlichen Bildungsschicht 1750–1819." In *Bildungsbürgertum im 19. Jahrhundert*. Vol. 3. *Lebensführung und ständische Vergesellschaftung*, edited by M. Rainer Lepsius. Stuttgart: Klett-Cotta, 1992.

———. *Vormärz. Der monarchische Staat und das Bürgertum*. Munich: Deutscher Taschenbuch Verlag, 1985.

Hau, Michael Grover. *The Cult of Health and Beauty in Germany. A Social History, 1890–1930*. Chicago: The University of Chicago Press, 2003.

Hauck, Karl. *Geschichte der Stadt Mannheim zur Zeit ihres Ueberganges an Baden*. Leipzig: Breitkopf & Härtel, 1899.

Haug, Wolfgang Fritz. *Kritik der Wahrenästhetik*. Frankfurt am Main: Suhrkamp, 1971.

Heimers, Manfred Peter. "Die Strukturen einer barocken Residenzstadt—München zwischen Dreißigjährigem Krieg und dem Vorabend der Französischen Revolution." In *Geschichte der Stadt München*, edited by Richard Bauer. Munich: Beck, 1992.

Hein, Dieter. "Bürgertum in Karlsruhe und Mannheim 1780–1820." In *Vom alten zum neuen Bürgertum. Die mitteleuropäische Stadt im Umbruch 1780–1820. Historische Zeitschrift. Beihefte (Neue Folge) 14*, edited by Lothar Gall. Munich: Oldenbourg, 1991.

———. "Soziale Konstituierungsfaktoren des Bürgertums." In *Stadt und Bürgertum im Übergang von der traditionalen zur modernen Gesellschaft. Historische Zeitschrift, Beiheft 16*, edited by Lothar Gall. Munich: R. Oldenbourg, 1993, 151–81.

Heindl, Waltraud. *Gehorsame Rebellen. Bürokratie und Beamte in Österreich 1780 bis 1848*. Vienna: Böhlau, 1991.

Helm, Dietrich. *Die Cholera in Lübeck. Epidemieprophylaxie und -bekämpfung im 19. Jahrhundert*. Neumünster: Karl Wachholtz Verlag, 1979.

Hennenberg, Fritz. *300 Jahre Leipziger Oper. Geschichte und Gegenwart*. Munich: Langen Müller, 1993.

Henze, Wilhelm. "Leibesübungen und Körpererziehung in der Gründungszeit der Universität Göttingen." In *Von den ritterlichen Exercitien zur modernen Bewegungskultur. 250 Jahre Leibesübungen und Sport an der Universität Göttingen*, edited Wolfgang Buss. Duderstadt: Mecke Druck und Verlag, 1989.

Herrmann, Ulrich. "Familie, Kindheit, Jugend." In *Handbuch der deutschen Bildungsgeschichte*. Vol. 3. *1800–1870. Von der Neuordnung Deutschlands bis zur Gründung des Deutschen Reiches*, edited by Karl-Ernst Jeismann and Peter Lundgreen. Munich: Beck, 1987.

Hertz, Deborah. *Jewish High Society in Old Regime Berlin*. New Haven: Yale University Press, 1988.

Herzig, Arno. "Die Juden in Hamburg 1780–1860." In *Die Geschichte der Juden in Hamburg*. Vol. 2. *Die Juden in Hamburg 1590 bis 1990*, edited by Arno Herzig. Hamburg: Dölling, 1991.

Heydick, Lutz. *Leipzig. Historischer Führer zu Stadt und Land.* Leipzig: Urania, 1990.

Hirsch, Erhard. " 'Zierde und Inbegriff des XVIII. Jahrhundert.' Der Dessau-Wörlitzer Kulturkreis im Spiegel der zeitgenössischen Urteile." In *Philanthropismus und Dessauer Aufklärung. Studien über den Philanthropismus und die Dessauer Aufklärung. Vorträge zur Kulturgeschichte des Dessau-Wörlitzer Kulturkreises.* Wissenschaftliche Beiträge der Martin-Luther-Universität Halle-Wittenberg 1970/3 (A 8). Halle, 1970.

Honneth, Axel. *The Struggle for Recognition. The Moral Grammar of Social Conflicts*. Cambridge: Polity Press, 1995.

Huerkamp, Claudia. *Der Aufstieg der Ärzte im 19. Jahrhundert. Vom gelehrten Stand zum professionellen Experten. Das Beispiel Preußens.* Göttingen: Vandenhoeck & Ruprecht, 1985.

———. "Medizinische Lebensreform im späten 19. Jahrhundert. Die Naturheilbewegung in Deutschland als Protest gegen die naturwissenschaftliche Universitätsmedizin." *Vierteljahrsschrift für Sozial- und Witschaftsgeschichte* 73 (1986).

Hufert, John. *Bewegungsdiätetik. Ein Paradigma auf der Grundlage von Krüger, Feuchtersleben und Zdarsky*. Ahrensburg: Czwalina, 1987.

Hull, Isabel V. *Sexuality, State, and Civil Society in Germany, 1700–1815.* Ithaca: Cornell University Press, 1996.

Hultberg, Helge. *Den ældre Henrich Steffens 1811–1845.* Kopenhagen: Retzels Boghandel, 1981.

Ibbeken, Rudolf. *Preußen 1807–1813. Staat und Volk als Idee un Wirklichkeit.* Berlin: Grote, 1970.

Irion, Jean M. "Historical Overview of Aquatic Rehabilitation." In *Aquatic Rehabilitation*, edited by Richard G. Ruoti, David M. Morris, and Andrew J. Cole. Philadelphia: Lippincott, 1997, 3–13.

Israëls, Han. *Schreber. Vater und Sohn. Eine Biographie*. Munich: Verlag Internationale Psychoanalyse, 1989.

Jacobs, Jürgen and Markus Krause. *Der deutsche Bildungsroman. Gattungsgeschichte vom 18. bis zum 20. Jahrhundert.* Munich: Beck, 1989.

Jäger, Goerg and Heinz-Elmar Tenorth. "Pädagogisches Denken." In *Handbuch der deutschen Bildungsgegschichte.* Vol. 3. *1800–1870. Von der Neuordnung Deutschlands bis zur Gründung des Deutschen Reiches*, edited by Karl-Ernst Jeismann and Peter Lundgreen. Munich: Beck, 1987.

Janke, Wolfgang. "Anerkennung. Fichtes Grundlegung des Rechstgrundes." In *Selbstbehauptung und Anerkennung. Spinoza—Kant—Fichte—Hegel*, edited by Helmut Girndt. Sankt Augustin: Academia Verlag, 1990.

Janson, Helmut. "45 Lesegesellschaften um 1800 bis heute." In *Harmonie-Almanach.* Bonn: Stein-Verlag, 1963.

Jeismann, Karl-Ernst. *Das preußische Gymnasium in Staat und Gesellschaft.* 2 vols. Stuttgart: Klett-Cotta, 1996.

———. "Einleitung. Zur Bedeutung der 'Bildung' im 19. Jahrhundert." In *Handbuch der deutschen Bildungsgegschichte.* Vol. 3. *1800–1870. Von der Neuordnung Deutschlands bis zur Gründung des Deutschen Reiches*, edited by Karl-Ernst Jeismann and Peter Lundgreen. Munich: Beck, 1987.

———. "Schulpolitik, Schulverwaltung, Schulgesetzgebung." In *Handbuch der deutschen Bildungsgegschichte.* Vol. 3. *1800–1870. Von der Neuordnung Deutschlands bis zur Gründung des Deutschen Reiches*, edited by Karl-Ernst Jeismann and Peter Lundgreen. Munich: Beck, 1987.

Jung-Köhler, Evi. *Verlust und Chance. Hamburg 1842. Stadtmodernisierung beim Wiederaufbau nach dem grossen Brand.* Hamburg: Verein für Hamburgische Geschichte, 1991.

Kant, Marion. "Nachwort." In Franz Anton Roller, *Systematisches Lehrbuch der bildenden Tanzkunst und körperlichen Ausbildung von der Geburt an bis zum vollendeten Wachsthume des Menschen. Ausgearbeitet für das gebildete Publikum, zur Belehrung bei der körperlichen Erziehung und als Unterricht für Diejenigen, welche sich zu ausübenden Künstlern und zu nützlichen Lehrern dieser Kunst bilden wollen* (1843). Leipzig: Zentralantiquariat der DDR, 1989.

Kaplan, Marion. *The Making of the Jewish Middle Class. Women, Family, and Identity in Imperial Germany.* Oxford: Oxford University Press, 1991.

Kaschuba, Wolfgang. "Deutsche Bürgerlichkeit nach 1800. Kultur als symbolische Praxis." In *Bürgertum im 19. Jahrhundert.* Vol. 2. *Wirtschaftsbürger und Bildungsbürger*, edited by Jürgen Kocka. Göttingen: Vandenhoeck & Ruprecht, 1995.

Käthner, Martina and Elke Kleinau. "Höhere Töchterschulen um 1800." In *Geschichte der Mädchen- und Frauenbildung.* Vol. 1. *Vom Mittelalter bis zur Aufklärung*, edited by Elke Kleinau and Claudia Opitz. Frankfurt am Main: Campus-Verlag, 1996.

Kazmaier, Martin. *Tübinger Spaziergänge.* Pfullingen: Neske, 1977.

Keiler, Uwe. "Die Lorinserschrift und die dazu erstellten Gutachten unter besonderer Berücksichtigung der Leibeserziehung." PhD diss., University of Mainz, 1978.

Kemp, Peter. *Die Familie Strauß. Geschichte einer Musikerdynastie.* Stuttgart: Verlags-Anstalt, 1987.

Kersting, Christa. *Die Genese der Pädagogik im 18. Jahrhundert. Campes "Allgemeine Revision " im Kontext der neuzeitlichen Wissenschaft.* Weinheim: Deutscher Studien Verlag, 1992.

Kirchner, Hans-Martin. *Friedrich Thiersch. Ein liberaler Kulturpolitiker und Philhellene in Bayern.* Munich: Hieronymus, 1996.

Kleindienst-Cachay, Christa. *Die Verschulung des Turnens. Bedingungen und Folgen der Institutionalisierung der Leibesübungen in den öffentlichen Schulen.* Schorndorf: Karl Hoffmann, 1980.

Kneschke, Emil. *Leipzig seit 100 Jahren.* Säcularchronik einer werdenden Großstadt. Ein Beitrag zur Sozialgeschichte seiner Heimath. Leipzig: Hartknoch, 1870.

Kocka, Jürgen. "Bürgertum und Bürgerlichkeit als Probleme der deutschen Geschichte vom späten 18. bis zum frühen 20. Jahrhundert." In *Bürger und Bürgerlichkeit im 19. Jahrhundert*, edited by Jürgen Kocka. Göttingen: Vandenhoeck & Ruprecht, 1987.

———, ed. *Bildungsbürgertum im 19. Jahrhundert.* Vol. 4. *Politischer Einfluß und gesellschaftliche Formation.* Stuttgart: Klett-Cotta, 1989.

Koebner, Thomas. "Versuch über den literarischen Spaziergang." In *Das achtzehnte Jahrhundert. Facetten einer Epoche. Festschrift für Rainer Gruenter*, edited by Wolfgang Adam. Heidelberg: Hitzeroth, 1988.

König, Gudrun M. *Eine Kulturgeschichte des Spazierganges. Spuren einer bürgerlichen Praktik 1780–1850.* Vienna: Böhlau, 1996.

Kosch, Wilhelm. *Deutsches Theater-Lexikon. Biographisches und bibliographisches Handbuch.* Vol. 1. Klagenfurt: Ferd. Kleinmayr, 1953.

Koselleck, Reinhart. "Einleitung—Zur anthropologischen und semantischen Struktur der Bildung." In *Bildungsbürgertum im 19. Jahrhundert.* Vol. 2. *Bildungsgüter und Bildungswissen*, edited by Reinhart Koselleck. Stuttgart: Klett-Cotta, 1990.

———. *Preußen zwischen Reform und Revolution. Allgemeines Landrecht, Verwaltung und soziale Bewegung von 1791 bis 1848.* Munich: Deutscher-Taschenbuch-Verlag, 1989.

———, ed. *Bildungsbürgertum im 19. Jahrhundert.* Vol. 2. *Bildungsgüter und Bildungswissen.* Stuttgart: Klett-Cotta, 1990.

Krauß, Martin. *Armenwesen und Gesundheitsfursorge in Mannheim vor der Industrialisierung, 1750-1850/60.* Sigmaringen: Jan Thorbecke Verlag, 1993.

Krebber, Sabine. *Der Spaziergang in der Kunst. Eine Untersuchung des Motivs in der Kunst des 18. und 19. Jahrhunderts.* Frankfurt am Main: Lang, 1990.

Krehnke, Walter. *Der Gang der Cholera in Deutschland seit ihrem ersten Auftreten bis heute.* Berlin: Schoetz, 1937.

Kroker, Ernst. *Die Gesellschaft Harmonie in Leipzig 1776 bis 1926. Zum hundertfünfzigjährigen Bestehen der Gesellschaft.* Leipzig: Teubner, 1926.

Krüger, Michael. *Einführung in die Geschichte der Leibeserziehung und des Sports.* Vol. 2. *Leibeserziehung im 19. Jahrhundert. Turnen fürs Vaterland.* Schorndorf: Verlag Karl Hofmann, 1993.

———. *Körperkultur und Nationsbildung. Die Geschichte des Turnens in der Reichsgründungsära—eine Detailstudie über die Deutschen.* Schorndorf: Verlag Karl Hofmann, 1996.

Kudlick, Catherine J. *Cholera in Post-Revolutionary Paris. A Cultural History.* London: University of California Press, 1996.

Kuhnert, Reinhold. *Urbanität auf dem Lande. Badereisen nach Pyrmont im 18. Jahrhundert.* Göttingen: Vandenhoeck & Ruprecht, 1984.

Kümmel, Werner Friedrich. "Der Homo litteratus und die Kunst, gesund zu leben. Zur Entfaltung eines Zweiges der Diätetik im Humanismus." In *Mitteilungen. Kommission für Humanismusforschung* 11 (1984): 67-85.

———. "Tafelmusik aus medizin- und musikhistorischer Sicht." In *Ernährung und Ernährungslehre im 19. Jahrhundert*, edited by Edith Heischkel-Artelt. Göttingen: Vandenhoeck & Ruprecht, 1976.

Kunze, Lydia. "Die physische Erziehung der Kinder." PhD diss., University of Marburg, 1971.

Labisch, Alfons. *Homo Hygienicus. Gesundheit und Medizin in der Neuzeit.* Frankfurt am Main: Campus Verlag, 1992.

Lachmund, Jens and Gunnar Stollberg. *Patientenwelten. Krankheit und Medizin vom späten 18. bis zum frühen 20. Jahrhundet im Spiegel vom Autobiographien.* Opladen: Leske + Budrich, 1995.

Lämmer, Manfred. "Vorwort." In Johann Christoph Friedrich GutsMuths, *Turnbuch für die Söhne des Vaterlandes. Beigebunden: Katechismus der Turnkunst.* Wiesbaden: Sändig, 1973.

Landfester, Manfred. *Humanismus und Gesellschaft im 19. Jahrhundert. Untersuchungen zur politischen und gesellschaftlichen Bedeutung der humanistischen Bildung in Deutschland.* Darmstadt: Wissenschaftliche Buchgesellschaft, 1988.

Lange, Walter. *Der Tunnel 1831 bis 1931.* Leipzig: Verlag Deutsche Buchwerkstätten, 1931.

Langenfeld, Hans and Josef Ulfkotte, ed. *Unbekannte Briefe von Friedrich Ludwig Jahn und Hugo Rothenstein als Quellen zur Frühgeschichte des Turnens.* Oberwerries: WTB, 1990.

Lehmann, Sibylle. *Das fürstliche Schauspielhaus in Bad Pyrmont. Die Funktion eines Kurtheaters im 19. Jahrhundert.* Göttingen: Hubert & Co, 1994.

Lehmann, Hartmut. *Pietismus und weltliche Ordnung in Württemberg vom 17. bis zum 20. Jahrhundert.* Stuttgart: W. Kohlhammer Verlag, 1969.

Lempa, Heikki. *Bildung der Triebe. Der deutsche Philanthropismus (1768–1788).* Turku: Turun yliopisto, 1993.

Lenoir, Timothy. *The Strategy of Life. Teleology and Mechanics in Nineteenth Century German Biology.* Dordrecht: D. Reidel Publishing Company, 1982.

Lepsius, M. Rainer, ed. *Bildungsbürgertum im 19. Jahrhundert.* Vol. 3. *Lebensführung und ständische Vergesellschaftung.* Stuttgart: Klett-Cotta, 1992.

Lesky, Erna. *Die Wiener medizinische Schule im 19. Jahrhundert.* Graz; Köln: Verlag Hermann Böhlaus Nachfolger, 1978.

———. "Introduction." In Johann Peter Frank, *A System of Complete Medical Police.* Selections. Baltimore: Johns Hopkins University Press, 1976.

———. "Van Swietens Hypochondrie. Zur Berufskrankheit der Gelehrten und zur Musiktherapie." *Clio Medica* 8 (1973): 171–90.

Lichtenstein, Ernst. *Zur Entwicklung des Bildungsbegriffs vom Meister Eckart bis Hegel.* Heidelberg: Quelle & Meyer, 1966.

Lindemann, Mary. *Health & Healing in Eighteenth-Century Germany*. Baltimore: Johns Hopkins University Press, 1996.

Loetz, Francisca. *Vom Kranken zum Patienten. Medikalisierung und medizinische Vergesellschaftung am Beispiel Badens 1750–1850*. Stuttgart: Franz Steiner, 1993.

Lukas, Gerhard. *Gerhard Ulrich Anton Vieth. Sein Leben und Werk*. Berlin: Sportverlag, 1964.

MacKaman, Douglas Peter. *Leisure Settings. Bourgeois Culture, Medicine, and the Spa in Modern France*. Chicago: University of Chicago Press, 1998.

Maentel, Thorsten. "Zwischen weltbürgerlicher Aufklärung und stadtbürgerlicher Emanzipation. Bürgerliche Geselligkeitskultur um 1800." In *Bürgerkultur im 19. Jahrhundert. Bildung, Kunst und Lebenswelt*, edited by Dieter Hein and Andreas Schulz. Munich: Beck, 1996.

Mahler, Bruno. "Die Leibesübungen in den Ritterakademien." PhD diss., University of Erlangen, 1921.

Makowski, Ilse. *Emanzipation oder "Harmonie"—zur Geschichte der gleichnahmigen Mannheimer Lesegesellschaft in der ersten Hälfte des 19. Jahrhunderts*. Munich: Saur, 1988.

Mani, Nikolaus. "Die wissenschaftliche Ernährungslehre." In *Ernährung und Ernährungslehre im 19. Jahrhundert*, edited by Edith Heischkel-Artelt. Göttingen: Vandenhoeck & Ruprecht, 1976.

Marchand, Suzanne L. *Down from Olympus. Archaeology and Philhellenism in Germany, 1750–1970*. Princeton: Princeton University Press, 1996.

Markiewicz, Barbara. "Hegels Tod." In *Die 'Jahrbücher für wissenschaftliche Kritik.' Hegels Berliner Gegenakademie*, edited by Christoph Jamme. Stuttgart-Bad Cannstatt: Fromman-Holzboog, 1994.

Martens, Wolfgang. *Die Botschaft der Tugend. Die Aufklärung im Spiegel der deutschen moralischen Wochenschriften*. Stuttgart: Metzler, 1971.

Maurer, Michael. *Die Biographie des Bürgers. Lebensformen und Denkweisen in der formativen Phase des deutschen Bürgertums (1680–1815)*. Göttingen: Vandenhoeck & Ruprecht, 1996.

Mayer, Gerhart. *Der deutsche Bildungsroman. Von der Aufklärung bis zur Gegenwart*. Stuttgart: J.B. Metzlersche Verlagsbuchhandlung, 1992.

McAleer, Kevin. *Dueling. The Cult of Honor in Fin-de-Siècle Germany*. Princeton: Princeton University Press, 1994.

McCagg, William O. *A History of Habsburg Jews, 1670–1918*. Bloomington and Indianapolis: Indiana University Press, 1989.

McMillan, Daniel Alexander. " '. . . die höchste und heiligste Pflicht . . .' Das Männlichkeitsideal der deutschen Turnbewegung 1811–1871." In *Männergeschichte—Geschlechtergeschichte. Männlichkeit im Wandel der Moderne*, edited by Thomas Kühne. Frankfurt: Campus Verlag, 1996.

———. "Germany Incarnate. Politics, Gender, and Sociability in the Gymnastics Movement, 1811–1871." PhD diss., Columbia University, 1997.

Mehrdorf, Wilhelm. "Geschichte des Bades Pyrmont." In *Chronik von Bad Pyrmont*. Bad Pyrmont: Stadt Bad Pyrmont, 1985.

Mester, Ludwig. *Die Körpererziehung an den Universitäten. Eine historisch-systematische Untersuchung über die Bedeutung der körperlichen Übungen für das Universitätsleben der Reformation, der Aufklärung und das Neuhumanismus*. Langensalza: Julius Beltz, 1931.

Michalski, Raoul Wenzel. "Die Hamburger Presse und die "Judenfrage" 1819–1849." In *Die Hamburger Juden in der Emanzipationsphase (1780–1870)*, edited Peter Freimark and Arno Herzig. Hamburg: Hans Christians Verlag, 1989.

Moretti, Franco. *The Way of the World. The Bildungsroman in European Culture*. London: Verso, 1987.

Mosse, George. *Die Nationalisierung der Massen. Politische Symbolik und Massenbewegungen in Deutschland von den Napoleonischen Kriegen bis zum Dritten Reich*. Frankfurt am Main: Ullstein, 1976.

Neuendorff, Edmund. *Geschichte der neueren deutschen Leibesübung vom Beginn des 18. Jahrhunderts bis zur Gegenwart*. 4 vols. Dresden: Limpert, 1932.

Neumann, Hannes. *Die deutsche Turnbewegung in der Revolution 1848/49 und in der amerikanischen Emigration*. Schorndorf bei Stuttgart: Hofmann, 1968.

Nipperdey, Thomas. *Deutsche Geschichte 1800-1866. Bürgerwelt und starker Staat*. Munich: Beck, 1984.

———. "Verein als soziale Struktur in Deutschland im späten 18 und frühen 19. Jahrhundert." In Idem, *Gesellschaft, Kultur, Theorie. Gesammelte Aufsätze zur neueren Geschichte*. Göttingen: Vandenhoeck & Ruprecht, 1976.

Nitschke, August. *Bewegungen in Mittelalter und Renaissance. Kämpfe, Spiele, Tänze, Zeremoniell und Umgangsformen*. Düsseldorf: Schwann, 1987.

Oberdorf, Bernd. *Geselligkeit und Realisierung von Sittlichkeit. Die Theorieentwicklung Friedrich Schleiermachers bis 1799*. Berlin: Walter de Gruyter, 1995.

Oxenius, Katharina. *Vom Promenieren zum Spazieren. Zur Kulturgeschichte des Pariser Parks*. Tübingen: Tübinger Vereinigung für Volkskunde, 1992.

Paulsen, Friedrich. *Geschichte des gelehrten Unterrichts auf den deutschen Schulen und Universitäten vom Ausgang des Mittelalters bis zur Gegenwart. Mit besonderer Rücksicht auf den klassischen Unterricht*. Vol. 2. Leipzig: Gruyter & Co., 1921.

Pemmer, Hans. "Der Graben und seine Bewohner." *Jahrbuch des Vereins für Geschichte der Stadt Wien* 14 (1958): 114–32.

Pemmer, Hans and Nini Lackner. *Der Prater*. Wien: Jugend und Volk, 1974.

Perrot, Michelle, ed. *A History of Private Life*. Vol. 4. *From the Fires of Revolution to the Great War*. Cambridge: Harvard University Press, 1990.

Pertz, Georg Heinrich. *Das Leben des Ministers Freiherrn vom Stein*. Vol 3. *1812 bis 1814*. Berlin: Reimer, 1851.

Petermann, Kurt. "Nachwort." In Johann Pasch, *Beschreibung wahrer Tanz-Kunst, Nebst einigen Anmerckungen über Herrn J.C.L.P.P. zu G. Bedencken gegen das Tanzen (1707)*. Munich: Reimer Verlag, 1978.

———. *Tanzbibliographie. Verzeichnis der in deutscher Sprache veröffentlichten Schriften und Aufsätze zum Bühnen-, Gesellschafts-, Kinder-, Volks- und Turniertanz sowie zur Tanzwissenschaft, Tanzmusik und zum Jazz*. 5 vols. Munich: Verl. Dokumentation Saur, 1978-1987.

Pfeifer, Klaus. *Christoph Wilhelm Hufeland. Mensch und Werk*. Halle: Niemeyer, 1968.

Pigeaud, Jackie. "La Renaissance hippocratique au XVIIIème siècle." In *Hippokratische Medizin und antike Philosophie*, edited by Renate Wittern and Pierre Pellegrin. Hildesheim: Olms, 1996.

Pinloche, Auguste. *Geschichte des Philanthropismus*. Leipzig: Brandstetter, 1896.

Poliakov, Léon. *Geschichte des Antisemitismus*. Vol. 6. *Emanzipation und Rassenwahn*. Worms: Verlag Georg Heintz, 1987.

Porter, Roy. "Introduction." In *The Popularization of Medicine 1650–1850*, edited by Roy Porter. London: Routledge, 1992.

———, ed. *Patients and practitioners. Lay perceptions of medecine in pre-industrial society*. Cambridge: Cambridge University Press, 1985.

Poten, Bernhard von. *Geschichte des Militär-Erziehungs- und Bildungswesens in den Landen deutscher Zunge*. 5 vols. Berlin: Hofmann & Co., 1889–1897.

Prüsener, Marlies. "Lesegesellschaften im 18. Jahrhundert." *Archiv für Geschichte des Buchwesens* 13 (1973): 370–594.

Rasmus, G. *Dr. Adolf Werner in seinem Wirken auf dem Felde der Gymnastik*. Dessau, 1848.

Rather, J. "The 'Six Things Non-Natural': A Note on the Origins and Fate of a Doctrine and a Phrase." *Clio Medica* 3 (1968): 337–47.

Raupach, Angela. "Zum Verhältnis von Politik und Ökonomie im Kameralismus. Ein Beitrag zur sozialen Theoriebildung in Deutschland in ihrer Genese als Polizei." PhD diss., University of Hamburg, 1982.

Reder, Dirk-Alexander. "'Natur und Sitte verbieten uns, die Waffen der Zerstörung zu führen . . .' Patriotische Frauen zwischen Frieden und Krieg" In *Kriegsbereitschaft und Friedensordnung in Deutschland 1800–1814*, edited by Jost Düffler. Jahrbuch für historische Friedensforschung. 3. Jahrgang 1994.

Reinhold, Josef. "Jüdischer Messebesuch und Wiederansiedlung von Juden in Leipzig im 18. und frühen 19. Jahrhundert." In *Judaica Lipsensia. Zur Geschichte der Juden in Leipzig*, edited by Manfred Unger. Leipzig: Edition Leipzig, 1994.

Rethschuhlte, Clemens. *Daniel Gottlob Moritz Schreber. Seine Erziehungslehre und sein Beitrag zur Körperbehindertenhilfe im 19. Jahrhundert. Genese und historische Einordnung*. Heidelberg: Edition Schindele, 1995.

Richarz, Monika. "Einleitung." In *Jüdisches Leben in Deutschland. Selbstzeugnisse zur Sozialgeschichte 1780–1871*. Augsburg: Deutsche Verlags-Anstalt, 1976.

Richter, Joachim Burkhard. *Hans Ferdinand Maßmann. Altdeutscher Patriotismus im 19. Jahrhundert*. Berlin: Walter de Gruyter, 1992.

Riley, James C. *The Eighteenth-Century Campaign to Avoid Disease*. London: MacMillan, 1987.

Risse, Guenter. "Kant, Schelling, and the search for a Philosophical 'Science' of Medicine in Germany." *Journal of the History of Medicine* 27 (1972): 145–58.

Rohrbacher, Stefan. *Gewalt im Biedermeier. Antijüdische Ausschreitungen in Vormärz und Revolution (1815–1848/49)*. Frankfurt am Main: Campus, 1993.

Roth, Klaus. "Selbstbehauptung und Anerkennung bei G.W.F. Hegel." In *Selbstbehauptung und Anerkennung. Spinoza—Kant—Fichte—Hegel*, edited by Helmut Girndt. Sankt Augustin: Academia Verlag, 1990.

Rotschuh, Karl, ed. *Konzepte der Medizin in Vergangenheit und Gegenwart*. Stuttgart: Hippokrates-Verlag, 1978.

Ruppert, Wolfgang. *Bürgerlicher Wandel. Die Geburt der modernen deutschen Gesellschaft im 18. Jahrhundert*. Frankfurt am Main: Fischer, 1984.

Sachs, Curt. *Eine Weltgeschichte des Tanzes*. Berlin: Dietrich Reimer & Ernst Vohsen, 1933.

Saftien, Volker. *Ars Saltandi. Der europäische Gesellschaftstanz im Zeitalter der Renaissance und des Barock*. Hildesheim: Olms, 1994.

Sanislo, Teresa, "Models of Manliness and Femininity: The Physical Culture of the Enlightenment and Early National Movement in Germany 1770–1819." PhD diss., University of Michigan, 2001.

Schaarschmidt, Ilse. "Die Bedeutungswandel der Worte 'bilden' und 'Bildung' in der Literaturperiode von Gottsched bis Herder." In Franz Rauhut and Ilse Schaarschmidt, *Beiträge zur Geschichte des Bildungsbegriffs*. Weinheim: Beltz, 1965.

Schäfer-Schmidt, Ilona. "Die Entwicklung der Kuranlagen in Bad Pyrmont." In *Kurstädte in Deutschland. Zur Geschichte einer Baugattung*, edited by Rolf Bothe. Berlin: Frölich & Kaufmann, 1984.

Schipperges, Heinrich. "Krankwerden und Gesundsein bei Novalis." In *Romantik in Deutschland. Ein interdisziplinäres Symposion*, edited by Richard Brinkmann. Stuttgart: J.B. Metzlersche Verlagsbuchhandlung, 1978.

Schlawe, Fritz. *Friedrich Theodor Vischer*. Stuttgart: J.B. Metzlersche Buchhandlung, 1959.

Schmucker, Alf-Rüdiger and Sebastian Kolb, *Die Museumsgesellschaft Tübingen—ein Mittelpunkt kultureller Geselligkeit*. Tübingen: Museumsgesellschaft Tübingen, 1992.

Schneider, Carl. *Die Hamburger Turnerschaft von 1816, von ihrer Begründung bis zur Gegenwart*. Hamburg: Hamburger Turnerschaft, 1891.

Schneider, Barbara. *Johannes Schulze und das preußische Gymnasium*. Frankfurt am Main: Peter Lang, 1989.

Schneidert, Otto. *Johann Strauss und die Stadt an der schönen Donau*. Berlin: VEB Lied der Zeit/Musikverlag, 1982.

Schorske, Carl E. *Fin-de-siècle Vienna : politics and culture.* New York: Knopf, 1980.

Schröder, Willi. *Burschenturner im Kampf um Einheit und Freiheit.* Berlin: Sportverlag, 1967.

———. *Johann Christoph GutsMuths. Leben und Wirken des Schnepfenthaler Pädagogen.* Sankt Augustin: Academia Verlag, 1996.

Schwanitz, Hans Joachim. *Die Theorie der praktischen Medizin zu Beginn des 19. Jahrhunderts. Eine historische und wissenschaftstheoretische Untersuchung anhand des 'Journals der practischen Arzneykunde und Wundarzneykunde' von Ch. W. Hufeland.* Köln: Pahl-Rugenstein, 1979.

Schwarzmaier, Michael. *Friedrich Immanuel Niethammer, ein bayerischer Schulreformator.* Vol. 1. *Niethammers Leben und Wirken bis zum Jahre 1807.* (1937). Aalen: Scientia, 1974.

Seibert, Peter. *Der Literarische Salon. Literatur und Geselligkeit zwischen Aufklärung und Vormärz.* Stuttgart: Verlag J.B. Metzler, 1993.

Seidler, Eduard. *Lebensplan und Gesundheitsführung. Franz Anton Mai und die medizinische Aufklärung in Mannheim.* Mannheim: Boehringer, 1979.

Sheehan, James. *German History, 1770–1866.* Oxford: Clarendon Press, 1989.

Sobania, Michael. "Vereinsleben und Formen bürgerlicher Assoziationen im 19. Jahrhundert." In *Bürgerkultur im 19. Jahrhundert. Bildung, Kunst und Lebenswelt,* edited by Dieter Hein and Andreas Schulz. Munich: Beck, 1996.

Sommer, Hermann. *Zur Kur nach Ems. Ein Beitrag zur Geschichte der Badereise von 1830 bis 1914.* Stuttgart: Steiner, 1999.

Springer, Elisabeth. *Geschichte und Kulturleben der Wiener Ringstrasse.* Wiesbaden: Franz Steiner Verlag, 1979.

Steudel, Johannes. "Therapeutische und soziologische Funktion der Mineralbäder im 19. Jahrhundert" In *Der Arzt und der Kranke in der Gesellschaft des 19. Jahrhunderts,* edited by Walter Artelt and Walter Ruegg. Stuttgart: Ferdinand Enke Verlag, 1967.

Strohmeyer, Hannes. "Von den 'sex res non naturales' zur 'Leibeserziehung.' (Ein Beitrag zur Begriffsgeschichte von 'Leibeserziehung')." In *Sportwirklichkeit. Beiträge zur Didaktik, Geschichte und Soziologie des Sports,* edited by Reinhard Bachleitner and Sepp Redl. Wien: Österreichischer Bundesverlag, 1981.

Suhr, Dieter. "Dialektik der Anerkennung in Hegels bürgerlicher Gesellschaft." In *Selbstbehauptung und Anerkennung. Spinoza—Kant—Fichte—Hegel,* edited by Helmut Girndt. Sankt Augustin: Academia Verlag, 1990.

Tanzer, Gerhard. *Spectacle müssen seyn. Die Freizeit der Wiener im 18. Jahrhundert.* Vienna: Böhlau, 1992.

Tornow, Ingo. *Das Münchner Vereinswesen in der ersten Hälfte des 19. Jahrhunderts. Mit einem Ausblicke auf die zweite Jahrhunderthälfte.* Munich: UNI-Druck, 1977.

Toury, Jacob. *Soziale und politische Geschichte der Juden in Deutschland 1847–1871. Zwischen Revolution, Reaktion und Emanzipation.* Düsseldorf: Droste Verlag, 1977.

Trepp, Anne-Charlott. *Sanfte Männlichkeit und selbständige Weiblichkeit. Frauen und Männer im Hamburger Bürgertum zwischen 1770 und 1840*. Göttingen: Vandenhoeck & Ruprecht, 1996.

Tribe, Keith. *Governing Economy. The Reformation of German Economic Discourse 1750–1840*. Cambridge: Cambridge University Press, 1988.

Triml, Raimund. "Die erste Cholera-Epidemie in Wien in den Jahren 1831 und 1832." PhD diss., University of Vienna, 1992.

Tuchman, Arleen Marcia. *Science, Medicine, and the State in Germany. The Case of Baden, 1815–1871*. Oxford: Oxford University Press, 1993.

Überhorst, Horst, ed. *Geschichte der Leibesübungen*. Vol. 3.1. *Leibesübungen und Sport in Deutschland von der Anfängen bis zum ersten Weltkrieg*. Berlin: Bartels & Wernitz, 1980.

Varrentrapp, Conrad. *Johannes Schulze und das höhere preußische Unterrichtswesen in seiner Zeit*. Leipzig: Teubner, 1889.

Vierhaus, Rudolf. "Der Aufstieg des Bürgertums vom späten 18. Jahrhundert bis 1848/49." In *Bürger und Bürgerlichkeit im 19. Jahrhundert*, edited by Jürgen Kocka. Göttingen: Vandenhoeck & Ruprecht, 1987.

———. "Bildung." In *Geschichtliche Grundbegriffe*. Vol. 1, edited by Otto Brunner, Werner Conze, and Reinhart Koselleck. Stuttgart: Klett-Cotta, 1972.

Wagner, Hermann. "Zur Geschichte des Turnwesens in Oesterreich." *Deutsche Turn-Zeitung* 10 (1884): 86–88.

———. "Zur Geschichte des Turnwesens in Oesterreich." *Deutsche Turn-Zeitung* 12 (1884): 105–8.

Walter, Friedrich. *Geschichte Mannheims vom Übergang an Baden (1802) bis zur Gründung des Reiches*. Vol. 2. *Mannheim in Vergangenheit und Gegenwart*. Frankfurt am Main: Weidlich, 1907.

Waszek, Norbert. *The Teaching of Cameralism, "Staatswissenschaften." and Economics in Early Nineteenth-Century Germany. A Case Study (University of Berlin) in Its National Context*. Fachbereich Wirtschaftswissenschaften Universität Hannover. Diskussionspapier Nr. 103, Juni 1987. Hannover, 1987.

Weidig, Ursula. "GutsMuths-Bibliographie." In *Festschrift zum 200. Geburtstage von Johann Christoph Friedrich GutsMuths*. s.l.: Ministerrat der Deutschen Demokratischen Republik, 1959.

Weiss, Melitta. *Medieval Dietetics. Food and Drink in Regimen Sanitatis Literature from 800 to 1400*. Frankfurt am Main: Lang, 1995.

Welke, Martin. "Gemeinsame Lektüre und frühe Formen von Gruppenbildungen im 17. und 18. Jahrhundert. Zeitungslesen in Deutschland." In *Lesegesellschaften und bürgerliche Emanzipation. Ein europäischer Vergleich*, edited by Otto Dann. Munich: Beck, 1981.

Wellmann, Angelika. *Der Spaziergang. Stationen eines poetischen Codes*. Würzburg: Königshausen & Neumann, 1991.

Wiesing, Urban. *Kunst oder Wissenschaft? Konzeptionen der Medizin in der deutschen Romantik*. Stuttgart: Fromman-Holzboog, 1995.

Wildt, Klemens. *Daten zur Sportgeschichte*. Vol. 2. *Europa von 1750 bis 1894*. Schorndorf bei Stuttgart: Hofmann, 1972.

Wilhelmy, Petra. *Der Berliner Salon im 19. Jahrhundert (1780–1914)*. Berlin: Walter de Gruyter, 1989.

Witzmann, Reingard. *Der Ländler in Wien. Ein Beitrag zur Entwicklungsgeschichte des Wiener Walzers bis in die Zeit des Wiener Kongresses*. Wien: Arbeitsstelle für den Volkskundeatlas in Österreich, 1976.

Wölfel, Kurt. "Andeutende Materialien zu einer Poetik des Spaziergangs. Von Kafkas Frühwerk zu Goethes 'Werther.'" In *Zur Geschichtlichkeit der Moderne in Theorie und Deutung*. Ulrich Fülleborn zum 60. Geburtstag, edited by Theo Elm and Gerd Hemmerich. Munich: Wilhelm Fink Verlag, 1982.

Wurst, Karin, *Fabricating Pleasure. Fashion Entertainment, and Cultural Consumption in Germany, 1780–1830.* Detroit: Wayne State University Press, 2005.

Zeidler, Johannes. *Die deutsche Turnsprache bis 1819. Untersuchungen zur Geschichte der deutschen Sprache*. Halle: Niemeyer, 1942.

Zerback, Ralf. "Unter der Kuratel des Staates. Die Stadt zwischen dem Gemeindeedikt von 1818 und der Gemeindeordnung von 1869." In *Geschichte der Stadt München*, edited by Richard Bauer. Munich: Beck, 1992.

Zunkel, Friedrich. "Ehre." In *Geschichtliche Grundbegriffe* Vol. 2, edited by Otto Brunner, Werner Conze, and Reinhart Koselleck. Stuttgart: Kett-Cotta, 1975.

Zwahr, Hartmut. "Leipzig im Übergang zur bürgerlichen Gesellschaft (1763–1871)." In *Neues Leipzigisches Geschicht-Buch*. Leipzig: Fachbuchverlag, 1990.

# Index

# About the Author

Heikki Lempa is an Assistant Professor of Modern European History at Moravian College, Bethlehem, Pennsylvania. His interests are in cultural history, the history of everyday life, emotions, education, and the history of masculinity. The book, *Bildung der Triebe. Der deutsche Philanthropismus (1768-1788)*, discussed the rise of modern education in Germany. His recent articles include "The Spa: Emotional Economy and Social Classes in Nineteenth-Century Pyrmont" in *Central European History* and "Patriarchalism and Meritocracy. Evaluating Students in Late Eighteenth-Century Schnepfenthal" in *Paedagogica Historica*.

www.ingramcontent.com/pod-product-compliance
Ingram Content Group UK Ltd.
Pitfield, Milton Keynes, MK11 3LW, UK
UKHW012036150926
475560UK00001B/34